GONADOTROPIN

Edited by **Jorge Vizcarra**

Gonadotropin
http://dx.doi.org/10.5772/2918
Edited by Jorge Vizcarra

Contributors

Jorge Vizcarra, Clay A. Lents, C. Richard Barb, Gary J. Hausman, Rosaria Meccariello, Rosanna Chianese, Silvia Fasano, Riccardo Pierantoni, María Ester Celis, Mark A. Crowe, Michael P. Mullen, Dara J. Cooke, Mark A. Crow

Published by InTech

Janeza Trdine 9, 51000 Rijeka, Croatia

Copyright © 2013 InTech

Notice

Publishing Process Manager Dimitri Jelovcan
Technical Editor InTech Prepress, Novi Sad
Cover InTech Design team

Additional hard copies can be obtained from orders@intechopen.com

Gonadotropin, Edited by Jorge Vizcarra
p. cm.
ISBN 978-953-51-1006-4

For EU product safety concerns:
IN TECH d.o.o., Prolaz Marije Krucifikse Kozulić 3, 51000 Rijeka, Croatia,
info@intechopen.com or visit our website at intechopen.com.

Meet the editor

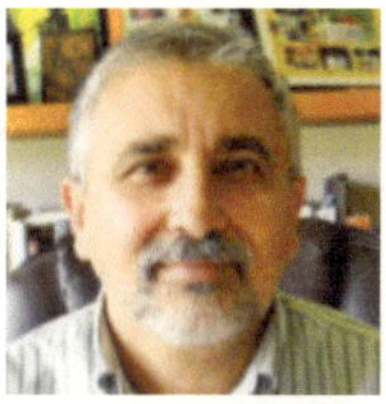

Dr. Vizcarra obtained his Bachelor degree in his home country as an Ingeniero Agrónomo at the University of Uruguay in 1981. He subsequently obtained his Master and PhD degree at Oklahoma State University in 1991 and 1994, respectively. Currently, Dr. Vizcarra is an Associate Professor at the Department of Food and Animal Science at Alabama A&M University. Dr. Vizcarra has published over 150 papers in various peer-reviewed scientific journals, proceedings, abstracts, and GeneBank. He has been a contributing expert in several multimedia educational programs and book chapters. Dr. Vizcarra also teaches face-to face and distance education courses including Reproductive Physiology, Statistics, Human Anatomy and Physiology, Poultry Science, and Graduate Seminar.

Contents

Preface

It is widely recognized that proper gonadal function depends on the coordinated action of multiple factors influencing the synthesis and secretion of gonadotropin hormones. The term gonadotropin derives from the combination of gonas (from Greek *gonos* or "seed") and tropin (from Greek *trepein* or "to change"). Thus, gonadotropins are protein hormones that have the ability to change gonadal function. Although the word gonadotrophin is also used in scientific literature, the etymological derivation of this alternative spelling is different. Trophic (from Greek *trophe* or "nutrition") implies a nurturing action, a function that is not consistent with the nature these protein hormones. Thus, from a physiological point of view, the term gonadotropin better describes the main emphasis of this book.

The gonadotropin family includes luteinizing hormone (LH) and follicle-stimulating hormone (FSH) secreted from the pituitary gland. These hormones are composed of two dissimilar subunits: an alpha subunit and a beta subunit. Within species, the alpha subunits are nearly identical; however, the beta subunits are specific for each hormone. When the subunits are combined, to form a noncovalently associated heterodimer, the beta subunit provides a unique spatial conformation that ensures a high affinity interaction with their membrane receptors; thus, the biological specificity of each hormone. Each subunit is the product of separate genes. Genes are translated and subsequently glycosylated before packaging and secretion from the Golgi apparatus. Glycosylation is an enzymatic process that attaches poly- or oligosaccharides (glycans) to the different subunits. Thus, gonadotropins are also part of the glycoprotein hormone family that includes other hormones such as thyroid-stimulation hormone (TSH). In addition, some species also secrete chorionic gonadotropins during pregnancy. Chorionic gonadotropins are also heterodimeric glycoprotein than can have different degrees of LH and FSH biological activity in horses (eCG), humans (hCG), and other primates.

Synthesis and secretion of LH and FSH takes place in the gonadotropes of the pituitary gland (adenohypophysis). The hypothalamus, in turn, controls the secretion of gonadotropins by the pulsatile secretion of gonadotropin releasing hormone (GnRH). Therefore, the neuroendocrine linkage of the hypothalamic-pituitary-gonadal axis provides an integrated system responsible for proper reproductive performance, including gamete development and sex steroids secretion.

The scope and objective of this book is to provide researchers and graduate students with an updated review of the control mechanisms associated with the synthesis and secretion of gonadotropins. From a practical point of view, the book also provides relevant information that integrates reproductive performance of domestic species. A dedicated panel of authors was assembled to address these topics, aiming to provide a cutting edge platform to those interested in reproductive physiology and endocrinology.

The book is organized in eight chapters. The first four chapters are dedicated to the control of gonadotropin secretion via GnRH and GnRH isoforms, Kisspeptin, Endocannabinoids and neuropeptide–glutamic acid-isoleucine. A series of three interrelated chapters summarize the regulation of gonadotropin secretion in cattle, and an additional chapter is devoted to the functions of gonadotropin-related structural features.

Putting this book together has been an enjoyable task. I would like to thank all the authors for their patience throughout the editorial process, and most importantly for their valuable contribution.

Dr. Jorge Vizcarra
Department of Food and Animal Science, Alabama A&M University,
USA

Chapter 1

Contribution of Chicken GnRH-II and Lamprey GnRH-III on Gonadotropin Secretion

Jorge Vizcarra

Additional information is available at the end of the chapter

http://dx.doi.org/10.5772/47863

1. Introduction

Proper gonadal function in mammals depends on gonadotropins secreted from the pituitary gland in a pulsatile manner. The hypothalamus, in turn, controls the secretion of gonadotropins by the pulsatile secretion of gonadotropin releasing hormone (GnRH) into the portal circulation of the pituitary. The idea of brain control over the hypophysis was first postulated by Geoffrey Harris during the late 1940s and early 1950s (Harris, 1948). The evidence available at that time indicated that stimulation of the central nervous system, but not direct stimulation of the pars distalis or neural lobe, caused the release of adenohypophysial hormones. During the 1950s and 1960s, trophic substances were extracted from the brain of different species (Guillemin, 2005). These releasing factors obtained from the median eminence affected secretions of the pars distalis. The search for these releasing factors was lead by McCann, Schally and Guillemin (Guillemin and Rosenberg, 1955; McCann and Fruit, 1957; Rumsfeld and Porter, 1962; Saffran et al., 1955).

Andrew Schally and his team isolated and synthesized for the first time the decapeptide GnRH, after the extraction of more than 250,000 pig hypothalami (Matsuo et al., 1971; Wade, 1978). Initially Schally and coworkers postulated that one hypothalamic hormone LH-RH/FSH-RH or simply GnRH controls the secretion of both LH and FSH from the pituitary gland (Schally et al., 1971). The terms luteinizing hormone-releasing hormone, and gonadotropin-releasing hormone have been widely adopted, and most journals allow the use of both names and abbreviations (Schally, 2000). In addition to GnRH, the occurrence of other two GnRH isoforms was first reported in chickens more than 10 years after of Dr. Schally's initial report (King and Millar, 1982; Miyamoto et al., 1982; Miyamoto et al., 1984). To date, several structural variants of GnRH have been identified in diverse vertebrates (Barran et al., 2005; Millar et al., 2004). These isoforms have various functions, including paracrine, autocrine, neuroendocrine, and neurotransmitter/neuromodulatory roles in the central and peripheral nervous systems (King and Millar, 1995; Millar and King, 1987; Sealfon et al., 1997; Skinner et al., 2009).

	1	2	3	4	5	6	7	8	9	10
Mammal (mGnRH)	**pGlu-**	**His-**	**Trp-**	**Ser-**	Tyr-	Gly-	Leu-	Arg-	**Pro-**	**Gly**
Chicken-I (cGnRH-I)	**pGlu-**	**His-**	**Trp-**	**Ser-**	Tyr-	Gly-	Leu-	Gln-	**Pro-**	**Gly**
Chicken-II (cGnRH-II)	**pGlu-**	**His-**	**Trp-**	**Ser-**	His-	Gly-	Trp-	Tyr-	**Pro-**	**Gly**
Lamprey-III (lGnRH-III)	**pGlu-**	**His-**	**Trp-**	**Ser-**	His-	Asp-	Trp-	Lys-	**Pro-**	**Gly**

Table 1. Amino acid (AA) sequence of GnRH isoforms. The bolded regions represent the conserved NH3- and COOH- terminal residues. The numbers represent the relative position of each AA in the GnRH peptide (1 represents the N-terminal AA)

The nomenclature used to distinguish different GnRH isoforms between mammalian and non-mammalian species have been described using a variety of phylogenic and genomic synteny analyses (Kim et al., 2011; Millar et al., 2004; Roch et al., 2011; Tostivint, 2011). For the purpose of this book chapter, we adopted the nomenclature based on the species in which they were first discovered, depicted in Table 1, and described elsewhere (Millar et al., 2004).

In addition to the classically described mammalian form of GnRH (for extensive review see (Barb et al., 2001; Clarke, 2002; Esbenshade et al., 1990; Kaiser et al., 1997; McCann et al., 2002; Millar, 2005; Millar et al., 2008)), chicken GnRH-II (cGnRH-II) and lamprey GnRH-III (lGnRH-III) are of particular significance because they may coordinate the control of LH and FSH secretion in some vertebrate species.

2. GnRH receptors

The coordination of gonadotropin secretion is also modulated by the interaction of the GnRH peptide with its receptors. The GnRH receptor (GnRHR) has the characteristic feature of a classical seven-transmembrane G-protein-coupled receptor (Millar, 2003, 2005; Neill, 2002). Four vertebrate GnRHR lineages have been proposed using genome synteny and phylogenic analyses; nonmammalian type I, nonmammalian type II, nonmammalian type III/mammalian type II, and mammalian type I (Kim et al., 2011). For the purpose of this book chapter, we refer to the type I and type II GnRHRs as the mammalian type I and mammalian type II GnRH receptor, respectively.

There is evidence that in the rhesus monkey (*Macaca mulatta*) and the marmoset (*Callithrix jacchus*), the type I GnRHR has high affinity for mGnRH and lower affinity for cGnRH-II, and the type II GnRHR has high affinity for cGnRH-II and lower affinity for mGnRH (Millar et al., 2001; Neill, 2002). In fact, when COS-1 or COS-7 cells were transfected with the type II GnRHR, the potency was high for cGnRH-II and low for mGnRH. Nonetheless, in vivo and in vitro work in rhesus monkey (Densmore and Urbanski, 2003; Okada et al., 2003) and pigs

(Neill et al., 2002), using specific type I GnRHR antagonists (Antide and Cetrorelix) suggest that cGnRH-II can also stimulate gonadotropin secretion via the type I GnRHR (Neill et al., 2004).

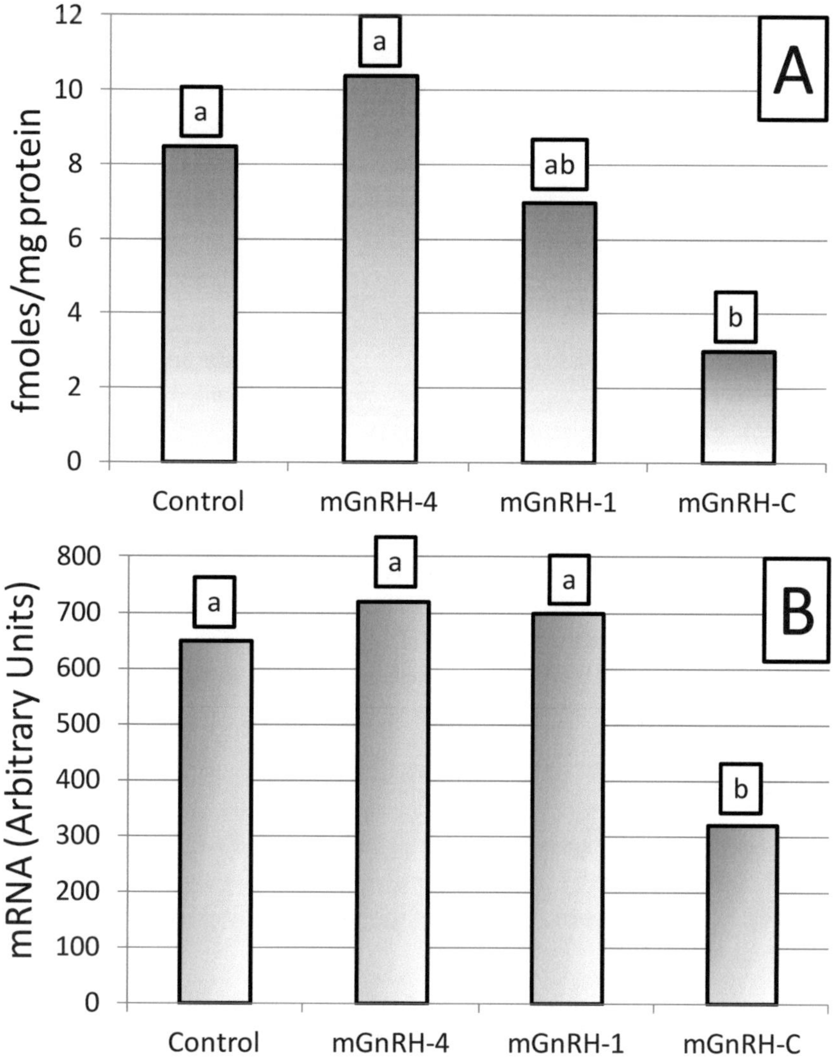

Figure 1. Concentrations of the type I GnRHR (A) and expression of the mRNA for the type I GnRHR (B) in the pituitary gland of anestrous cows that were treated for 13 days with 2 μg of mGnRH infused (i.v.) continuously during 1 h (mGnRH-C), during 5 min once every hour (mGnRH-1), or during 5 min once every fourth hour (mGnRH-4) or with saline (control). Different letters indicate significant differences ($P < 0.1$ for A and $P < 0.05$ for B). Adapted from (Vizcarra et al., 1997).

In the pig, as well as other mammals, type I GnRHRs are characterized by the absence of a carboxyl-terminal tail (Kakar et al., 1992; Millar et al., 2004; Neill et al., 2004; Tsutsumi et al., 1992; Weesner and Matteri, 1994). The tail-less type I GnRHR is associated with a resistance to rapid desensitization and ligand-induced internalization (Blomenrohr et al., 1999). When COS-1 cells expressing the type I receptor were incubated with a maximal dose of a mGnRH agonist, [^{3}H]-inositol phosphate (IP) accumulated for 90 min indicating the failure of mGnRH desensitization during the experimental period (Neill, 2002). From a practical standpoint, we have demonstrated that administration of mGnRH at different frequencies differentially regulates the concentrations and the expression of the type I GnRHR (Vizcarra et al., 1997). Concentrations and expression of the type I GnRHR were reduced when mGnRH was infused continuously compared with those in control cows (Figure 1). However, when mGnRH was given as a pulse every hour or every fourth hour, concentration and expression of the type I GnRHR were not different from those in control cows. Our data indicates that pulsatile mGnRH does not influence concentrations of the type I GnRHR or type I GnRHR mRNA, but continuous infusion of mGnRH dramatically reduces the concentrations and expression of the type I GnRHR in the pituitary gland (Vizcarra et al., 1997).

The type II GnRHR has only 41% identity with the type I receptor and in contrast to the type I GnRHR, the type II receptor has a C-terminal cytoplasmic tail that is important for cell surface expression and agonist binding. The type II GnRHR has been cloned in several vertebrate species; whereas the type I GnRHR has been identified only in mammals (Kim et al., 2011). The tail of the type II GnRHR is phosphorylated upon agonist-binding followed by internalization and desensitization of the receptor (Blomenrohr et al., 1999). As with the type I receptor, the type II couples to the Gqα protein and, consequently, mediates the intracellular production of inositol trisphosphate (Cabrera-Vera et al., 2003; Millar and Newton, 2010). In contrast to the type I GnRHR, desensitization of the type II GnRHR in rhesus monkeys takes about 60 minutes, reflecting the properties of the cytoplasmic tail (Neill, 2002).

3. Chicken GnRH-II

Phylogenic evidence indicates that cGnRH-II (initially isolated from the chicken brain) is an ancient form of GnRH that has been structurally conserved for over 100 million years of evolution, suggesting that its neural functions may have an important significance (Powell et al., 1994; Rastogi et al., 1998).

In birds, two forms of GnRH (cGnRH-I and cGnRH-II; Table 1) have been reported (King and Millar, 1982; Miyamoto et al., 1982; Miyamoto et al., 1984) and only indirect measurements of the GnRH pulse generator is available by measuring plasma LH concentrations in frequent samples or in pituitary extracts (Chou and Johnson, 1987; Sharp and Gow, 1983; Wilson and Sharp, 1975). In addition, we have reported the episodic nature of gonadotropin secretion in the mature fowl (Vizcarra et al., 2004). Gonadotropin secretion in chickens is characterized by a pulsatile pattern with LH pulses being more frequent and having greater amplitude than FSH pulses (Figure 2). Furthermore, we observed that there was a lack of synchrony between the episodic release of LH and FSH. Only 23% of the LH pulses were associated with FSH episodes, suggesting that in the adult male fowl LH and FSH secretion are regulated independently (Vizcarra et al., 2004).

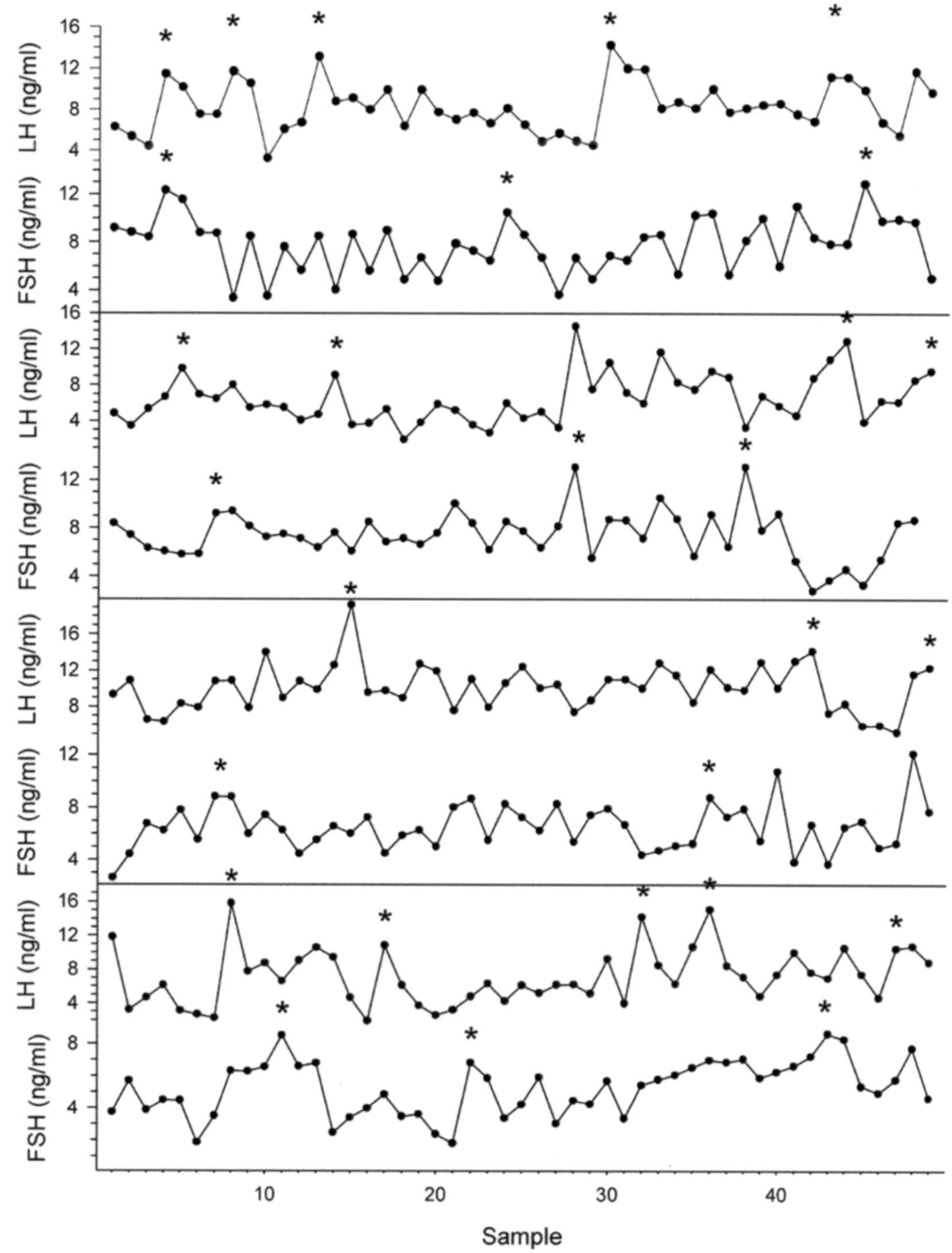

Figure 2. Pulsatile secretion of LH and FSH in plasma of four birds. Blood samples were obtained every 10-min for 8 h. Asterisks indicate the presence of a pulse of LH or FSH, as determined by Pulsar. Adapted from (Vizcarra et al., 2004)

Both cGnRH-I and -II stimulates gonadotropin release *in vivo* and *in vitro* in the chicken (Hattori et al., 1986). However, cGnRH-II was not found in the median eminence of the white-crowned sparrow (*Zonotrichia leucophrys gambelii*), suggesting that in these species cGnRH-II does not regulate pituitary gonadotropin secretion (Meddle et al., 2006). Although concentrations of FSH in small cockerels were not affected by cGnRH-I challenge (Krishnan et al., 1993), most of the evidence indicates that cGnRH-I is the prime regulator of gonadotropin release in chickens (Katz et al., 1990; Sharp et al., 1990). Active immunization against cGnRH-I but not against cGnRH-II was associated with decreased concentration of LH in laying hens (Sharp et al., 1990). We also evaluated the effect of active immunization against cGnRH-I and cGnRH-II in adult broiler breeder males (Vizcarra et al., 2000). At 10 weeks of age, males (10 per treatment), received a primary immunization against cGnRH-I, cGnRH-II, BSA, or were not immunized. Peptides were conjugated to BSA and emulsified in Freund's incomplete adjuvant and diethylaminoethyl-dextran. Booster immunizations were given at 3, 6 and 14 weeks after the primary immunization. Titers were increased in cGnRH-I but not in cGnRH-II treated birds compared with BSA immunized males (Figure 3). Concentrations of LH and FSH in frequent samples were not affected by treatment; however, testis weight was significantly decreased in cGnRH-I birds compared to the other treatments (Figure 4).

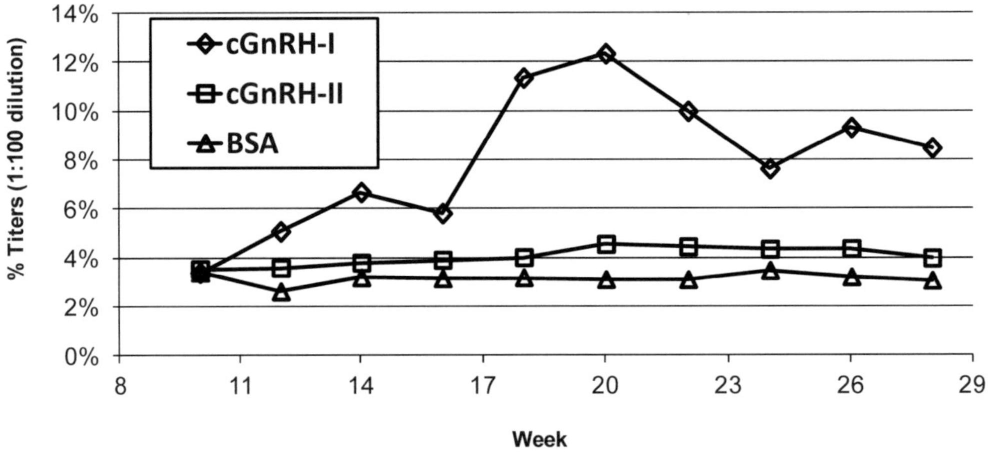

Figure 3. Antibody titers of male broiler breeders immunized against cGnRH-I, cGnRH-II, and BSA. Titers were increased ($P < 0.05$) in cGnRH-I but not in cGnRH-II treated birds compared with BSA immunized males.

There is evidence of a behavioral role attributed to cGnRH-II in birds that may be independent from cGnRH-I. Intracerebroventricular (ICV) infusion of cGnRH-II induced copulation solicitation in the female white-crowned sparrow, and social interactions in the house sparrow (*Passer domesticus*) may be regulated by cGnRH-II (Maney et al., 1997; Stevenson et al., 2008). In the mature male Zebra finch (*Taeniopygia guttata*) the number of cGnRH-II neurons is significantly reduced during the non-breeding season as compared with the breeding season (Perfito et al., 2011). A similar behavioral role of cGnRH-II has been reported in mice (Kauffman and Rissman, 2004a). However, this information is questionable due to the lack of a functional cGnRH-II peptide and the lack of a functional type II GnRHR in mice (Stewart et al., 2009).

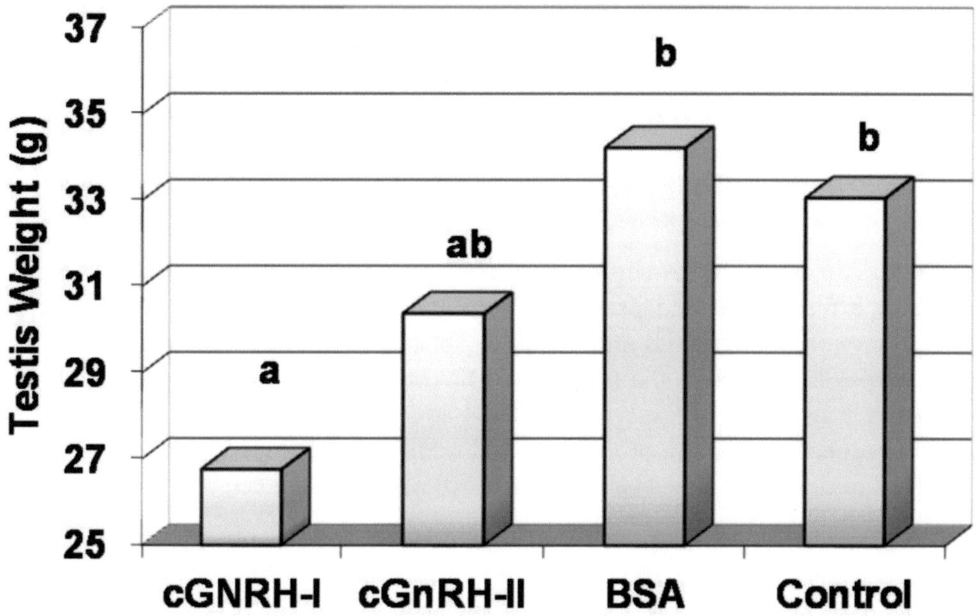

Figure 4. Testis weight of male broiler breeders immunized against cGnRH-I, cGnRH-II, BSA, and not immunized (Control) birds. Different letters indicate significant differences ($P < 0.05$)

Among primates, the rhesus monkey (*Macaca mulatta*), is one of the few species studied to date that posses a functional cGnRH-II peptide and type II GnRHR (Stewart et al., 2009). In these species, cGnRH-II is expressed in the hypothalamic median eminence (Urbanski et al., 1999), and has the ability to stimulate gonadotropin secretion (Lescheid et al., 1997). The rhesus hypothalamic cells that express mGnRH and cGnRH-II have a differential distribution pattern. In contrast to mGnRH, the axonal projections of cGnRH-II have a direct input in the neural lobe of the pituitary gland, raising the possibility that both forms of GnRH may play different physiological roles in the regulation of gonadotropin secretion (Urbanski et al., 1999). When cultured pituitary cells form male rhesus monkeys were incubated with cGnRH-II, LH and FSH were significantly increased. However, the *in vitro* effect of cGnRH-II on gonadotropin secretion was less potent than that of mGnRH (Okada et al., 2003). In contrast, *in vivo* exogenous doses of mGnRH and cGnRH-II in female rhesus monkeys were equally potent at stimulating LH release with little effect on FSH secretion (Densmore and Urbanski, 2003). In males and females rhesus monkeys, cGnRH-II mRNA expression in the mediobasal hypothalamus (MBH) significantly increased in adult animals compared with prepubertal macaques (Latimer et al., 2001). Since the MBH is associated with the pre-ovulatory LH surge and overall reproductive development (Spies et al., 1977), it is possible that cGnRH-II may play a role in the onset of puberty and sexual behavior.

Estrogen significantly increases cGnRH-II expression in the MBA (Densmore and Urbanski, 2004), while the same steroid significantly decreases mGnRH expression (Densmore and Urbanski, 2004; El Majdoubi et al., 1998). The positive and negative feedback mechanism of estrogen on the reproductive axis may be explained by the presence of the two GnRH isoforms present in the brain of the rhesus monkey. As noted above, few primate species are known to possess a functional cGnRH-II peptide and associated type II GnRH receptor. For instance, in the Chimpanzee (*Pan troglodytes*) the genes encoding the cGnRH-II peptide and the type II GnRH receptor contains a premature stop codon (Ikemoto and Park, 2006; Stewart et al., 2009); therefore there is a disruption of the ligand and the receptor. Information on regard to the GnRH-II system obtained in the rhesus monkey should not be generalized to other primate species.

Although human posses a functional cGnRH-II peptide, the type II GnRH receptor is disrupted by a frame shift and premature stop codon (Pawson et al., 2005). The type II GnRHR gene remains active and an alternative splicing (GnRHR-II-reliquum) is expressed in gonadotropes that contains the type I GnRHR (Millar et al., 1999; Pawson et al., 2005). Simultaneous transfection of the type I GnRHR and GnRHR-II-reliquum into COS-7 cells resulted in reduced expression of the type I GnRHR, suggesting a modulator role of the GnRHR-II reliquum on the type I GnRH receptor (Pawson et al., 2005).

In the Musk shrew (*Suncus murinus*), cGnRH-II was identified by HPLC and radioimmunoassay (RIA), and the presence of a functional peptide subsequently reported (Dellovade et al., 1993; Rissman and Li, 1998; Stewart et al., 2009). Although there is evidence that the type II GnRHR may mediate behavioral effects of cGnRH-II in the Musk shrew (Kauffman et al., 2005), a functional type II GnRHR has not been reported (Stewart et al., 2009). Nevertheless, ICV infusion of cGnRH-II but not mGnRH stimulated sexual behavior in nutritionally challenged female musk shrews (Temple et al., 2003). When musk shrews were exposed to different levels of caloric intake, cGnRH-II mRNA expression was modulated by feed intake (Kauffman et al., 2006; Kauffman and Rissman, 2004b). These data suggest a role of GnRH-II in both feeding and sexual behavior.

Among domestic animals, the pig is the only relevant livestock species that expresses both a functional mGnRH and cGnRH-II peptide and the associated cognate functional type I and type II GnRHR (Stewart et al., 2009). In bovine and ovine species the cGnRH-II peptide and the type II GnRHR receptor are functionally inactivated (Morgan et al., 2006) and in equine species, the type II GnRHR is functionally inactivated (Stewart et al., 2009).

Very little information on the effect of cGnRH-II on gonadotropin secretion is available in pigs. Treatment of pig pituitary cells with nanomolar concentrations of cGnRH-II consistently stimulated a 15-20 fold increase in LH secretion, while FSH secretion was more variable, ranging from none to a 4-fold stimulation (Neill et al., 2002).

We conducted studies to evaluate the effect of active immunization against cGnRH-II on gonadotropin secretion and testicular function in boars (Bowen et al., 2006). A synthetic cGnRH-II peptide, where the common pGlu-His-Trp-Ser sequence at the N-terminal was suppressed (see table 1) and a Cys residue was incorporated, was used in the conjugation process. Antibody titers were detectable in GnRH-II immunized animals four weeks after primary immunization (bottom panel Figure 5). Titers continued to increase as booster immunizations were given with limited to no cross-reactivity between mGnRH and cGnRH-II. No mGnRH specific antibodies were detected in control animals. Antibody titers against mGnRH were measured to determine if cGnRH-II antibodies recognized mGnRH. None of the animals produced antibodies that recognized mGnRH. However, when a plasma sample from a cow previously immunized against mGnRH was used, antibody titers were significantly higher (Figure 5; inset upper panel). None of the animals produced antibodies that recognized mGnRH, indicating that animals immunized against cGnRH-II produced antibodies that recognized only their own specific amino acid sequence. Active immunization against cGnRH-II significantly decreased gonadotropin secretion when compared with control barrows (Figure 6). These data suggest that the two GnRHs and GnRHRs systems, along with differences in signaling pathways, provide the potential for differential gonadotropin secretion in pigs.

GnRH antagonists, of which thousands have been formulated, cause an immediate and rapid reversible suppression of gonadotropin secretion. The principal mechanism of action of GnRH antagonists is competitive receptor occupancy of GnRHRs (Herbst, 2003; Huirne and Lambalk, 2001). The first generation of mGnRH antagonists contained replacements for His at position 2 and for Trp at position 3 (Huirne and Lambalk, 2001). The inhibitory activity increased after incorporation of a D-amino acid at position 6, but increased histamine-releasing activity resulted in anaphylactic reactions. The third generation antagonists have low histamine-releasing potency by replacing the D-amino acid at position 6 by neutral D-ureidoalkyl amino acids (Huirne and Lambalk, 2001). In pigs a third-generation antagonist (Cetrorelix) has been used in vivo and in vitro (Neill, 2002; Zanella et al., 2000). The ability of cetrorelix to inhibit [3H]-IP accumulation in response to cGnRH-II was evaluated in COS-1 cells that were transfected with the type II GnRHR. Increased concentrations of cGnRH-II in the media resulted in no inhibition of IP, and when cetrorelix was tested for agonist activity with the type II GnRHR, no activity was observed even at large doses (Neill, 2002). These data suggest that cetrorelix is a potent and specific antagonist to the type I GnRH receptor.

Daily intramuscular (i.m.) doses of cetrorelix decreased gonadotropin secretion in intact and castrated boars and gilts (Wise et al., 2000; Zanella et al., 2000; Ziecik et al., 1989). Administration of low doses (5 μg/kg of body weight; BW) of cetrorelix resulted in a decline of LH but had no effect on FSH concentrations, while doses of 10 μg/kg BW of cetrorelix were sufficient to inhibit FSH secretion (Wise et al., 2000; Zanella et al., 2000). Larger doses (20 μg, 50 μg, and 1 mg/kg BW) of cetrorelix also resulted in a significant decrease in LH concentrations with varied responses in FSH secretion (Moran et al., 2002; Wise et al., 2000; Ziecik et al., 1989). The lack of a consistent reduction of FSH secretion in pigs treated with the type I GnRHR antagonist may be associated with the presence of two GnRHs and two GnRH receptors, together with the differences in their signaling in swine species.

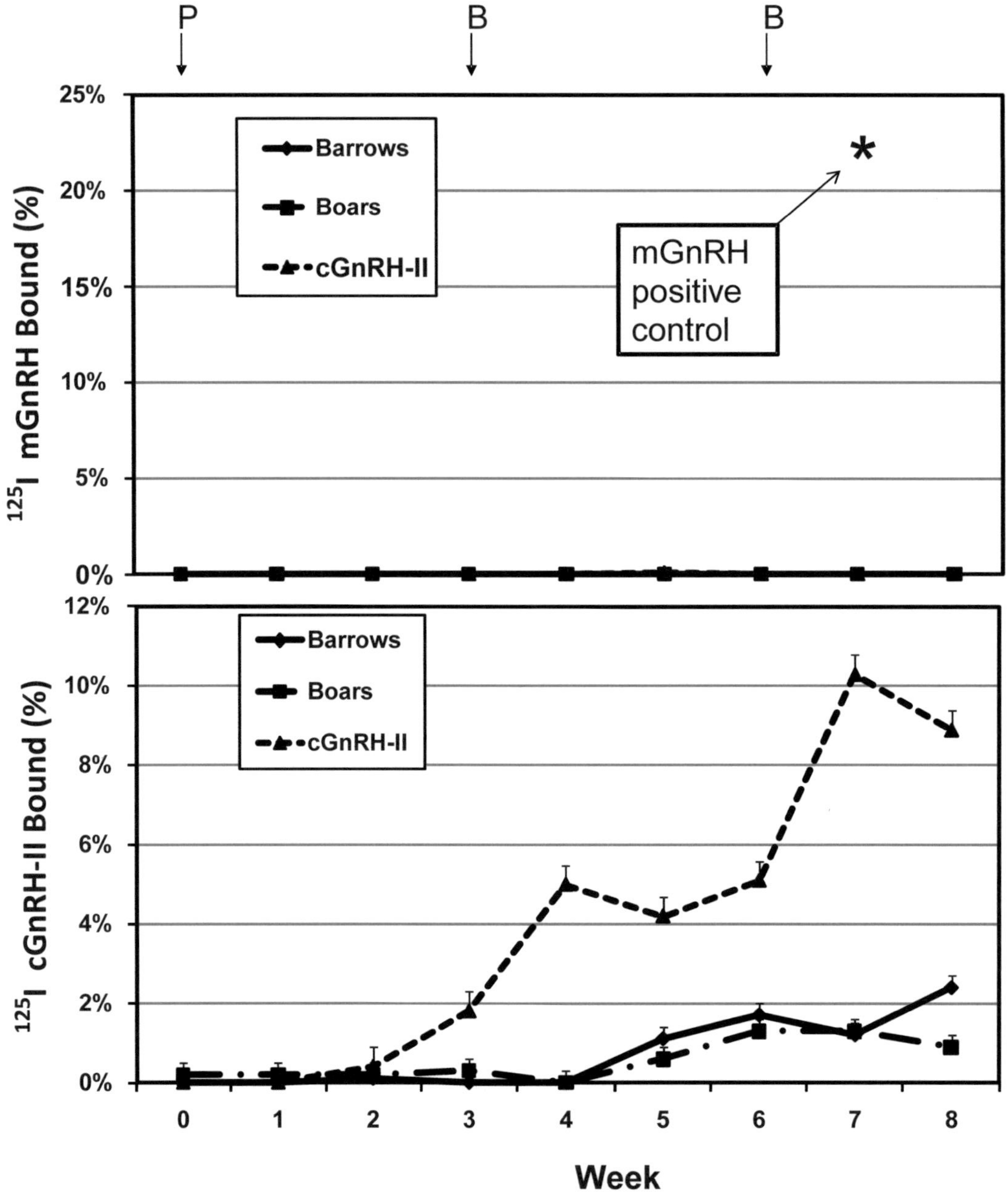

Figure 5. Effect of immunization on antibody titers against mGnRH and cGnRH-II in control barrows and boars immunized against BSA, and intact pigs immunized against cGnRH-II (n = 12/treatment). Antibody titers increased in animal immunized against cGnRH-II after the first booster immunization. Arrows indicate the times at which primary (P) and booster (B) immunizations were given. Plasma from a cow previously immunized against mGnRH (Vizcarra et al., 2011) was used as a positive control (inset). Adapted from (Bowen et al., 2006).

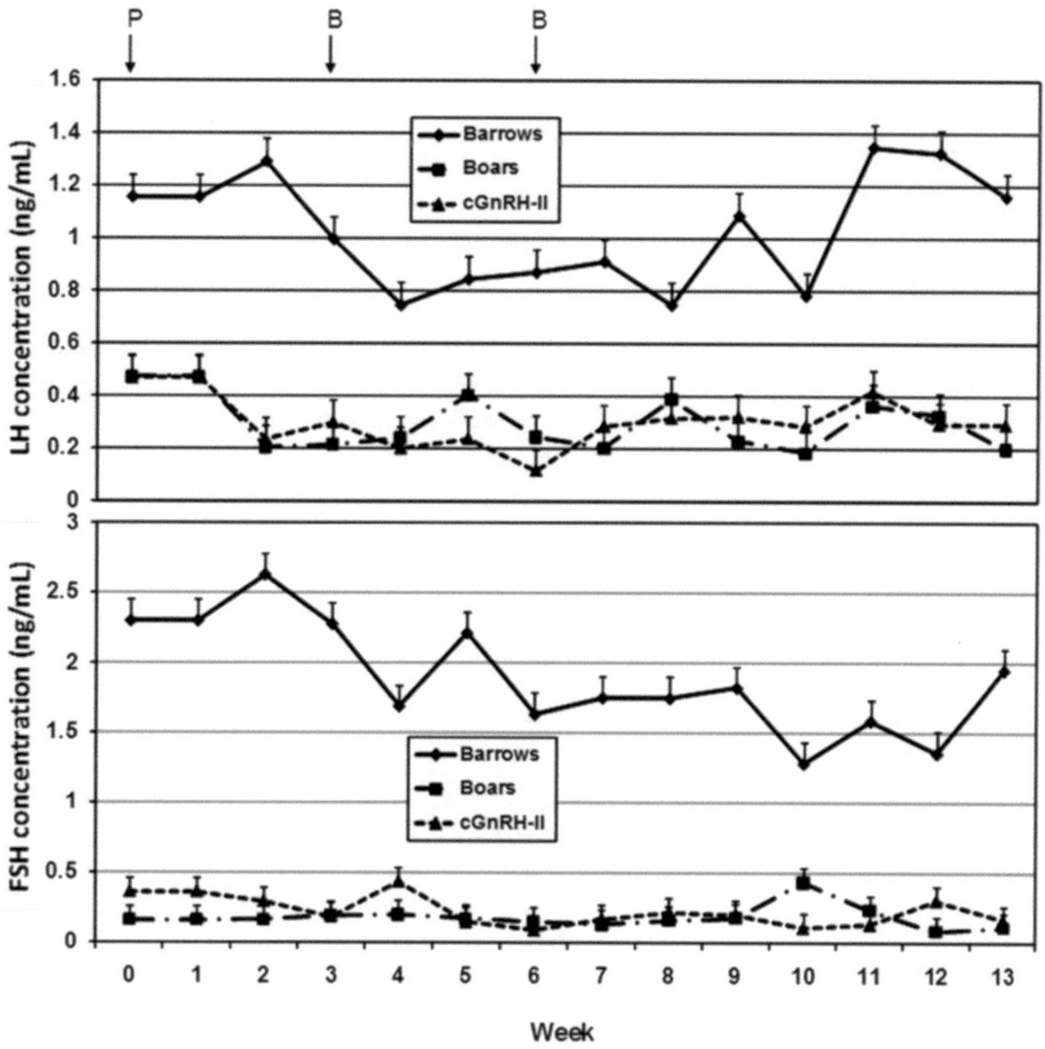

Figure 6. Concentrations of LH and FSH in weekly samples of control barrows and boars immunized against BSA, and intact pigs immunized against cGnRH-II (n= 12/treatment). There was a treatment effect for LH ($P < 0.01$) and a treatment x week interaction for FSH ($P < 0.03$), resulting in gonadotropin concentrations that were greater in control barrows compared with boars and cGnRH-II pigs. Arrows indicate the time at which primary (P) and booster (B) immunizations were given. Adapted from (Bowen et al., 2006).

Antagonist for the type II GnRHR have also been developed and tested in cells expressing rat GnRH (Maiti et al., 2003), human endometrial cells (Fister et al., 2007), and mice (Kim et al., 2009). However, all of these species have lost a functional type II GnRHR (Stewart et al., 2009) and data from these experiments are questionable. A type II GnRHR knockdown swine is being developed (Desaulniers et al., 2011). This animal model may provide new cues on the relative contribution of the type II GnRHR in pigs.

Taken together, GnRH-II is the most ancient and conserved member of the GnRH family, it is expressed in several vertebrates, and has the ability to control gonadotropin secretion in species that have a functional GnRH-II and type II GnRHR.

4. Lamprey GnRH-III

Sower and coworkers (Sower et al., 1993), reported the isolation of lGnRH-III from the sea lamprey (*Petromyzon marinus*). Although lGnRH-III is not a natural ligand of the type I or type II GnRHR, the lGnRH-III receptor shares different characteristics of both type I and type II GnRHRs (Silver et al., 2005; Silver and Sower, 2006). The presence of lGnRH-III (or a related analog) have been reported in brain extracts from humans, sheep, cows and rats (Dees et al., 1999; Hiney et al., 2002; Yahalom et al., 1999; Yu et al., 2000), suggesting a biological activity of this GnRH isoform in several species. However, to date, the gene expression of lGnRH-III has not been reported in mammalian species. There are indications that lGnRH-III might have antiproliferative effects on different types of cancer. Several GnRH analogs are used to treat various forms of cancer (Schally et al., 2001). Among these isoforms, lGnRH-III has a substantial antiproliferative effect on several cancer cell lines (Heredi-Szabo et al., 2006; Lovas et al., 1998; Mezo et al., 1997; Palyi et al., 1999),

The physiologic role played by lGnRH-III on gonadotropin secretion in mammalian species is controversial. Although lGnRH-III is a weak GnRH agonist, early research in mammalian species suggested that lGnRH-III can selectively stimulate the secretion of FSH without changing concentration of LH.

In rodents, lGnRH-III significantly increased FSH concentrations in a dose-dependent manner when using anterior pituitaries at 10^{-9} to 10^{-4} *M* concentrations. In contrast, LH concentrations were affected only when the highest doses of lGnRH-III (10^{-6} to 10^{-4} *M*) were used (Yu et al., 1997). Intravenous (i.v.) infusion of lGnRH-III also increased FSH without changes in LH concentrations (Yu et al., 1997). Subsequently, data from the same laboratory reported the isolation of a FSH-releasing factor (RF) obtained from the stalk-median eminence of rats. The FSHRF was associated with lGnRH-III, and had the ability to interact with a putative receptor to selectively release FSH (McCann et al., 2001; Yu et al., 2002; Yu et al., 2000). These data and that from other non-traditional sources (McCann and Yu, 2001) suggest that lGnRH-III is a potent and specific FSH-releasing peptide. However, other lines of research have raised questions about the ability of lGnRH-III to selectively secrete FSH in rodents (see below).

The presence of lGnRH-III in the brain of rats was identified by immunocytochemistry (Dees et al., 1999), and subsequently localized in the dorsomedial preoptic area (POA) of the brain and colocalized with mGnRH (Hiney et al., 2002). However, lGnRH-III was not detected in rats and other rodents by reverse-phase-HPLC followed by RIA, or by performing two successive HPLC steps to prevent the coelution of GnRH peptides (Gautron et al., 2005; Montaner et al., 1999; Montaner et al., 2001). When rats were infused (i.v.) with doses of lGnRH-III or mGnRH, gonadotropin secretion was increased in a dose-dependent manner with a greater increase in LH than FSH concentrations. The potency of lGnRH-III was 180 to 650 fold weaker than that of mGnRH (Kovacs et al., 2002). Similarly, when rat pituitary cells were perfused with lGnRH-III or mGnRH (10^{-9} to 10^{-6} *M*), lGnRH-III was 1,000 fold less active in releasing LH than mGnRH (Lovas et al., 1998). Moreover, when rat pituitary cells were perfused with doses (10^{-7} to 10^{-5} *M*) of lGnRH-III, gonadotropin secretion was increased without any indication of a selective secretion of FSH (Kovacs et al., 2002). These data is in agreement with *in vitro* results obtained from rat hemipituitaries incubated with doses (10^{-9} to 10^{-7} *M*) of lGnRH-III (Montaner et al., 2001). The contradictory results obtained by different laboratories, may be explained by experimental condition, the influence of the presence or absence of steroid in the *in vivo* models, and data interpretation (Kovacs et al., 2002).

Undoubtedly, more research is needed to clarify the existence of lGnRH-III or a FSHRF that may be involved in the differential secretion of gonadotropins in mammals. In addition to the information provided above, other areas of investigation have stressed the need to reconsider the traditional conjecture that a single GnRH molecule controls reproduction (Igarashi and McCann, 1964; McCann et al., 1983; Padmanabhan and McNeilly, 2001). Briefly, lesions to the median eminence (ME) of castrated male rats suppressed LH but not FSH pulses, while animals with posterior to mid-ME lesions had no FSH pulses but maintained LH episodic releases (Marubayashi et al., 1999). Similarly, ablation of the dorsal anterior hypothalamus of ovariectomized rats suppressed FSH pulses but not LH (Lumpkin et al., 1989). These results raise the possibility that another form of GnRH may contribute nontraditionally to the control of reproductive function or may take part in an important neuroendocrine role. The nature of episodic FSH secretion in portal blood cannot be accounted completely by changes in GnRH secretion (Padmanabhan et al., 1997). When male rats were administered GnRH antiserum and/or GnRH antagonists, pulsatile FSH release was maintained while LH was abolished, giving further credence to the view that reproductive function may be regulated by more than one GnRH neuronal system (Culler and Negro-Vilar, 1987). We have observed that GnRH pulse frequency and amplitude differentially regulates LH and FSH gene transcription and serum concentrations of LH and FSH in cattle (Vizcarra et al., 1997). However, this mechanism of FSH secretion does not preclude the existence of other GnRH releasing factors. It is also possible that the concerted action of local pituitary factors and peripheral steroids could lead to a pulsatile FSH pattern. For instance activins, inhibins, and follistatins may provide an autocrine-paracrine regulation of FSH release at the pituitary level (Baird et al., 1991; DePaolo et al., 1991; Mather et al., 1992; Nett et al., 2002; Padmanabhan et al., 2002; Padmanabhan et al., 1997; Padmanabhan and McNeilly, 2001).

Data obtained in the late 1990's, using the rat model, inspired other laboratories to investigate the use of lGnRH-III in domestic species. Since this peptide was able to selectively stimulate FSH secretion in rats, several researches evaluated the potential use of lGnRH-III in different livestock species. Using similar techniques as those reported in rats, lGnRH-III (or a closely related peptide), was also extracted from sheep stalk-median eminence using a Sephadex G-25 column (Lumpkin et al., 1987; Yu et al., 2000), and from bovine brain samples using HPLC (Yahalom et al., 1999). However, as noted above, the gene expression of lGnRH-III has not been reported in mammalian species. The ability of lGnRH-III (obtained from bovine midbrain tissue) to release LH was evaluated in cultured rat pituitary cells. The potency of lGnRH-III was only about 2% of that of mGnRH, suggesting that lGnRH-III is a weak agonist of mGnRH (Yahalom et al., 1999). When lGnRH-III (0.25 and 0.5 mg) was infused (i.v.) during the luteal phase of the estrous cycle of crossbred heifers, FSH concentrations were increased without changes in LH concentrations. At higher doses (2.0 and 8.0 mg) both FSH and LH were increased compared with basal concentrations. In contrast, a dose of 0.5 mg of lGnRH-III elicited a significant increase in LH with no changes in FSH secretion at day 20 of the estrous cycle. Authors suggested that the selectivity of lGnRH-III in cattle depends on the dosage and the stage of the estrous cycle (Dees et al., 2001).

In sharp contrast to the observations described above, no differential gonadotropin secretion was reported in ovariectomized cows (exposed to different steroid replacement therapy) when infused with doses (0.055, to 1.1 mg/kg BW) of lGnRH-III. Higher doses (4.4 mg/kg BW) released LH but not FSH. Similarly, *in vitro* doses (10^{-7} to 10^{-6} *M*) of lGnRH-III elicited a non-selective increase of LH and FSH, while lower doses (10^{-9} to 10^{-8} *M*) were not associated with gonadotropin secretion in bovine adenohypophyseal cells (Amstalden et al., 2004).

A clear and unbiased interpretation of the discordant results observed in cattle (Amstalden et al., 2004; Dees et al., 2001) is difficult. Reagents (RIAs) used in both laboratories to evaluate LH and FSH were provided by the National Hormone and Pituitary Program. Thus, it is unlikely that differences can be attributed to the ability of a particular RIA to detect FSH concentrations (Amstalden et al., 2004). The ovariectomized cow model, with estradiol and progesterone replacement therapy, used in one experiment (Amstalden et al., 2004) may provide a better animal model compared with intact cows. As noted above, it is well established that ovarian follicular peptides such as actvin, inhibin and follistain regulate FSH secretion; therefore, intact animals could be influenced by ovarian secretions that may act as a confounding factor.

Along the same lines described for rats and cattle, there is contradictory evidence on the involvement of lGnRH-III on gonadotropin secretion in pigs. Infusion (i.m.) of lGnRH-III in barrows differentially stimulated FSH secretion within 1 h after treatment (Kauffold et al., 2005). On the other hand, when boars were actively immunized against lGnRH-III, concentrations of both LH and FSH were decreased without any evidence of a differential regulation of gonadotropin secretion (Bowen et al., 2006). We (Barretero-Hernandez et al., 2010) also evaluated the effect of infusion (i.v.) of different doses of lGnRH-III on the release of LH and FSH in pigs. Barrows were used to evaluate the effect of 0.1, 1.0 or 10.0 μg/kg BW of exogenous lGnRH-III on LH and FSH secretion (Figure 7). Blood samples were taken at 10-min intervals for 6 h, starting 2 h before treatments were applied. Relative concentrations of FSH after lGnRH-III infusion did not influence mean concentration of FSH at any of the doses; however, 10.0 μg/kg BW had a significant effect on LH secretion. We conclude that lGnRH-III is a weak GnRH agonist, and at high doses, lGnRH-III has the ability to release LH but not FSH in barrows. Similar findings were also obtained in gilts that were infused (i.m.) with a synthetic lGnRH-III product (Brussow et al., 2010).

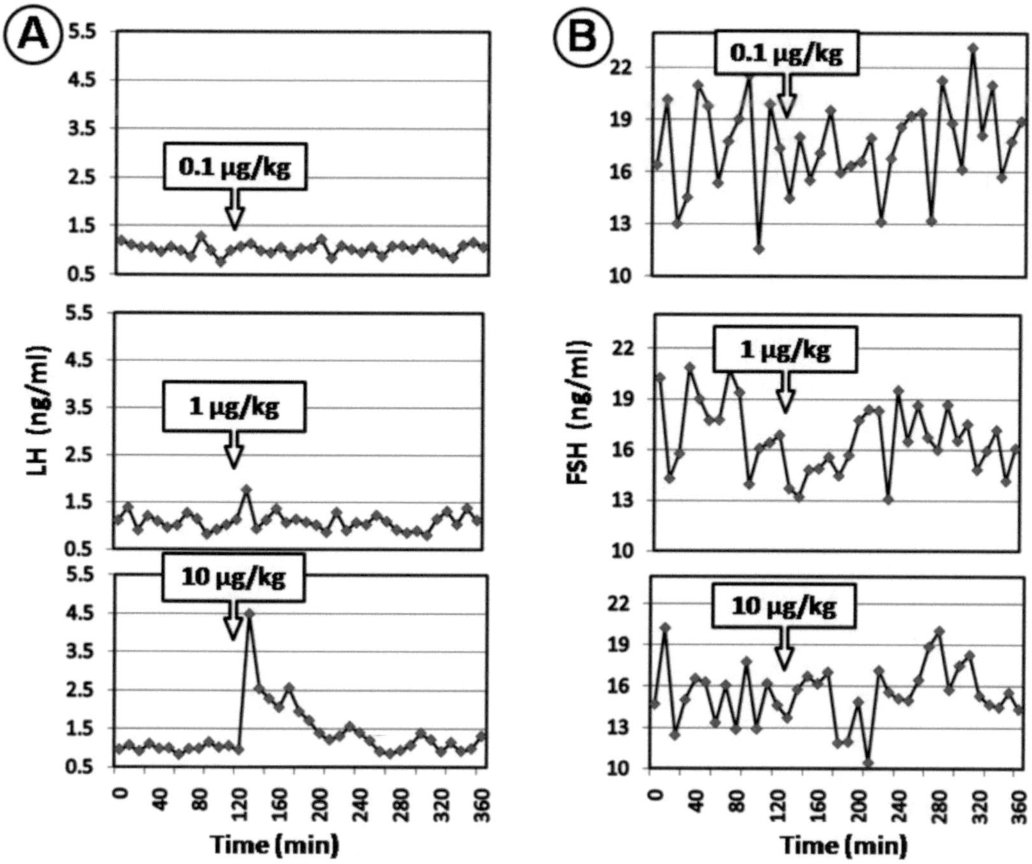

Figure 7. Mean concentrations of LH (A) and FSH (B) in serum at 10-min intervals before and after (arrows) 0.1, 1.0 or 10 µg of lGnRH-III were given intravenously. Only a dose of 10 µg/kg BW elicited a significant LH increase that was considered to be associated with exogenous lGnRH-III infusion (n = 6 animals per treatment). Adapted from (Barretero-Hernandez et al., 2010).

Taken together, the gene expression of lGnRH-III and its receptor has not been reported in mammalian species. Although early work in rats, cows and pigs suggested a selective release of FSH via lGnRH-III, the bulk of the evidence does not support a contribution of lGnRH-III on the selective release of FSH. It is possible that a different peptide (closely related to lGnRH-III) may be associated with FSH release.

Author details

Jorge Vizcarra
Alabama A&M University, USA

5. References

Amstalden, M., D. A. Zieba, M. R. Garcia, R. L. Stanko, T. H. Welsh, Jr., W. H. Hansel, and G. L. Williams. 2004. Evidence that lamprey GnRH-III does not release FSH selectively in cattle. Reproduction 127: 35-43.

Baird, D. T., B. K. Campbell, G. E. Mann, and A. S. McNeilly. 1991. Inhibin and oestradiol in the control of FSH secretion in the sheep. Journal of Reproduction and Fertility 43: 125-138.

Barb, C. R., R. R. Kraeling, and G. B. Rampacek. 2001. Nutritional regulators of the hypothalamic-pituitary axis in pigs. Reproduction (Cambridge, England) Supplement 58: 1-15.

Barran, P. E., R. W. Roeske, A. J. Pawson, R. Sellar, M. T. Bowers, K. Morgan, Z. L. Lu, M. Tsuda, T. Kusakabe, and R. P. Millar. 2005. Evolution of constrained gonadotropin-releasing hormone ligand conformation and receptor selectivity. J Biol Chem 280: 38569-38575.

Barretero-Hernandez, R., J. A. Vizcarra, A. Bowen, and M. Galyean. 2010. Lamprey GnRH-III releases luteinizing hormone but not follicle stimulating hormone in pigs. Reproduction in Domestic Animals 45: 983-987.

Blomenrohr, M., A. Heding, R. Sellar, R. Leurs, J. Bogerd, K. A. Eidne, and G. B. Willars. 1999. Pivotal role for the cytoplasmic carboxyl-terminal tail of a nonmammalian gonadotropin-releasing hormone receptor in cell surface expression, ligand binding, and receptor phosphorylation and internalization. Molecular Pharmacology 56: 1229-1237.

Bowen, A., S. Khan, L. Berghman, J. D. Kirby, R. P. Wettemann, and J. A. Vizcarra. 2006. Immunization of pigs against chicken gonadotropin-releasing hormone-II and lamprey gonadotropin-releasing hormone-III: effects on gonadotropin secretion and testicular function. Journal of Animal Science 84: 2990-2999.

Brussow, K. P., F. Schneider, A. Tuchscherer, and W. Kanitz. 2010. Influence of synthetic lamprey GnRH-III on gonadotropin release and steroid hormone levels in gilts. Theriogenology 74: 1570-1578.

Cabrera-Vera, T. M., J. Vanhauwe, T. O. Thomas, M. Medkova, A. Preininger, M. R. Mazzoni, and H. E. Hamm. 2003. Insights into G protein structure, function, and regulation. Endocrine Reviews 24: 765-781.

Chou, H. F., and A. L. Johnson. 1987. Luteinizing hormone secretion from anterior pituitary cells of the cockerel: evidence for an ultradian rhythm. Poultry Science 66: 732-740.

Clarke, I. J. 2002. Two decades of measuring GnRH secretion. Reproduction (Cambridge, England) Supplement 59: 1-13.

Culler, M. D., and A. Negro-Vilar. 1987. Pulsatile follicle-stimulating hormone secretion is independent of luteinizing hormone-releasing hormone (LHRH): pulsatile replacement of LHRH bioactivity in LHRH-immunoneutralized rats. Endocrinology 120: 2011-2021.

Dees, W. L., J. K. Hiney, S. A. Sower, W. H. Yu, and S. M. McCann. 1999. Localization of immunoreactive lamprey gonadotropin-releasing hormone in the rat brain. Peptides 20: 1503-1511.

Dees, W. L., R. K. Dearth, R. N. Hooper, S. P. Brinsko, J. E. Romano, H. Rahe, W. H. Yu, and S. M. McCann. 2001. Lamprey gonadotropin-releasing hormone-III selectively releases follicle stimulating hormone in the bovine. Domest Anim Endocrinol 20: 279-288.

Dellovade, T. L., J. A. King, R. P. Millar, and E. F. Rissman. 1993. Presence and differential distribution of distinct forms of immunoreactive gonadotropin-releasing hormone in the musk shrew brain. Neuroendocrinology 58: 166-177.

Densmore, V. S., and H. F. Urbanski. 2003. Relative effect of gonadotropin-releasing hormone (GnRH)-I and GnRH-II on gonadotropin release. The Journal of Clinical Endocrinology and Metabolism 88: 2126-2134.

Densmore, V., and H. Urbanski. 2004. Effect of 17beta-estradiol on hypothalamic GnRH-II gene expression in the female rhesus macaque. Journal of Molecular Endocrinology 33: 145-153.

DePaolo, L. V., T. A. Bicsak, G. F. Erickson, S. Shimasaki, and N. Ling. 1991. Follistatin and activin: a potential intrinsic regulatory system within diverse tissues. Proceedings of the Society for Experimental Biology and Medicine. Society for Experimental Biology and Medicine New York, N.Y 198: 500-512.

Desaulniers, A. T., A. M. Voss, R. A. Cederberg, C. Lee, G. A. Mills, M. D. Snyder, and B. R. White. 2011. 6 Production of gonadotropin-releasing hormone II receptor knockdown swine. Reproduction, Fertility and Development 24: 114-114.

El Majdoubi, M., A. Sahu, and T. M. Plant. 1998. Effect of estrogen on hypothalamic transforming growth factor alpha and gonadotropin-releasing hormone gene expression in the female rhesus monkey. Neuroendocrinology 67: 228-235.

Esbenshade, K. L., A. J. Ziecik, and J. H. Britt. 1990. Regulation and action of gonadotrophins in pigs. Journal of Reproduction and Fertility 40: 19-32.

Fister, S., A. R. Gunthert, G. Emons, and C. Grundker. 2007. Gonadotropin-releasing hormone type II antagonists induce apoptotic cell death in human endometrial and ovarian cancer cells in vitro and in vivo. Cancer Research 67: 1750-1756.

Gautron, J. P., C. Gras, and A. Enjalbert. 2005. Molecular polymorphism of native gonadotropin-releasing hormone (GnRH) is restricted to mammalian GnRH and [hydroxyproline9] GnRH in the developing rat brain. Neuroendocrinology 81: 69-86.

Guillemin, R., and B. Rosenberg. 1955. Humoral hypothalamic control of anterior pituitary: a study with combined tissue cultures. Endocrinology 57: 599-607.

Guillemin, R. 2005. Hypothalamic hormones a.k.a. hypothalamic releasing factors. J Endocrinol 184: 11-28.

Harris, G. W. 1948. Neural control of the pituitary gland. Physiological Reviews 28: 139-179.

Hattori, A., S. Ishii, and M. Wada. 1986. Effects of two kinds of chicken luteinizing hormone-releasing hormone (LH-RH), mammalian LH-RH and its analogs on the release of LH and FSH in Japanese quail and chicken. Gen Comp Endocrinol 64: 446-455.

Herbst, K. L. 2003. Gonadotropin-releasing hormone antagonists. Current Opinion in Pharmacology 3: 660-666.

Heredi-Szabo, K., R. F. Murphy, and S. Lovas. 2006. Is lGnRH-III the most potent GnRH analog containing only natural amino acids that specifically inhibits the growth of human breast cancer cells? Journal of Peptide Science. 12: 714-720.

Hiney, J. K., S. A. Sower, W. H. Yu, S. M. McCann, and W. L. Dees. 2002. Gonadotropin-releasing hormone neurons in the preoptic-hypothalamic region of the rat contain lamprey gonadotropin-releasing hormone III, mammalian luteinizing hormone-releasing hormone, or both peptides. Proceedings of the National Academy of Sciences of the United States of America 99: 2386-2391.

Huirne, J. A., and C. B. Lambalk. 2001. Gonadotropin-releasing-hormone-receptor antagonists. Lancet 358: 1793-1803.

Igarashi, M., and S. M. McCann. 1964. A Hypothalamic Follicle Stimulating Hormone-Releasing Factor. Endocrinology 74: 446-452.

Ikemoto, T., and M. K. Park. 2006. Comparative genomics of the endocrine systems in humans and chimpanzees with special reference to GNRH2 and UCN2 and their receptors. Genomics 87: 459-462.

Kaiser, U. B., P. M. Conn, and W. W. Chin. 1997. Studies of gonadotropin-releasing hormone (GnRH) action using GnRH receptor-expressing pituitary cell lines. Endocrine Reviews 18: 46-70.

Kakar, S. S., L. C. Musgrove, D. C. Devor, J. C. Sellers, and J. D. Neill. 1992. Cloning, sequencing, and expression of human gonadotropin releasing hormone (GnRH) receptor. Biochem Biophys Res Commun 189: 289-295.

Katz, I. A., R. P. Millar, and J. A. King. 1990. Differential regional distribution and release of two forms of gonadotropin-releasing hormone in the chicken brain. Peptides 11: 443-450.

Kauffman, A. S., and E. F. Rissman. 2004a. A critical role for the evolutionarily conserved gonadotropin-releasing hormone II: mediation of energy status and female sexual behavior. Endocrinology 145: 3639-3646.

Kauffman, A. S., and E. F. Rissman. 2004b. The evolutionarily conserved gonadotropin-releasing hormone II modifies food intake. Endocrinology 145: 686-691.

Kauffman, A. S., A. Wills, R. P. Millar, and E. F. Rissman. 2005. Evidence that the type-2 gonadotrophin-releasing hormone (GnRH) receptor mediates the behavioural effects of GnRH-II on feeding and reproduction in musk shrews. Journal of Neuroendocrinology 17: 489-497.

Kauffman, A. S., K. Bojkowska, A. Wills, and E. F. Rissman. 2006. Gonadotropin-releasing hormone-II messenger ribonucleic acid and protein content in the mammalian brain are modulated by food intake. Endocrinology 147: 5069-5077.

Kauffold, J., F. Schneider, W. Zaremba, and K. P. Brussow. 2005. Lamprey GnRH-III stimulates FSH secretion in barrows. Reproduction in Domestic Animals 40: 475-479.

Kim, D. K., J. S. Yang, K. Maiti, J. I. Hwang, K. Kim, D. Seen, Y. Ahn, C. Lee, B. C. Kang, H. B. Kwon, J. Cheon, and J. Y. Seong. 2009. A gonadotropin-releasing hormone-II antagonist induces autophagy of prostate cancer cells. Cancer Research 69: 923-931.

Kim, D. K., E. B. Cho, M. J. Moon, S. Park, J. I. Hwang, O. Kah, S. A. Sower, H. Vaudry, and J. Y. Seong. 2011. Revisiting the evolution of gonadotropin-releasing hormones and their receptors in vertebrates: secrets hidden in genomes. Gen Comp Endocrinol 170: 68-78.

King, J. A., and R. P. Millar. 1982. Structure of chicken hypothalamic luteinizing hormone-releasing hormone. II. Isolation and characterization. J Biol Chem 257: 10729-10732.

King, J. A., and R. P. Millar. 1995. Evolutionary aspects of gonadotropin-releasing hormone and its receptor. Cell Mol Neurobiol 15: 5-23.

Kovacs, M., J. Seprodi, M. Koppan, J. E. Horvath, B. Vincze, I. Teplan, and B. Flerko. 2002. Lamprey gonadotropin hormone-releasing hormone-III has no selective follicle-stimulating hormone-releasing effect in rats. Journal of Neuroendocrinology 14: 647-655.

Krishnan, K. A., J. A. Proudman, D. J. Bolt, and J. M. Bahr. 1993. Development of an homologous radioimmunoassay for chicken follicle-stimulating hormone and measurement of plasma FSH during the ovulatory cycle. Comp Biochem Physiol Comp Physiol 105: 729-734.

Latimer, V. S., S. G. Kohama, V. T. Garyfallou, and H. F. Urbanski. 2001. A developmental increase in the expression of messenger ribonucleic acid encoding a second form of gonadotropin-releasing hormone in the rhesus macaque hypothalamus. The Journal of Clinical Endocrinology and Metabolism 86: 324-329.

Lescheid, D. W., E. Terasawa, L. A. Abler, H. F. Urbanski, C. M. Warby, R. P. Millar, and N. M. Sherwood. 1997. A second form of gonadotropin-releasing hormone (GnRH) with characteristics of chicken GnRH-II is present in the primate brain. Endocrinology 138: 5618-5629.

Lovas, S., I. Palyi, B. Vincze, J. Horvath, M. Kovacs, I. Mezo, G. Toth, I. Teplan, and R. F. Murphy. 1998. Direct anticancer activity of gonadotropin-releasing hormone-III. J Pept Res 52: 384-389.

Lumpkin, M. D., J. H. Moltz, W. H. Yu, W. K. Samson, and S. M. McCann. 1987. Purification of FSH-releasing factor: its dissimilarity from LHRH of mammalian, avian, and piscian origin. Brain Research Bulletin 18: 175-178.

Lumpkin, M. D., J. K. McDonald, W. K. Samson, and S. M. McCann. 1989. Destruction of the dorsal anterior hypothalamic region suppresses pulsatile release of follicle stimulating hormone but not luteinizing hormone. Neuroendocrinology 50: 229-235.

Maiti, K., J. H. Li, A. F. Wang, S. Acharjee, W. P. Kim, W. B. Im, H. B. Kwon, and J. Y. Seong. 2003. GnRH-II analogs for selective activation and inhibition of non-mammalian and type-II mammalian GnRH receptors. Molecules and Cells 16: 173-179.

Maney, D. L., R. D. Richardson, and J. C. Wingfield. 1997. Central administration of chicken gonadotropin-releasing hormone-II enhances courtship behavior in a female sparrow. Hormones and Behavior 32: 11-18.

Marubayashi, U., W. H. Yu, and S. M. McCann. 1999. Median eminence lesions reveal separate hypothalamic control of pulsatile follicle-stimulating hormone and luteinizing hormone release. Proceedings of the Society for Experimental Biology and Medicine. Society for Experimental Biology and Medicine. New York, N.Y 220: 139-146.

Mather, J. P., T. K. Woodruff, and L. A. Krummen. 1992. Paracrine regulation of reproductive function by inhibin and activin. Proceedings of the Society for Experimental Biology and Medicine. Society for Experimental Biology and Medicine. New York, N.Y 201: 1-15.

Matsuo, H., Y. Baba, R. M. Nair, A. Arimura, and A. V. Schally. 1971. Structure of the porcine LH- and FSH-releasing hormone. I. The proposed amino acid sequence. Biochem Biophys Res Commun 43: 1334-1339.

McCann, S. M., and A. Fruit. 1957. Effect of synthetic vasopressin on release of adrenocorticotrophin in rats with hypothalamic lesions. Proceedings of the Society for Experimental Biology and Medicine. Society for Experimental Biology and Medicine. New York, N.Y 96: 566-567.

McCann, S. M., H. Mizunuma, W. K. Samson, and M. D. Lumpkin. 1983. Differential hypothalamic control of FSH secretion: a review. Psychoneuroendocrinology 8: 299-308.

McCann, S. M., S. Karanth, C. A. Mastronardi, W. L. Dees, G. Childs, B. Miller, S. Sower, and W. H. Yu. 2001. Control of Gonadotropin Secretion by Follicle-Stimulating Hormone-Releasing Factor, Luteinizing Hormone-Releasing Hormone, and Leptin. Archives of Medical Research 32: 476-485.

McCann, S. M., and W. H. Yu. 2001. FSH-releasing peptides. US Patent 6,300,471.

McCann, S. M., S. Karanth, C. A. Mastronardi, W. L. Dees, G. Childs, B. Miller, S. Sower, and W. H. Yu. 2002. Hypothalamic control of gonadotropin secretion. Progress in Brain Research 141: 151-164.

Meddle, S. L., S. Bush, P. J. Sharp, R. P. Millar, and J. C. Wingfield. 2006. Hypothalamic pro-GnRH-GAP, GnRH-I and GnRH-II during the onset of photorefractoriness in the white-crowned sparrow (Zonotrichia leucophrys gambelii). Journal of Neuroendocrinology 18: 217-226.

Mezo, I., S. Lovas, I. Palyi, B. Vincze, A. Kalnay, G. Turi, Z. Vadasz, J. Seprodi, M. Idei, G. Toth, E. Gulyas, F. Otvos, M. Mak, J. E. Horvath, I. Teplan, and R. F. Murphy. 1997. Synthesis of gonadotropin-releasing hormone III analogs. Structure-antitumor activity relationships. Journal of Medicinal Chemistry 40: 3353-3358.

Millar, R. P., and J. A. King. 1987. Structural and functional evolution of gonadotropin-releasing hormone. International Review of Cytology 106: 149-182.

Millar, R., D. Conklin, C. Lofton-Day, E. Hutchinson, B. Troskie, N. Illing, S. C. Sealfon, and J. Hapgood. 1999. A novel human GnRH receptor homolog gene: abundant and wide tissue distribution of the antisense transcript. J Endocrinol 162: 117-126.

Millar, R., S. Lowe, D. Conklin, A. Pawson, S. Maudsley, B. Troskie, T. Ott, M. Millar, G. Lincoln, R. Sellar, B. Faurholm, G. Scobie, R. Kuestner, E. Terasawa, and A. Katz. 2001. A novel mammalian receptor for the evolutionarily conserved type II GnRH. Proceedings of the National Academy of Sciences of the United States of America 98: 9636-9641.

Millar, R. P. 2003. GnRH II and type II GnRH receptors. Trends in Endocrinology and Metabolism: TEM 14: 35-43.

Millar, R. P., Z. L. Lu, A. J. Pawson, C. A. Flanagan, K. Morgan, and S. R. Maudsley. 2004. Gonadotropin-releasing hormone receptors. Endocrine Reviews 25: 235-275.

Millar, R. P. 2005. GnRHs and GnRH receptors. Anim Reprod Sci 88: 5-28.

Millar, R. P., A. J. Pawson, K. Morgan, E. F. Rissman, and Z. L. Lu. 2008. Diversity of actions of GnRHs mediated by ligand-induced selective signaling. Frontiers in Neuroendocrinology 29: 17-35.

Millar, R. P., and C. L. Newton. 2010. The year in G protein-coupled receptor research. Molecular Endocrinology Baltimore, Md 24: 261-274.

Miyamoto, K., Y. Hasegawa, T. Minegishi, M. Nomura, Y. Takahashi, M. Igarashi, K. Kangawa, and H. Matsuo. 1982. Isolation and characterization of chicken hypothalamic luteinizing hormone-releasing hormone. Biochem Biophys Res Commun 107: 820-827.

Miyamoto, K., Y. Hasegawa, M. Nomura, M. Igarashi, K. Kangawa, and H. Matsuo. 1984. Identification of the second gonadotropin-releasing hormone in chicken hypothalamus: evidence that gonadotropin secretion is probably controlled by two distinct gonadotropin-releasing hormones in avian species. Proceedings of the National Academy of Sciences of the United States of America 81: 3874-3878.

Montaner, A. D., J. M. Affanni, J. A. King, J. J. Bianchini, G. Tonarelli, and G. M. Somoza. 1999. Differential distribution of gonadotropin-releasing hormone variants in the brain of Hydrochaeris hydrochaeris (Mammalia, Rodentia). Cell Mol Neurobiol 19: 635-651.

Montaner, A. D., L. Mongiat, V. A. Lux-Lantos, M. K. Park, W. H. Fischer, A. G. Craig, J. E. Rivier, D. Lescheid, D. Lovejoy, C. Libertun, N. M. Sherwood, and G. M. Somoza. 2001. Structure and biological activity of gonadotropin-releasing hormone isoforms isolated from rat and hamster brains. Neuroendocrinology 74: 202-212.

Moran, F. M., J. J. Ford, C. J. Corbin, S. M. Mapes, V. C. Njar, A. M. Brodie, and A. J. Conley. 2002. Regulation of microsomal P450, redox partner proteins, and steroidogenesis in the developing testes of the neonatal pig. Endocrinology 143: 3361-3369.

Morgan, K., R. Sellar, A. J. Pawson, Z. L. Lu, and R. P. Millar. 2006. Bovine and ovine gonadotropin-releasing hormone (GnRH)-II ligand precursors and type II GnRH receptor genes are functionally inactivated. Endocrinology 147: 5041-5051.

Neill, J. D. 2002. GnRH and GnRH receptor genes in the human genome. Endocrinology 143: 737-743.

Neill, J. D., L. W. Duck, and L. C. Musgrove. 2002. Potential regulatory role for GnRH II in gonadotropin secretion: molecular characterization of a GnRH II receptor from pig pituitary. Proceedings of the Society for Neuroscience Abstract 74.9.

Neill, J. D., L. C. Musgrove, and L. W. Duck. 2004. Newly recognized GnRH receptors: function and relative role. Trends in Endocrinology and Metabolism: TEM 15: 383-392.

Nett, T. M., A. M. Turzillo, M. Baratta, and L. A. Rispoli. 2002. Pituitary effects of steroid hormones on secretion of follicle-stimulating hormone and luteinizing hormone. Domest Anim Endocrinol 23: 33-42.

Okada, Y., A. Murota-Kawano, S. S. Kakar, and S. J. Winters. 2003. Evidence that gonadotropin-releasing hormone (GnRH) II stimulates luteinizing hormone and follicle-stimulating hormone secretion from monkey pituitary cultures by activating the GnRH I receptor. Biology of Reproduction 69: 1356-1361.

Padmanabhan, V., K. McFadden, D. T. Mauger, F. J. Karsch, and A. R. Midgley, Jr. 1997. Neuroendocrine control of follicle-stimulating hormone (FSH) secretion. I. Direct evidence for separate episodic and basal components of FSH secretion. Endocrinology 138: 424-432.

Padmanabhan, V., and A. S. McNeilly. 2001. Is there an FSH-releasing factor? Reproduction 121: 21-30.

Padmanabhan, V., F. J. Karsch, and J. S. Lee. 2002. Hypothalamic, pituitary and gonadal regulation of FSH. Reproduction (Cambridge, England) Supplement 59: 67-82.

Palyi, I., B. Vincze, S. Lovas, I. Mezo, J. Pato, A. Kalnay, G. Turi, D. Gaal, R. Mihalik, I. Peter, I. Teplan, and R. F. Murphy. 1999. Gonadotropin-releasing hormone analogue conjugates with strong selective antitumor activity. Proceedings of the National Academy of Sciences of the United States of America 96: 2361-2366.

Pawson, A. J., S. Maudsley, K. Morgan, L. Davidson, Z. Naor, and R. P. Millar. 2005. Inhibition of human type i gonadotropin-releasing hormone receptor (GnRHR) function by expression of a human type II GnRHR gene fragment. Endocrinology 146: 2639-2649.

Perfito, N., R. Zann, T. Ubuka, G. Bentley, and M. Hau. 2011. Potential roles for GNIH and GNRH-II in reproductive axis regulation of an opportunistically breeding songbird. Gen Comp Endocrinol 173: 20-26.

Powell, J. F., Y. Zohar, A. Elizur, M. Park, W. H. Fischer, A. G. Craig, J. E. Rivier, D. A. Lovejoy, and N. M. Sherwood. 1994. Three forms of gonadotropin-releasing hormone characterized from brains of one species. Proceedings of the National Academy of Sciences of the United States of America 91: 12081-12085.

Rastogi, R. K., D. L. Meyer, C. Pinelli, M. Fiorentino, and B. D'Aniello. 1998. Comparative analysis of GnRH neuronal systems in the amphibian brain. Gen Comp Endocrinol 112: 330-345.

Rissman, E. F., and X. Li. 1998. Sex differences in mammalian and chicken-II gonadotropin-releasing hormone immunoreactivity in musk shrew brain. Gen Comp Endocrinol 112: 346-355.

Roch, G. J., E. R. Busby, and N. M. Sherwood. 2011. Evolution of GnRH: diving deeper. Gen Comp Endocrinol 171: 1-16.

Rumsfeld, H. W., Jr., and J. C. Porter. 1962. ACTH-releasing activity of bovine posterior pituitaries. Endocrinology 70: 62-67.

Saffran, M., A. V. Schally, and B. G. Benfey. 1955. Stimulation of the release of corticotropin from the adenohypophysis by a neurohypophysial factor. Endocrinology 57: 439-444.

Schally, A. V., A. Arimura, A. J. Kastin, H. Matsuo, Y. Baba, T. W. Redding, R. M. Nair, L. Debeljuk, and W. F. White. 1971. Gonadotropin-releasing hormone: one polypeptide regulates secretion of luteinizing and follicle-stimulating hormones. Science 173: 1036-1038.

Schally, A. V. 2000. Use of GnRH in preference to LH-RH terminology in scientific papers. Human Reproduction 15: 2059-2061.

Schally, A. V., A. M. Comaru-Schally, A. Nagy, M. Kovacs, K. Szepeshazi, A. Plonowski, J. L. Varga, and G. Halmos. 2001. Hypothalamic hormones and cancer. Frontiers in neuroendocrinology 22: 248-291.

Sealfon, S. C., H. Weinstein, and R. P. Millar. 1997. Molecular mechanisms of ligand interaction with the gonadotropin-releasing hormone receptor. Endocrine Reviews 18: 180-205.

Sharp, P. J., and C. B. Gow. 1983. Neuroendocrine control of reproduction in the cockerel. Poultry Science 62: 1671-1675.

Sharp, P. J., R. T. Talbot, G. M. Main, I. C. Dunn, H. M. Fraser, and N. S. Huskisson. 1990. Physiological roles of chicken LHRH-I and -II in the control of gonadotrophin release in the domestic chicken. J Endocrinol 124: 291-299.

Silver, M. R., N. V. Nucci, A. R. Root, K. L. Reed, and S. A. Sower. 2005. Cloning and characterization of a functional type II gonadotropin-releasing hormone receptor with a lengthy carboxy-terminal tail from an ancestral vertebrate, the sea lamprey. Endocrinology 146: 3351-3361.

Silver, M. R., and S. A. Sower. 2006. Functional characterization and kinetic studies of an ancestral lamprey GnRH-III selective type II GnRH receptor from the sea lamprey, Petromyzon marinus. J Mol Endocrinol 36: 601-610.

Skinner, D. C., A. J. Albertson, A. Navratil, A. Smith, M. Mignot, H. Talbott, and N. Scanlan-Blake. 2009. Effects of gonadotrophin-releasing hormone outside the hypothalamic-pituitary-reproductive axis. Journal of Neuroendocrinology 21: 282-292.

Sower, S. A., Y. C. Chiang, S. Lovas, and J. M. Conlon. 1993. Primary structure and biological activity of a third gonadotropin-releasing hormone from lamprey brain. Endocrinology 132: 1125-1131.

Spies, H. G., R. L. Norman, S. K. Quadri, and D. K. Clifton. 1977. Effects of estradiol-17beta on the induction of gonadotropin release by electrical stimulation of the hypothalamus in rhesus monkeys. Endocrinology 100: 314-324.

Stevenson, T. J., G. E. Bentley, T. Ubuka, L. Arckens, E. Hampson, and S. A. MacDougall-Shackleton. 2008. Effects of social cues on GnRH-I, GnRH-II, and reproductive physiology in female house sparrows (Passer domesticus). Gen Comp Endocrinol 156: 385-394.

Stewart, A. J., A. A. Katz, R. P. Millar, and K. Morgan. 2009. Retention and silencing of prepro-GnRH-II and type II GnRH receptor genes in mammals. Neuroendocrinology 90: 416-432.

Temple, J. L., R. P. Millar, and E. F. Rissman. 2003. An evolutionarily conserved form of gonadotropin-releasing hormone coordinates energy and reproductive behavior. Endocrinology 144: 13-19.

Tostivint, H. 2011. Evolution of the gonadotropin-releasing hormone (GnRH) gene family in relation to vertebrate tetraploidizations. Gen Comp Endocrinol 170: 575-581.

Tsutsumi, M., W. Zhou, R. P. Millar, P. L. Mellon, J. L. Roberts, C. A. Flanagan, K. Dong, B. Gillo, and S. C. Sealfon. 1992. Cloning and functional expression of a mouse gonadotropin-releasing hormone receptor. Molecular Endocrinology Baltimore, Md 6: 1163-1169.

Urbanski, H. F., R. B. White, R. D. Fernald, S. G. Kohama, V. T. Garyfallou, and V. S. Densmore. 1999. Regional expression of mRNA encoding a second form of gonadotropin-releasing hormone in the macaque brain. Endocrinology 140: 1945-1948.

Vizcarra, J. A., R. P. Wettemann, T. D. Braden, A. M. Turzillo, and T. M. Nett. 1997. Effect of gonadotropin-releasing hormone (GnRH) pulse frequency on serum and pituitary concentrations of luteinizing hormone and follicle-stimulating hormone, GnRH receptors, and messenger ribonucleic acid for gonadotropin subunits in cows. Endocrinology 138: 594-601.

Vizcarra, J., M. Rhoads, C. Hsu, J. Washington, J. Morgan, J. Yang, H. Tang, J. Warren, and J. Kirby. 2000. Effect of immunization against chicken gonadotropin releasing hormone –I (cGnRH-I) and cGnRH-II on reproductive function in adult broiler breeder males. Poultry Sci 79: Abs 343.

Vizcarra, J. A., D. L. Kreider, and J. D. Kirby. 2004. Episodic gonadotropin secretion in the mature fowl: serial blood sampling from unrestrained male broiler breeders (Gallus domesticus). Biology of Reproduction 70: 1798-1805.

Vizcarra, J. A., S. L. Karges, and R. P. Wettemann. 2012. Immunization of beef heifers against gonadotropin-releasing hormone prevents luteal activity and pregnancy: effect of conjugation to different proteins and effectiveness of adjuvants. Journal of Animal Science (In Press).

Wade, N. 1978. Guillemin and Schally: The Years in the Wilderness. Science 200: 279-282.

Weesner, G. D., and R. L. Matteri. 1994. Rapid communication: nucleotide sequence of luteinizing hormone-releasing hormone (LHRH) receptor cDNA in the pig pituitary. Journal of Animal Science 72: 1911.

Wilson, S. C., and P. J. Sharp. 1975. Episodic release of luteinizing hormone in the domestic fowl. J Endocrinol 64: 77-86.

Wise, T., E. L. Zanella, D. D. Lunstra, and J. J. Ford. 2000. Relationships of gonadotropins, testosterone, and cortisol in response to GnRH and GnRH antagonist in boars selected for high and low follicle-stimulating hormone levels. Journal of Animal Science 78: 1577-1590.

Yahalom, D., A. Chen, N. Ben-Aroya, S. Rahimipour, E. Kaganovsky, E. Okon, M. Fridkin, and Y. Koch. 1999. The gonadotropin-releasing hormone family of neuropeptides in the brain of human, bovine and rat: identification of a third isoform. FEBS Lett 463: 289-294.

Yu, W. H., S. Karanth, A. Walczewska, S. A. Sower, and S. M. McCann. 1997. A hypothalamic follicle-stimulating hormone-releasing decapeptide in the rat. Proceedings of the National Academy of Sciences of the United States of America 94: 9499-9503.

Yu, W. H., S. Karanth, S. A. Sower, A. F. Parlow, and S. M. McCann. 2000. The similarity of FSH-releasing factor to lamprey gonadotropin-releasing hormone III (l-GnRH-III). Proceedings of the Society for Experimental Biology and Medicine. Society for Experimental Biology and Medicine New York, N.Y 224: 87-92.

Yu, W. H., S. Karanth, C. A. Mastronardi, S. Sealfon, C. Dean, W. L. Dees, and S. M. McCann. 2002. Lamprey GnRH-III acts on its putative receptor via nitric oxide to release follicle-stimulating hormone specifically. Experimental Biology and Medicine Maywood, N.J 227: 786-793.

Zanella, E. L., D. D. Lunstra, T. H. Wise, J. E. Kinder, and J. J. Ford. 2000. GnRH antagonist inhibition of gonadotropin and steroid secretion in boars in vivo and steroid production in vitro. Journal of Animal Science 78: 1591-1597.

Ziecik, A. J., K. L. Esbenshade, and J. H. Britt. 1989. Effects of a gonadotrophin-releasing hormone antagonist on gonadotrophin secretion and gonadal development in neonatal pigs. J Reprod Fertil 87: 281-289.

Chapter 2

Role of Adipose Secreted Factors and Kisspeptin in the Metabolic Control of Gonadotropin Secretion and Puberty[1]

Clay A. Lents, C. Richard Barb and Gary J. Hausman

Additional information is available at the end of the chapter

http://dx.doi.org/10.5772/48802

1. Introduction

1.1. Adipose tissue as an endocrine organ

Recent investigations from many species continue to reinforce and validate adipose tissue as an endocrine organ that impacts physiological mechanisms and whole-body homeostasis. Factors secreted by adipose tissue or "adipokines" continue to be discovered and are linked to important physiological roles (Ahima, 2006) including the innate immune response (Schäffler & Schöolmerich, 2010). In a number of recent experiments transcriptional profiling demonstrated that 5,000 to 8,000 adipose tissue genes were differentially expressed during central stimulation of the melanocortin 4 receptor (Barb et al., 2010a) and several conditions such as fasting (Lkhagvadorj et al., 2009) and feed restriction (Lkhagvadorj et al., 2010). In contrast, 300 to 1,800 genes were differentially expressed in livers in these three studies (Barb et al., 2010a; Lkhagvadorj et al., 2009, 2010). This degree of differential gene expression in adipose depots reflects the potential influence of adipose tissue as a secretory organ on multiple systems in the body. Furthermore, advances in the study of adipose tissue gene expression include high throughput technologies in transcriptome profiling and deep sequencing of the adipose tissue microRNA transcriptome (review, Basu et al., 2012).

Recent proteomic studies of human and rat adipocytes have revealed the true scope of the adipose tissue secretome (Chen et al., 2005; Kheterpal et al., 2011; Lehr et al., 2012; Lim et al., 2008; Zhong et al., 2010). With refined and advanced proteomics techniques, these studies have revealed that many of the adipose tissue secreted factors identified at the gene level do indeed encode secreted proteins (Chen et al., 2005; Kheterpal et al., 2011; Lehr et al., 2012;

[1] Mention of trade names or commercial products in this publication is solely for the purpose of providing specific information and does not imply recommendation or endorsement by the U.S. Department of Agriculture.

Lim et al., 2008; Zhong et al., 2010). The presence of an N-terminal secretion signal peptide validates secreted proteins in conditioned media (Renes et al., 2009). In many of these studies, the presence or absence of a signal peptide was used to validate or identify truly secreted adipocyte proteins (Chen et al., 2005; Lehr et al., 2012; Lim et al., 2008; Zhong et al., 2010). In these studies, the percentage of total apparent secreted proteins that were considered secreted (+ signal peptide) ranged from 39 to 75% and the total number of secreted proteins ranged from 164 to 263 (Chen et al., 2005; Lehr et al., 2012; Lim et al., 2008; Zhong et al., 2010). However, the signal peptide approach could underestimate the adipocyte derived proteins present in the extracellular space (review, Renes et al., 2009). For instance, a blocking strategy has been used to distinguish between true secreted proteins and proteins that simply "leak" from the cell (review, Renes et al., 2009). Continued development and refinement of proteomic approaches in the study of the adipose tissue secretome will ultimately confirm the endocrine status of adipose tissue.

1.2. Adipose tissue as a modulator of gonadotropin secretion

Adipose tissue plays a role in whole-body homeostasis by acting as an endocrine organ, which was clearly demonstrated with the discovery of leptin. Evidence indicates a strong link between neural influences and adipocyte expression and secretion of leptin and other adipokines such as other cytokines (interleukins), neurotrophic factors (ciliary neurotrophic factor, CNTF; brain-derived neurotrophic factor, BDNF), insulin-like growth factor (IGF–I, and –II), binding protein (IGFBP-5), and neuropeptides such as neuropeptide Y (NPY) and nesfatin-1 (Table 1). Developmental changes in these relationships are considered important for onset of puberty. Leptin augments secretion of gonadotropins which are essential for initiation and maintenance of normal reproductive function, by acting centrally at the hypothalamus to regulate the gonadotropin-releasing hormone (GnRH) and neuronal activity. The effects of leptin on GnRH are mediated through interneuronal pathways involving NPY, proopiomelanocortin (POMC) and kisspeptin. Increased infertility associated with diet induced obesity or central leptin resistance are likely mediated through the kisspeptin-GnRH pathway. Furthermore, leptin regulates reproductive function by altering the sensitivity of the pituitary gland to GnRH. Other putative metabolic signals are circulating long chain fatty acid which can signal nutrient availability to the central nervous system (CNS) and alter feed intake and glucose availability.

2. Free Fatty Acids (FFA)

2.1. Long-chain fatty acids act in the CNS

The control of appetite and metabolism in response to changes in nutrient availability occurs in part at the level of the hypothalamus (Barb et al., 1999, 2001a; Woods et al., 1998). Thus, macronutrients, such as carbohydrates and lipids, play a role in regulating peripheral concentrations of leptin and insulin (Ahima et al., 1996), which in turn has a direct effect on appetite and energy expenditure primarily through the hypothalamus (Barb et al., 2006; Woods et al., 1998). Levin et al. (1999) reported that hypothalamic neurons may directly detect nutrients. To that extent, treatment with a fatty acid synthase inhibitor reduced food

Regulatory – secreted factors			Receptors
adiponectin	IFNG	IL-5	ADIPOR2
adipsin	IGFBP-1	IL-6	BMPR2
agouti	IGFBP-3	IL-8	EDNRB
ANG	IGFBP-4	leptin	ESR1
ANGPTL2, ANGPTL4	IGFBP-5	PAI-1	FGFR1, FGFR4
RBP1, RBP4	IGFBP-7	RANTES	GNRHR2
APO-A1	IL-10	RTN	IFNGR1
APO-CIII	IL-12	TGF- β, TGF-β3	IGF-IR, IGF-IIR
APO-E	IL-15	THBS1	IL-4R, IL-10R
APO-R1	IL-18	TNFα	PGRMC1
BDNF	IL-1A	VEGFC	INSR
bFGF	IL-1B	visfatin	NGFR
CNTF	IL-1RN	CTGF	OB-rb
IGF-I, IGF-II	IL-4	NPY	THRA, THRA2, TSHR
Chemokine ligands 2, 3, 4, 12	Compliment component 1, 2, 4A, 6X, C7	TGF-α	EGFR
BMP-4, BMP-15	CTRP4, CIQTN4	MCP-1	LDLR
RLN	PDGFD	NUCB2, nesfatin-1	LHCGR
LPL			TLR 4
			AGTR1

Abbreviations: ADIPOR2 = adiponectin receptor 2, AGTR1 = angeotensin II receptor, ANG = angiotensin, ANGPTL = angiopoietin-like protein, APO = apolipoprotein, BDNF = brain-derived neurotrophic factor, bFGF = basic fibroblast growth factor, BMP = bone morphogenic protein, BMPR2 = bone morphogenic protein receptor 2, CIQTN4 = complement-c1q tumor necrosis factor-related protein 4, CNTF = ciliary neurotrophic factor, CTGF = connective tissue growth factor, CTRP4 = complement-c1q tumor necrosis factor-related protein 4, EDNRB = endothelin receptor type B, EGFR = epidermal growth factor receptor, ESR1 = estrogen receptor 1, GNRHR2 = gonadotropin-releasing hormone receptor 2, IFNG = interferon gamma, IGF = insulin-like growth factor, IGF-IR = IGF-I receptor, IGFBP = insulin-like growth factor binding protein, IL = interleukin, INSR = insulin receptor, LDLR = low density lipoprotein receptor, LHCGR = luteinizing hormone-choriogonadotropin receptor, LPL = lipoprotein lipase, MCP-1 = monocyte chemoattractant protein-1, NGFR = nerve growth factor receptor, NPY = neuropeptide Y, OB-rb = long form leptin receptor, NUCB2 = nucleobindin 2, PAI-1 = plasminogen activator inhibitor-1, PDGFD = platelet derived growth factor D, PGRMC1 = progesterone receptor membrane component 1, RANTES = chemokine (c-c motif) ligand 5, RBP = retinol binding protein, RLN = relaxin, TGF = transforming growth factor, RTN = reticulon, THR = thyroid hormone receptor, TLR = toll-like receptor, TNF = tumor necrosis factor, TSHR = thyroid-stimulating hormone receptor, VEGFC = vascular endothelial growth factor C.

References: Barb et al., 2010a; Basu et al., 2012; Chen et al., 2005; Hausman & Hausman, 2004; Hausman et al., 2009; Lehr et al., 2012; Lim et al., 2008; Lkhagvadorj et al., 2009, 2010; Renes et al., 2009; Zhong et al., 2010

Table 1. List of representative genes and proteins reported to be expressed by adipose tissue of humans, large animals, and rats.

intake and body weight in mice by reducing expression of NPY in the hypothalamus via a malonyl-Coenzyme A mechanism, which supports the idea that lipid metabolism in the CNS plays a role in the control of appetite (Loftus et al., 2000). Furthermore, long-chain Furthermore, long-chain fatty acyl CoAs (LC-CoAs), such as oleyl-CoA, can activate ATP-sensitive K^+ channels in non-neuronal cells (Larsson et al., 1996). Circulating fatty acids gain rapid access to the brain, where they equilibrate with neuronal LC-CoAs (J.C. Miller et al., 1987; Rapaport, 1996). They are then further metabolized via mitochondria β-oxidation or incorporated into phospholipids (J.C. Miller et al., 1987; Rapaport, 1996). Obici et al. (2002) hypothesized that fatty acids may signal nutritional status to selective neurons in the CNS and activate a feedback loop designed to curtail further influx of nutrients into the circulation. To that extent, Obici and coworkers (2002) reported that intracerebroventricular (i.c.v.) administration of the long-chain fatty acid, oleic acid, suppressed glucose production and feed intake. In addition, this was accompanied by a reduction in hypothalamic expression of NPY. This neuronal circuit plays a role in maintaining energy homeostasis by switching fuel sources from carbohydrates to lipids and by limiting circulating endogenous and exogenous nutrients. Disruption of this circuit may play a role in obesity, type 2 diabetes and other endocrine abnormalities (for a review, see Obici, 2009), which are often accompanied by gonadotropin insufficiency.

2.2. Regulation of gonadotropin secretion by long-chain fatty acids

In the pig, feed deprivation results in a rapid mobilization of FFA from peripheral fat depots, but maintenance of euglycemia suggests increased hydrolysis of triglycerides and FFA oxidation resulting in a glucose sparing effect (Barb et al., 1997). We previously reported that metabolic response to acute feed deprivation occurred more rapidly in prepubertal gilts compared to mature gilts, likely because prepubertal gilts have a higher metabolic rate, smaller energy reserves and thus a greater nutrient intake requirement for growth (Barb et al., 1997). In mature animals, chronic feed restriction resulted in cessation of estrous cycles and lower concentrations of plasma insulin, increased levels of FFA and reduced LH pulse frequency compared to controls (Armstrong & Britt, 1987). This brings into question, therefore, if alterations in serum concentrations of FFA influence hypothalamic-pituitary function. To address this matter, prepubertal gilts received intravenous (i.v.) injection of a lipid emulsion which consisted of the following fatty acids: linoleic (65.87%), oleic (17.7%), palmitic (8.8%), linolenic (4.2%) and stearic (3.43%) acid. The fatty acid content of the lipid emulsion was comparable to that present in the circulation of the pig (Cera et al., 1989). Lipid emulsion injection enhanced the LH response to GnRH (Barb et al., 1991), whereas infusion of lipid emulsion at 1 hour intervals increased serum LH pulse amplitude without effecting LH pulse frequency (Barb et al., 1991). Dispersed cells of the anterior pituitary gland of the pig were cultured to determine whether the effects of FFA *in vivo* occur at the pituitary without the benefit of input from the CNS. The long-chain fatty acids, oleic and linoleic acids increased basal LH release. In contrast oleic acid suppressed the GnRH-induced release of LH (Figure 1). The response for linoleic acid was equivocal (Barb et al., 1995). These events seem to be mediated at the plasma membrane because oleic and linoleic acids did not block the forskolin-induced release of LH (Barb et al., 1995). These results may explain the altered neuroendocrine activity observed during periods of feed restriction and fast. To that extent, administration of oleic acid into the third ventricle suppressed food intake and hypothalamic expression of NPY in the rat (Obici et al., 2002).

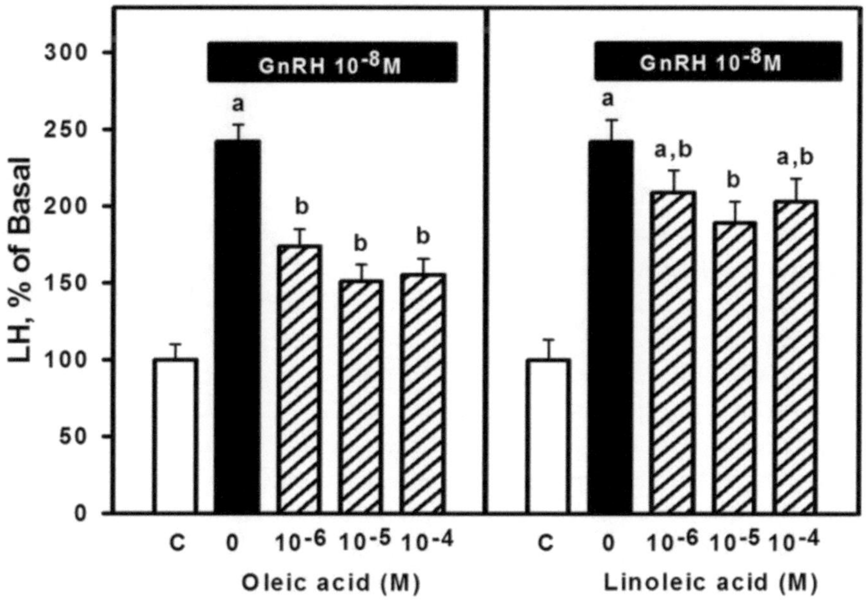

Figure 1. Anterior pituitary cells from prepubertal gilts (n = 11) were cultured in the presence of media alone (C, control wells; basal secretion in absence of any treatment) or gonadotropin releasing hormone (GnRH) at 10^{-8} M. Oleic or linoleic acid were included at 10^{-6} M, 10^{-5} M or 10^{-4} M in wells containing GnRH. Pituitary cells were exposed to oleic or linoleic acid for 30 min before the addition of GnRH. Media was collected 4 h after GnRH treatment. [a]Different from C (P < 0.03). [b]Different from GnRH alone (*P* < 0.03). Data from Barb et al. (1995).

An acute 28 h fast increased serum FFA concentrations, and decreased leptin pulse frequency but not mean concentrations of leptin in serum nor LH secretion in the ovariectomized prepubertal gilt (Barb et al., 2001b), while treatment with a competitive inhibitor of glycolysis suppressed LH secretion without affecting serum concentrations of leptin (Barb et al., 2001b). In contrast, short term feed restriction for 8 days decreased leptin secretion and LH pulse frequency in the mature ovariectomized gilt (Whisnant & Harrel, 2002). The ability of the pig to maintain euglycemia during acute fast may account for the failure of acute food deprivation to effect LH secretion (Barb et al., 1997). Although, leptin may serve as a metabolic signal which communicates metabolic status to the brain, the neuroendocrine response to acute energy deprivation may depend on age or mass of adipose tissue.

3. Nesfatin-1

3.1. Nesfatin-1 as an adipokine

While searching for new satiety factors, Oh-I et al. (2006) discovered a troglitazone- (PPARγ ligand) stimulated transcript expressed in SQ-5 (lung squamous carcinoma cell line) cells that was homologous to the nucleobindin 2 (NUCB2) gene, which codes for a DNA binding/EF hand/acidic protein (NEFA). The NUCB2 gene product is a 396 amino acid protein with several cleavage sites for prohormone convertase. Post-translational processing of the NUCB2 preprotein produces three cleavage products corresponding to amino acid residues 1-82, 85-163, and 166-396. Upon the observation that i.c.v. injection of the first 82 amino acid cleavage product suppressed feed intake resulting in reduced body and fat depot weights in mice, Oh-I et al. (2006) termed the protein nesfatin-1 for NEFA/nucleobindin2-encoded satiety- and fat-influencing protein-1.

Immediately upstream of the nesfatin-1 protein is a 26 amino acid signal sequence indicating that nesfatin-1 is likely a secreted factor that may have endocrine or paracrine action. Expression of NUCB2 mRNA is observed in predifferentiated 3T3-L1 cells (Oh-I et al., 2006; Ramanjaneya et al., 2010) and induction of differentiation resulted in a marked increase in expression of NUCB2 mRNA and secretion of nesfatin-1 into culture media (Ramanjaneya et al., 2010). Nesfatin-1 also is expressed and secreted from human and mouse adipose tissue explants (Ramanjaneya et al., 2010), with subcutaneous adipose tissue having greater expression of NUCB2/nesfatin-1 than omental adipose tissue (Ramanjaneya et al., 2010). Moreover, NUCB2 expression was greater in the adipocyte fraction of adipose tissue than in the stromal vascular fraction (Ramanjaneya et al., 2010) adding further support to the concept of nesfatin-1 as an adipose derived factor. Further studies are needed to define the precise roles of nesfatin-1, or the other NUCB2 gene products, in adipose tissue, but current evidence suggests involvement in chronic inflammatory response of adipose tissue associated with metabolic disease. Treating adipose tissue explants with energy partitioning hormones (insulin, dexamethasone) and cytokines, interleukin-6 (IL-6) and tumor necrosis factor α (TNFα), altered NUCB2 expression and nesfatin-1 secretion (Ramanjaneya et al., 2010). Furthermore, NUCB2 is involved in IL-1β stimulated release of soluble tumor necrosis factor receptor 1 to the extracellular space (Islam et al., 2006).

It is important to note that NUCB2 mRNA and nesfatin-1 protein have been found to be expressed in several endocrine cells and glands throughout the body including gastric glands of digestive tract (Stengel et al., 2009a; Zhang et al., 2010), islet cells of the pancreas (Gonzalez et al., 2009), and Leydig cells of the testes (Garcia-Galiano et al., 2012). This is indicative of the role nesfatin-1 plays in gastric emptying and nutrient absorption (Stengel et al., 2009b), glucose utilization (Gonzalez et al., 2011; Nakata et al., 2011; Su et al., 2010), and testosterone production (Garcia-Galiano et al., 2012). At present, it is unclear how these tissues may contribute to circulating concentrations of nesfatin-1; however, given that adipose tissue is the largest endocrine organ of the body, the contribution that fat depots would have to plasma concentrations of nesfatin-1 seems obvious. Concentrations of nesfatin-1 in the blood are, for the most part, positively correlated with body mass index (BMI) in healthy human subjects (Aydin et al., 2009; Li et al., 2010; Ogiso et al., 2011; Ramanjaneya et al., 2010) as are several single nucleotide polymorphisms within the NUBC2 gene (Zegers et al., 2011). Expression of nesfatin-1 in subcutaneous adipose tissue of mice is suppressed with fasting and increased when mice were fed a high fat diet (Ramanjaneya et al., 2010) indicating that nesfatin-1 concentrations in serum could be regulated by nutritional status. In point of fact, circulating concentrations of nesfatin-1 were less in patients with anorexia nervosa (Ogiso et al., 2011) and type 2 diabetes (Li et al., 2010). Together with the fact that nesfatin-1 crosses the blood-brain barrier via a nonsaturatable mechanism (Pan et al., 2007; Price et al., 2007), these data collectively indicate that nesfatin-1 is secreted from adipose tissue into the circulation and can enter the brain to regulate appetite.

3.2. Nesfatin-1 as a central regulator of food intake

The anorexogenic effects of nesfatin-1 are observed when nesfatin-1 is given either centrally (Shimizu et al., 2009) or peripherally (Stengel et al., 2009b). It is not clear, however, if suppression of appetite is entirely due to peripherally derived nesfatin-1 or the paracrine action of the protein produced within the hypothalamus. Expression of NUCB2/nesfatin-1 mRNA and protein has been demonstrated in several areas of the CNS. Within the hypothalamus, NUCB2/nesfatin-1 is expressed in nuclei that have important roles for control of appetite including the arcuate (ARC), paraventricular (PVN), lateral hypothalamic area and supraoptic nucleus (Brailoiu et al., 2007; Foo et al., 2008; Kohno et al., 2008; Oh-I et al., 2006). Areas of the brain stem that play pivotal roles in regulating energy homeostasis including the area postrema and the nucleus tractus solitaries (NTS) as well as the nucleus dorsalis of the vagus nerve all express NUCB2/nesfatin-1. Functional evidence that hypothalamic NUCB2/nesfatin-1 is involved in control of energy balance is derived from the observations that NUCB2/nesfatin-1 expression in the PVN is suppressed after fasting in adult and juvenile rats (Garcia-Galiano et al., 2010; Oh-I et al., 2006), and that refeeding activates nesfatin-1 neurons (as assessed by c-Fos) in the PVN (Kohno et al., 2008). Anorexigenic effects of nesfatin-1 require melanocortin receptors (Oh-I et al., 2006) and NPY neurons in hypothalamic slices of the ARC from mice were inhibited by nesfatin-1 *in vitro* (Price et al., 2008); although expression of NPY mRNA in the ARC of the rat *in vivo* was unchanged with nesfatin-1 treatment (Oh-I et al., 2006). Furthermore, alpha melanocyte-stimulating hormone treatment increased NUCB2 expression in the PVN (Oh-I et al., 2006) and nesfatin-1 has potent anorectic action in animals that are resistant to the effects of leptin (Oh-I et al., 2006; Su et al., 2010). This led to the initial thought that nesfatin-1 might be a down-stream effecter of the action of leptin; however, i.c.v. injection of nesfatin-1 antibodies did not block the anorectic effect of leptin in the rat (Oh-I et al., 2006). Instead, the anorexigenic actions of nesfatin-1 appear to be relayed through a mechanism independent from leptin. For instance, nesfatin-1 stimulates oxytocin cells in the PVN which in turn activate POMC neurons in the NTS of the brain stem (Maejima et al., 2009). Moreover, cholecystokinin (CCK) activates NUCB2/nesfatin-1 cell bodies in the PVN and NTS. The inhibition of food intake by CCK is mediated, at least partially, through NUCB2/nesfatin-1 neurons via a corticotrophin-releasing hormone (CRH) 2-receptor. Blocking the action of the CRH2 receptor with an antagonist ameliorated the suppressive effects of nesfatin-1 on food intake (Stengel et al., 2009b).

3.3. Nesfatin-1 as a neuroendocrine regulator of gonadotropin secretion

The neuroanatomical distribution of nesfatin-1 cell bodies in areas of the hypothalamus involved in integration of energy balance and reproduction (i.e., the ARC) and the fact that peripheral concentrations of nesfatin-1 reflect BMI suggest a role for nesfatin-1 in metabolic regulation of gonadotropin secretion. Hypothalamic expression of NUCB2/nesfatin-1 increases during the pubertal transition in the activity of the gonadotropic axis of rats (Garcia-Galiano et al., 2010). When young pubertal female rats were given i.c.v. injection of nesfatin-1, LH secretion increased two- to threefold; however, the effects of centrally administered nesfatin-1 on LH were much greater (9-fold increase) when rats were fasted for 48 h (Garcia-Galiano et al., 2010). The later observation is likely related to the fact that fasting or less severe but long-term nutrient restriction reduced NUCB2/nesfatin-1 expression in the brain and may explain a possible mechanism whereby fluctuations in energy balance impact gonadotropin secretion in a leptin independent manner. The stimulatory effects of i.c.v. nesfatin-1 on LH were not evident in adult female rats (Garcia-Galiano et al., 2010) suggesting nesfatin-1 plays an important role in regulating gonadotropin secretion during the pubertal transition; a period when increasing adiposity and sensitivity to adipokines is generally thought to be important for activation of the reproductive axis. Consistent with this is the fact that central infusion of nesfatin-1 antisense-morpholino oligonucleotides suppressed LH secretion and delayed puberty (as determined by absence of vaginal opening) in approximately 60% of peripubertal female rats but failed to alter ovulatory surges of LH in adult females (Garcia-Galiano et al., 2010). The effects of nesfatin-1 on LH and follicle-stimulating hormone (FSH) secretion may be sexually dimorphic as i.c.v. treatment with nesfatin-1 stimulated LH and FSH secretion in male rats that were fasted (Tadross et al., 2010). Moreover, nesfatin-1 stimulated release of GnRH from hypothalamic explants taken from male rats (Tadross et al., 2010).

Collectively these data indicated that nesfatin-1 is a protein hormone that participates in metabolic regulation of appetite and energy homeostasis. Reproductive function is sensitive to nutritional status and nesfatin-1 appears to have a role in conferring metabolic state to the gonadotropic axis, particularly during pubertal development. The mechanisms whereby this occurs have not been revealed yet, but likely involve action at the GnRH neuron. Whether this is a direct paracrine action of hypothalamic nesfatin-1 or an alteration in plasma concentrations of nesfatin-1 entering the brain is not known at present. Expression of nesfatin-1 in the testis and its role in regulating testosterone release (Garcia-Galiano et al., 2012) adds further complexity, and raises the possibility that nesfatin-1 can have indirect action on gonadotropin secretion through changes in gonadal steroid feed-back to the hypothalamus or anterior pituitary gland.

4. Leptin

4.1. Effects of leptin on the hypothalamic-pituitary axis

In the pig, presence of biologically-active leptin receptor (OB-rb) in the hypothalamus and pituitary (Lin et al., 2000) and the fact that leptin increased LH secretion from pig pituitary cells (Barb et al., 2004) and GnRH release from hypothalamic tissue (Figure 2; Barb et al., 2004) *in vitro* suggests that leptin acts through the hypothalamic-pituitary axis to modulate

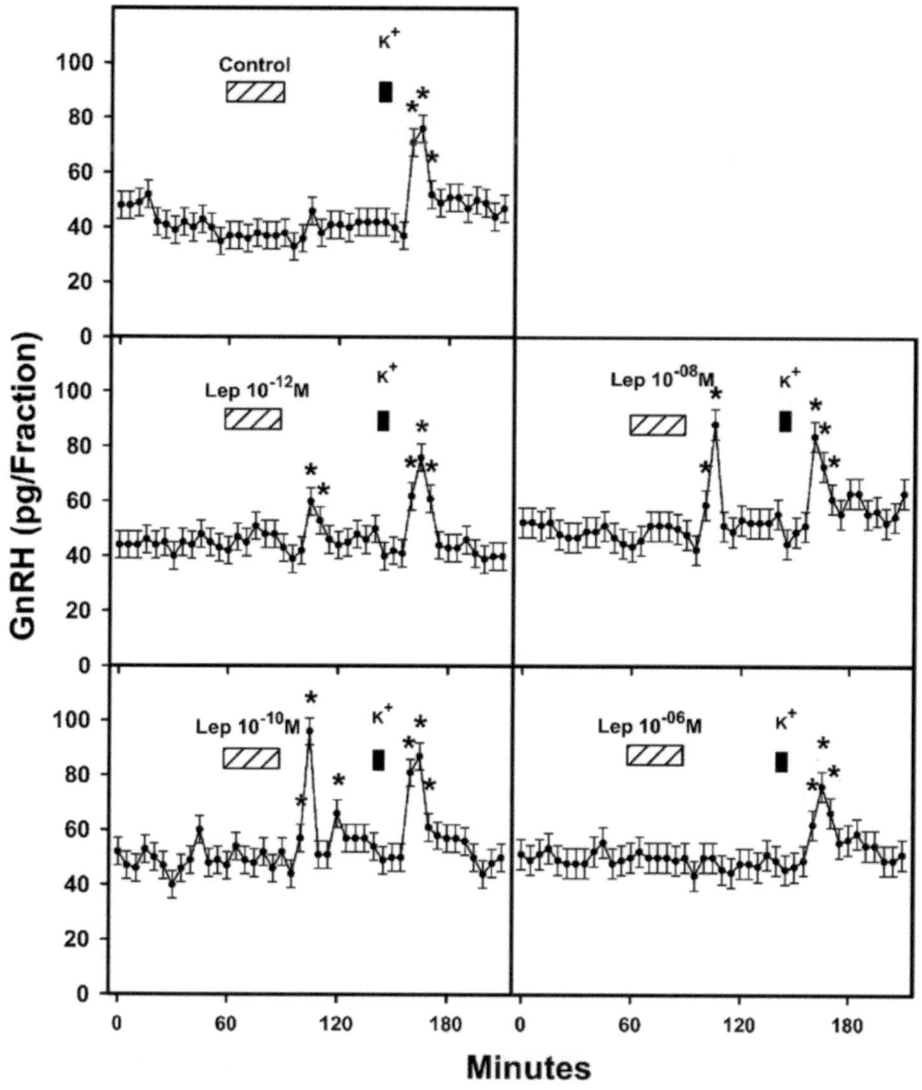

Figure 2. Hypothalamic explants (hypothalamic-preoptic area) were collected from ovariectomized prepubertal gilts and were placed in perfusion culture. Tissue was treated as shown with recombinant human leptin (Lep) at 10^{-12} M (n = 4), 10^{-10} M (n = 4), 10^{-8} M (n = 4), 10^{-6} M (n = 5) or control (n = 5). All fragments were exposed to K^+ (60 mM) to verify tissue viability. Effluent was continuously collected as 5-min fractions (500 µl). *Increased above baseline ($P < 0.05$). Data from Barb et al. (2004).

LH secretion. There is strong evidence from co-localization of leptin receptor mRNA with NPY gene expression that hypothalamic NPY is a potential target for leptin in the pig (Czaja et al., 2002). Moreover, central administration of NPY suppressed LH secretion and stimulated feed intake by reversing the inhibitory action of leptin (Barb et al., 2006). These results support the idea that leptin may serve as a metabolic signal in the activation of the reproductive axis.

Leptin treatment stimulated basal LH secretion directly from pig anterior pituitary cells in culture and GnRH release from hypothalamic-preoptic tissue explants from intact and ovariectomized prepubertal gilts on maintenance rations (Barb et al., 2004). Interestingly, i.c.v. administration of leptin failed to stimulate LH secretion in the well-fed intact prepubertal gilt (Barb et al., 2004). Obviously, hypothalamic explants are deprived of neuro-anatomical connections with other extra-hypothalamic tissues that may convey the heightened negative feedback action of estradiol on the GnRH pulse generator that occurs during pubertal development (Barb et al., 2010a), which may in part explain the failure of a LH response to i.c.v. administration of leptin in the pig.

Intracerebroventricular injection of leptin stimulated LH secretion in steroid-implanted castrated male sheep (D.W. Miller et al., 2002), and chronic i.c.v. administration of leptin stimulated LH secretion in the feed-restricted ovariectomized cow (Amstalden et al., 2002) and ewe (Henry et al., 2001). In contrast, chronic i.c.v. administration of leptin failed to stimulated LH secretion in well nourished ovariectomized ewes with no steroid replacement (Henry et al., 1999), and in intact ewe lambs (Morrison et al., 2001). *In vitro* studies demonstrated that leptin treatment stimulated basal and GnRH-mediated LH secretion from pituitary explants from fasted, but not control-fed cows, while having no effect on GnRH release from hypothalamic explants from either group of cows (Amstalden et al., 2003). Thus, metabolic state appears to be a primary determinant of the hypothalamic-pituitary response to leptin in ruminants.

4.2. The role of leptin in onset of puberty

Onset of puberty may be linked to attainment of a critical body weight or a minimum percentage of body fat (Frisch, 1984). Alternatively, metabolic mass and food intake or its correlated metabolic rate may be the triggering mechanism (Frisch, 1984). Initiation of puberty also may be influenced by metabolic factors of peripheral origin. In this regard, it has been postulated that metabolic signals are important in the initiation of puberty (Barb et al., 1997; Cameron et al., 1985). The discovery of leptin has improved our understanding of the relationship between adipose tissue and energy homeostasis (Campfield et al., 1995). Leptin treatment advanced sexual maturation in restricted and *ad lib* fed animals (Ahima et al., 1997; Barash et al., 1996). In addition, chronic leptin treatment not only reduced food intake and body weight in *ob/ob* (leptin deficient) mice, but also restored fertility (Barash et al., 1996). Serum leptin concentrations increased during puberty in the mouse (Chehab et al., 1997), heifer (Garcia et al., 2002) and pig (Qian et al., 1999) and, in the human female, age at first menarche was inversely related to serum leptin concentrations (Matkovic et al., 1997).

There exists, however, controversy as to the precise role of leptin in the onset of puberty. Several reports demonstrated that blood leptin concentrations remain relatively unchanged during pubertal development in the female mouse and rat (Ahima et al., 1998; Bronson, 2001; Cheung et al., 2001), while leptin administration failed to advance puberty onset in well nourished female mice (Cheung et al., 2001). Although, serum leptin concentrations increased during puberty in the gilt, other factors in addition to leptin may regulate onset of puberty. As indicated above, it is hypothesized that estradiol modulates the hypothalamic-pituitary axis response to leptin (Barb et al., 2004). Moreover, estradiol may regulate the pubertal related changes in Ob-rb gene expression (Figure 3). In the ovariectomized prepubertal gilt, estrogen-induced increase in leptin mRNA expression in adipose tissue occurred at the time of expected puberty but not in younger animals (Qian et al., 1999). This was associated with an increase in LH pulse frequency (Barb et al., 2010b) and an age dependent increase in hypothalamic OB-rb expression (Lin et al., 2001).

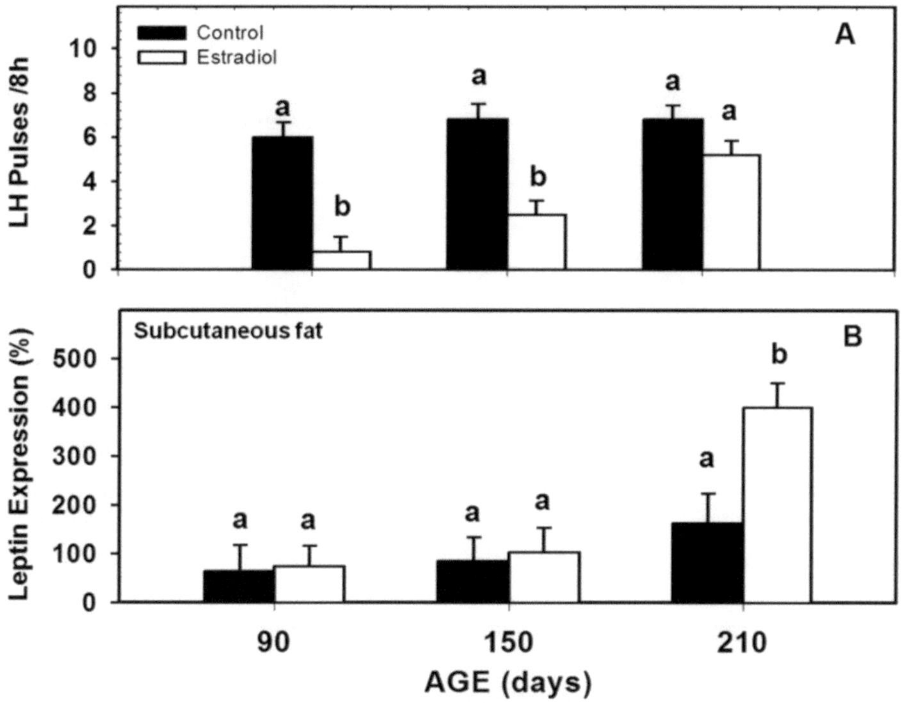

Figure 3. The frequency of luteinizing hormone (LH) pulses (A) and expression of leptin mRNA in subcutaneous (s.q.) adipose tissue (B) of ovariectomized (OVX) gilts. Gilts were OVX at 90, 150, or 210 d of age. Osmotic pumps were implanted s.q. and delivered control (vehicle; polypropylene glycol) or 0.19 mg of estradiol benzoate per kg of body weight daily for 7 d. Messenger RNA for leptin was quantified with RNA protection assays. Means without a common superscript are different; for (A) $^{a,b}P<$ 0.04 and for (B) $^{a,b}P < 0.01$. Data from Qian et al. (1999) and Barb et al. (2010b). Redrawn from Barb et al. (1999).

Several human studies, both cross-sectional and longitudinal, have demonstrated a sharp rise in serum leptin concentrations in young girls starting as early as age 7 and continuing to rise as they progressed through puberty at least age 15 (Ahmed et al., 1999; Blum et al., 1997; Garcia-Mayor et al., 1997). In contrast, in boys, leptin concentrations seem to increase transiently and then decline after Tanner stage 2 to prepubertal concentrations that are approximately one third of those observed in the late-pubertal girl. These changes in concentrations of leptin were paralleled by increasing body fat during female puberty and decreasing body fat during male puberty. Garcia-Mayor et al. (1997) reported in one cross-sectional study, that the rise in serum concentrations of leptin were well established 2 years prior to marked increases in serum LH and estradiol concentrations were detected. The authors (Garcia-Mayor et al., 1997) suggest this is consistent with the hypothesis that leptin concentrations reach a putative threshold which allows puberty to progress; as opposed to a critical factor that triggers puberty.

Matkovic et al. (1997) examined the idea that if the relationship between body fat and early menarche in humans is mediated by leptin, then leptin concentrations would be related to age at menarche. This study consisted of 343 healthy girls (Tunner stage 2 of puberty) between 8.3 and 13.1 years of age. Menstrual history, height and weight, body composition by dual-energy X-ray absorptiometry, and leptin were measured every 6 to 12 months during a 4-year period. Leptin concentration was highly correlated with body fat mass (r = 0.81). Greater leptin concentrations up to 12 ng/mL were associated with a decline in the age of menarche by approximately 1 month per 1 ng/mL increase in leptin. Furthermore, a group of girls who remained premenarcheal for the entire 4 years of the study had significantly lower leptin concentrations compared to the groups of girls who reached menarche during the study. Matkovic and coworkers (1997) concluded that a threshold blood concentration of leptin may be needed for establishment of normal menses. Furthermore, in a recent review, Kaplowitz (2008) reports that current data supports the idea that leptin plays a permissive role as opposed to a metabolic signal that initiates puberty.

In the prepubertal ruminant, short term feed restriction reduced adipose leptin gene expression and leptin secretion, but increased hypothalamic OB-rb expression (Amstalden et al., 2000; Dyer et al., 1997). This was associated with decreased serum insulin concentration, IGF-I concentration and LH pulse frequency (Amstalden et al., 2000; Morrison et al., 2001). In addition, serum leptin concentrations increased as did leptin gene expression in heifers during pubertal development, which coincided with increases in serum IGF-I concentrations and body weight (Garcia et al., 2002). In contrast to the prepubertal heifer (Amstalden et al., 2000), short-term fasting failed to reduce pulsatile LH secretion in the mature cow (Amstalden et al., 2002). This suggests that there is a heightened sensitivity of the hypothalamic-pituitary axis to variations in energy availability in the heifer. Previous reports demonstrated that inhibition of LH secretion by nutrient restriction in the ovariectomized ewe (Henry et al., 2001) or the ewe lamb (Morrison et al., 2001) was reversed by leptin treatment demonstrating a positive association between LH secretion and leptin. Although leptin treatment reversed the fasting mediated reduction in LH pulse frequency in prepubertal heifers as cited above, chronic administration of ovine leptin by subcutaneous injections twice daily to 12- to 13-month old heifers for 40 days (Maciel et al., 2004) or 3 i.v. leptin injections per hour for 5 hours at 5-week intervals during pubertal development (Zieba et al., 2004) were unable to accelerate LH pulse frequency or onset of puberty. In contrast to data obtained from the cow, it is proposed that the effect of leptin on LH secretion in the pig during pubertal development is associated with stage of sexual maturation and subsequent change in the negative feedback action of estradiol on LH secretion (see Figure 3 and Barb et al., 2004, 2010a).

5. Kisspeptin

5.1. Kisspeptin regulates gonadotropin secretion and pubertal development

Kisspeptin is a hypothalamic neuropeptide and a potent stimulator of gonadotropin secretion (Caraty et al., 2007; Lents et al., 2008; Navarro et al., 2004a, 2005) due to its action directly on GnRH neurons (Constantin et al., 2009; Herbison et al., 2010; Irwig et al., 2004) to stimulate release of GnRH into the hypophysial portal vessels (Messager et al., 2005; Smith et al., 2011). A substantial body of evidence has accumulated that demonstrates kisspeptin plays a pivotal role in the timing of the onset of puberty. Hypothalamic expression of kisspeptin-1 (KiSS-1) and the kisspeptin receptor (GPR54) are developmentally regulated with expression increasing near the expected time of puberty (Castellano et al., 2005; Navarro et al., 2004a; Shahab et al., 2005). Furthermore, expression of KiSS-1 in the ARC and the rostral preoptic area are differentially regulated by gonadal steroids (Estrada et al., 2006; Smith et al., 2005, 2007; Tomikawa et al., 2010). It has recently been shown that increased LH pulsatility during sexual maturation in the ewe is associated with a reduction in the suppressive effects of estradiol on KiSS-1 expression (Redmond et al., 2011). The fundamental importance of kisspeptin in the onset of puberty raises the question as to whether kisspeptin has a central role in the timing of pubertal events associated with metabolic state or body energy reserves.

5.2. Kisspeptin is sensitive to energy balance

Restricted feeding and fasting reduces hypothalamic expression of KiSS-1 in rodents (Castellano et al., 2005; Luque et al., 2007), sheep (Backholer et al., 2010a), and nonhuman primates (Wahab et al., 2011). Expression of KiSS-1 also is suppressed during negative energy balance associated with lactation (True et al., 2011; Yamada et al., 2007). These data demonstrate that kisspeptin neurons in the hypothalamus are an important component to how the reproductive axis senses nutritional state. Castellano et al. (2005) used long-term caloric restriction to inhibit the occurrence of puberty (as defined by absence of vaginal opening and suppressed gonadotropin and estradiol concentrations) in female rats. Treating these rats with kisspeptin rescued gonadotropin secretion and induced puberty (vaginal opening) in approximately 60% of the animals, indicating that kisspeptin may have a role in integrating the effects of energy balance with the pubertal transition in gonadotropin secretion.

Recent data from growth restricted castrate male lambs indicates that the nutritional control of gonadotropin release may also involve alterations in sensitivity to kisspeptin. At 4 weeks after weaning, castrate male lambs were randomly assigned to different diets so that they either continued to grow or maintained body weight. After 12 weeks of treatment, animals in each group were then assigned to receive either i.v. infusion of 0.77 μmoles of kisspeptin or saline control. Area under the LH curve (AUC) for the saline treated animals was similar for growth and restricted lambs; however, the kisspeptin-induced release of LH was greater and lasted longer, as indicated by AUC, in the growth restricted lambs than in the full growth lambs (Figure 4). Our findings in the growth restricted male lamb corroborate those of Castellano et al. (2005) in rats. These authors used prepubertal male and female rats that were fed either *ad libitum* or were fasted for 72 h. In fed animals, both prepubertal female and male rats demonstrated a 9 to 10 fold increase in LH concentrations in serum 15 minutes after i.c.v. injection of kisspeptin. In contrast, fasted rats demonstrated a much greater 50 to 60 fold increase in LH release. Moreover, the kisspeptin-stimulated release of GnRH from

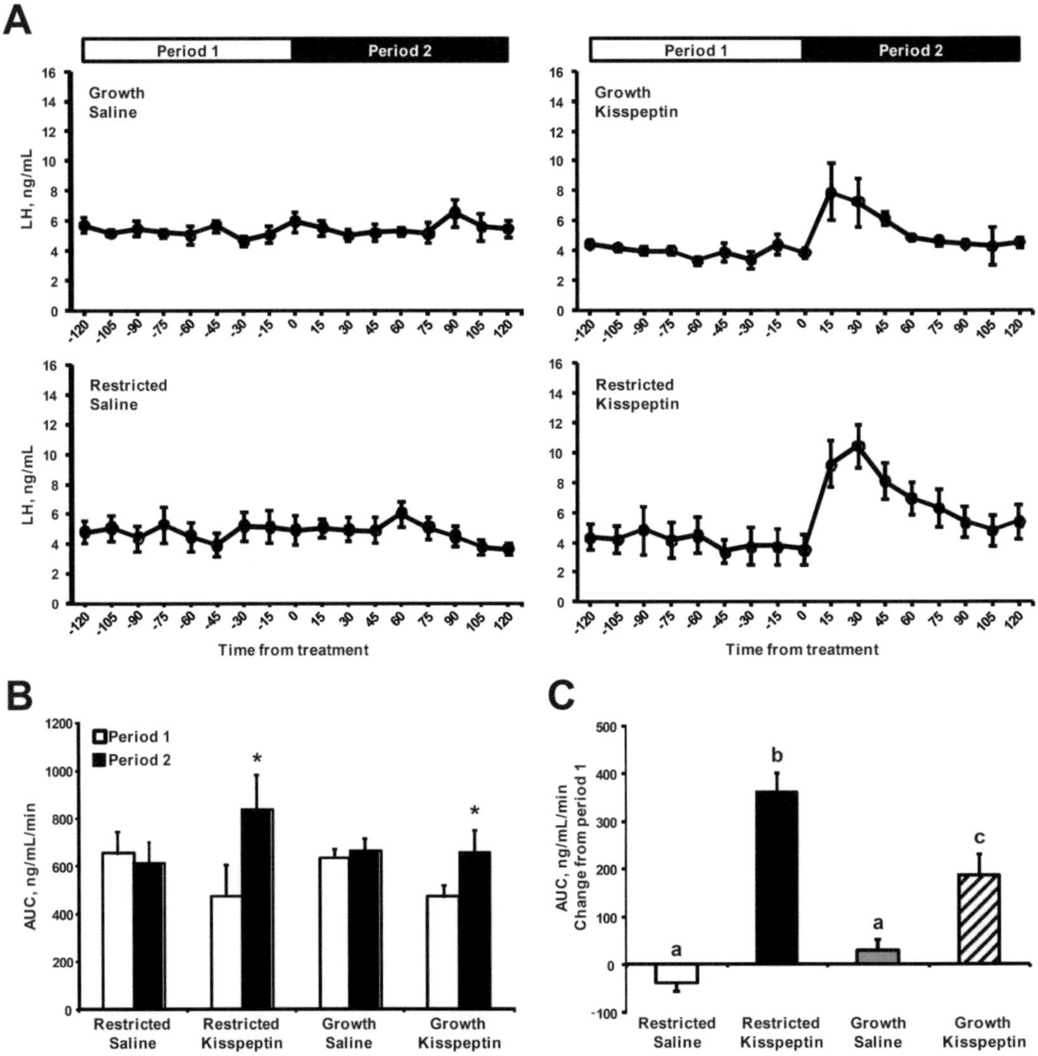

Figure 4. Four weeks after weaning, castrate male lambs (n = 16) were divided and assigned to either continue normal growth (growth) or to maintain body weight (restricted). After 12 weeks, animals in both groups received 0.77 μmoles of kisspeptin or saline as a single intravenous injection (time 0). A) Serum concentrations of luteinizing hormone (LH) during the 120 minutes before (period 1) and after (period 2) injection. B) Area under the curve (AUC) for each period (*$P < 0.05$). C) AUC in period 2 expressed as the change from period 1. [a,b,c]Means without a common superscript are different ($P < 0.05$). Data from C. A. Lents (unpublished).

hypothalamic explants collected from rats that were fasted for 72 h was greater than that from hypothalamic explants collected from *ad libitum* fed rats (Castellano et al., 2005). The increased responsiveness of the hypothalamus to kisspeptin and the subsequently greater release of LH in underfed animals are likely related to changes in expression of kisspeptin receptors. Expression of GPR54 mRNA in the hypothalamus was greater in fasted rats than in *ad libitum* fed controls (Castellano et al., 2005). Thus it appears that the pubertal transition in gonadotropin secretion involves not only increased expression and release of kisspeptin itself (Bentsen et al., 2010), but also a heightened sensitivity of the hypothalamus to the action of kisspeptin (Shahab et al., 2005). Both of these aspects can be modulated by metabolic state and are important for the overall tone of the kisspeptin system (Castellano et al., 2011; Roa et al., 2010).

5.3. Kisspeptin mediates the action of leptin on sexual development and gonadotropin secretion

The effect of energy balance on the kisspeptin system appears to be a consequence of the action of leptin. Expression of KiSS-1 in the ARC of the hypothalamus of *ob/ob* mice, which lack functional leptin, is significantly less when compared to expression in wild-type mice (Quennell et al., 2011; Smith et al., 2006); however, KiSS-1 expression in the anteroventral periventricular nucleus (AVPV) of *ob/ob* mice was similar to wild-type animals. This indicates that leptin acts on a specific population of kisspeptin cells within the ARC to modulate gonadotropin release. Leptin stimulated firing of kisspeptin neurons in hypothalamic slices of the ARC from guinea pigs (Qiu et al., 2011) and treating either *ob/ob* mice or *KiSS1*-Cre mice with leptin stimulated increased hypothalamic expression of kisspeptin mRNA in the ARC (Quennell et al., 2011; Smith et al., 2006) but not the AVPV (Cravo et al., 2011; Quennell et al., 2011; Smith et al., 2006). Leptin probably affects kisspeptin neurons in the ARC directly because kisspeptin cells localized within this hypothalamic area of guinea pigs (Qiu et al., 2011) and mice (Quennell et al., 2011; Smith et al., 2006) express leptin receptor mRNA. Moreover, second messengers that are important in signaling of leptin receptor (i.e., STAT-3) were expressed in kisspeptin cells in the ARC, but not within kisspeptin cells of the AVPV (Quennell et al., 2011). This indicates that increasing concentrations of leptin associated with greater body energy reserves may impact activity of the GnRH pulse generator through increasing the tone of the kisspeptin system via its action on kisspeptin neurons within the ARC.

The consequences of negative energy balance on KiSS-1 expression aren't fully offset by the positive effect of leptin. For example, leptin treatment did not fully reverse the lactation-induced reduction in KiSS-1 expression in rats (Xu et al., 2009). In a similar fashion, continuous i.c.v. infusion of leptin during a 72 h fast of ovariectomized ewes that were thin (made so with chronic nutritional restriction) rescued LH pulses (Backholer et al., 2010b) but KiSS-1 expression was only partially restored when compared with ewes that had greater body fat (Backholer et al., 2010a). Consequently, the suppressive effect of negative energy balance or nutrient deprivation on the gonadotropic axis via the KiSS-1 system likely involves more than simply altered leptin signaling alone. Other metabolic factors, such as insulin for example, are reflective of metabolic state or availability of food and likely have an important role in regulating the kisspeptin system to augment gonadotropin release.

The possibility that adipocyte derived factors may also inhibit gonadotropin release in undernourished subjects should not be dismissed. Adiponectin is secreted by adipose tissue in response to nutrient restriction and body weight loss. It activates adenosine monophosphate-activated protein kinase (AMPK) to stimulate glucose uptake and β-oxidation of free fatty acids (Gil-Campos et al., 2004). Receptors for adiponectin are expressed not only in the hypothalamus (Kos et al., 2007) but also the anterior pituitary gland (Rodriguez-Pacheco et al., 2007). Furthermore, mice that overexpress adiponectin have an infertile phenotype (Combs et al., 2004). This is indicative of a role for adiponectin in modulating gonadotropin secretion during periods when nutrient intake is insufficient to meet energy demands. Treating anterior pituitary cells *in vitro* (Rodriguez-Pacheco et al., 2007) or LβT2 cells (immortalized embryonic gonadotrope cell line) with adiponectin suppressed both basal and GnRH-stimulated LH release (Lu et al., 2008). When adiponectin was administered i.c.v. to male rats, mean concentrations of LH were decreased owing to a suppression of LH pulse amplitude (Cheng et al., 2011). The later observation would indicate that adiponectin could be functioning to suppress activity of the GnRH neuronal network in subjects experiencing reductions in energy balance. In line with this is the fact that adiponectin inhibits the release of GnRH from GT1-7 cells (immortalized hypothalamic cell line) via an AMPK pathway (Cheng et al., 2011; Wen et al., 2008). It may well be that increased secretion and activity of adiponectin in animals during food deprivation or nutrient restriction off-set, to some degree, the stimulatory action of exogenous leptin on KiSS-1 expression in the hypothalamus. It is yet to be determined, however, if the suppressive effects of adiponectin on GnRH/LH release involve changes in the hypothalamic kisspeptin system.

Expression of KiSS-1 in immortalized hypothalamic N6 cells was increased after treatment with NPY (Luque et al., 2007). This would suggest that neuronal pathways downstream of leptin can impact the kisspeptin system. In the ewe, 13 to 30% of kisspeptin neurons in the ARC are in close apposition to NPY fibers (Backholer et al., 2010a). Moreover, 30 to 40% of kisspeptin cells in the ARC were contacted by POMC fibers (Backholer et al., 2010a). Since both NPY and POMC expressing cells are direct targets for leptin's action, the effects of leptin on gonadotropin secretion may be mediated through kisspeptin neurons indirectly via NPY and POMC pathways. It is also noted that kisspeptin neuronal fibers are located in close apposition to approximately 7% of NPY cell bodies and 20% of POMC cell bodies in the ovine hypothalamus (Backholer et al., 2010a). This anatomical evidence implies that the reproductive axis can influence neuronal pathways to modulate appetite. In fact, i.c.v. injection of kisspeptin increased NPY mRNA and reduced POMC mRNA in the ARC of the hypothalamus of sheep (Backholer et al., 2010a). Thus, other factors that may drive NPY or POMC expression during conditions of underfeeding may further limit the ability of leptin to stimulate increased KiSS-1 expression in the hypothalamus.

5.4. Kisspeptin is involved in the reproductive pathobiology of diabetes and obesity

Metabolic disorders such as diabetes and obesity are accompanied by alterations in adipose tissue biology and impaired fertility. Given the impacts of leptin on the kisspeptin system in the hypothalamus, one could easily speculate that metabolic diseases that impinge upon circulating concentrations of leptin could have negative consequences for reproductive function via alterations in the hypothalamic expression of kisspeptin. Using the streptozotocin-induced diabetic male rat model, Castellano et al. (2006) observed that LH release was rescued when rats were treated with exogenous kisspeptin. Moreover, expression of KiSS-1 was reduced in the hypothalamus of these diabetic male rats. When the authors treated the diabetic rats with leptin, they found that KiSS-1 expression was restored along with increased concentrations of LH and testosterone in serum.

Obesity is an ever growing epidemic and patients that are obese present a number of pathologies. One of these is a reduction in the sensitivity to the action of leptin. Iwasa et al. (2010) observed that female rats which underwent intrauterine growth retardation during their growth as fetuses developed leptin resistance after birth. These leptin resistant female rats demonstrated delayed onset of puberty associated with reduced expression of KiSS-1 in the hypothalamus. Thus, infertility associated with obesity and central leptin resistance may be related to tone of the kisspeptin system within the hypothalamus. Navarro et al. (2004b) found kisspeptin treatment restored LH secretion in *fa/fa* Zucker rats; a genetic model for leptin resistance. Furthermore, diet induced leptin resistance in mice, resulting from prolonged feeding of a high fat diet, was associated with reduced KiSS-1 expression and LH concentrations in serum (Quennell et al., 2011). Therefore, infertility resulting from hypogonadotropism that arises in diabetic or obese patients is likely due to alterations in the expression and secretion of kisspeptin in the hypothalamus.

6. Conclusion

Adipose tissue expresses and secretes a wide array of regulatory factors that have diverse biological roles. These factors contribute to the regulation of energy homeostasis by acting on neural circuits within the hypothalamus. Gonadotropin-releasing hormone is secreted from hypothalamic neurons and acts on gonadotrope cells within the anterior pituitary gland to stimulate the synthesis and release of LH. Activity of this gonadotropic-axis is sensitive to metabolic state. Free fatty acids are released from adipose tissue to have a glucose sparing effect and can be directly sensed by neurons in the hypothalamus. Cyclic changes in availability of FFA associated with meal frequency act to sustain continued release of LH pulses over short periods of time, but chronically elevated FFA likely impairs reproductive function by decreasing the sensitivity of the pituitary gland to GnRH. Conversely, leptin can enhance pituitary GnRH sensitivity and increase LH secretion. Within the hypothalamus, leptin stimulates release of GnRH by acting through interneuronal pathways involving NPY, POMC, and kisspeptin. Other adipose derived factors such as adiponectin and nesfatin-1 can have negative or positive effects on LH release, respectively (figure 5). Metabolic control of puberty onset likely involves developmental changes in these relationships.

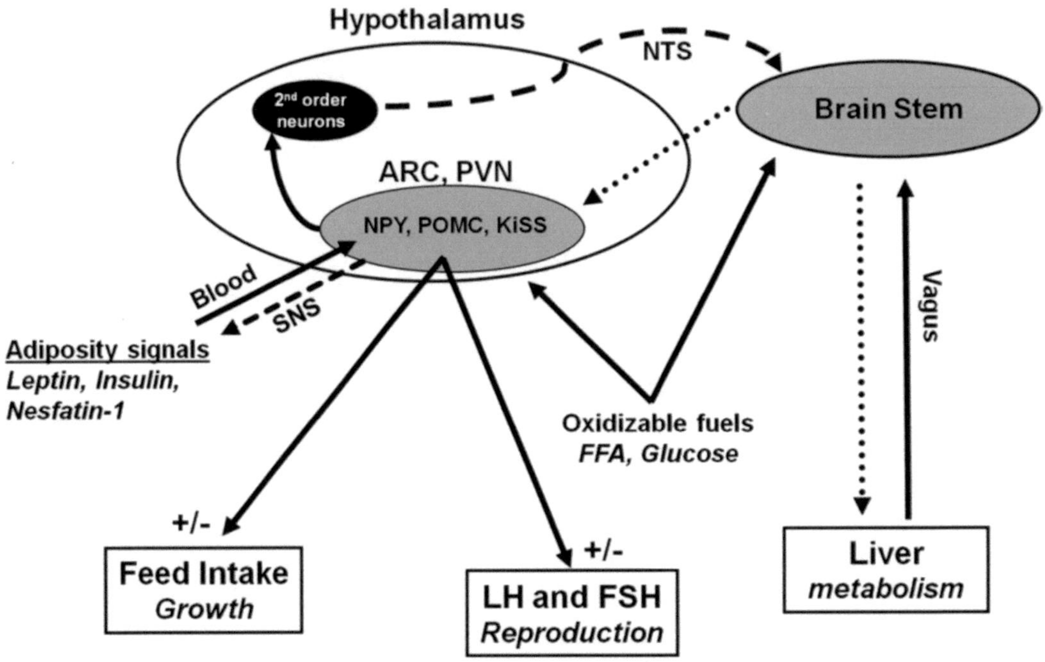

Figure 5. A proposed model for how metabolic signals, including adipokines such as leptin, affect gonadotropin secretion. Insulin fluctuates with consumption of meals at regular intervals to promote adipose accretion. Increased mass of adipose tissue is reflected in concentrations of adipokines such as leptin and nesfatin-1 that circulate in the blood to act as specific neural circuits within the hypothalamus. Leptin suppresses feed intake by modifying activity of POMC and NPY neurons in the arcuate (ARC) and paraventricular (PVN) nuclei, and stimulates release of gonadotropin hormones (LH and FSH). Many neurons in these areas of the hypothalamus express leptin receptor and directly innervate adipose tissue, thus constituting a hypothalamic-adipose neuroendocrine axis involving the sympathetic nervous system (SNS). Leptin directly activates kisspeptin (KiSS) cell bodies to stimulate GnRH release and to cause an upregulation of LH pulses. Nesfatin-1, which also stimulates LH release, suppresses food intake by acting through second order neurons to modulate activity of POMC systems in the nucleus tractus solitaries (NTS) of the hind brain as well as the nucleus dorsalis of the vagus nerve; thus altering liver function, which results in shifting availability of oxidizable fuels. Elevated free fatty acids (FFA) have a glucose sparing affect and can be directly sensed by neurons in the hypothalamus to sustain continued release of LH pulses over a short period.

Author details

Clay A. Lents*

United States Department of Agriculture[2] (USDA), Agricultural Research Service (ARS), U.S. Meat Animal Research Center (USMARC), Clay Center, Nebraska, USA

* Corresponding Author

Richard C. Barb and Gary J. Hausman
United States Department of Agriculture[2] (USDA), Agricultural Research Service (ARS), Richard B. Russell Research Center (RRC), Athens, Georgia, USA

Acknowledgement

The authors thank Linda Parnell for assistance in manuscript preparation. This project was supported by Agriculture and Food Research Initiative Competitive Grant no. 2005-35203-16852 (C.A. Lents) from the USDA National Institute of Food and Agriculture.

Abbreviations

ADIPOR2	adiponectin receptor 2	KiSS-1	kispeptin-1
AGTR1	angeotensin II receptor	LC-CoAs	long-chain fatty acyl CoAs
AMPK	adenosine monophosphate-activated protein kinase	LDLR	low density lipoprotein receptor
		LH	luteinizing hormone
ANG	angiotensin	LHA	lateral hypothalamic area
ANGPTL	angiopoietin-like protein	LHCGR	luteinizing hormone-choriogonadotropin receptor
APO	apolipoprotein		
ARC	arcuate	LPL	lipoprotein lipase
ARS	Agricultural Research Service	LβT2	immortalized embryonic gonadotrope cell line
AUC	Area under curve		
AVPV	anteroventral periventricular nucleus	MCP-1	monocyte chemoattractant protein-1
BDNF	brain-derived neurotrophic factor	N6	neuronal 6 cells
		NEFA	DNA binding/EF hand/acidic amino acid rich protein
bFGF	basic fibroblast growth factor		
BMI	body mass index	NGFR	nerve growth factor receptor
BMP	bone morphogenic protein	NPY	neuropeptide Y
BMPR2	bone morphogenic protein receptor 2	NTS	nucleus tractus solitaries
		NUCB2	nucleobindin 2
CCK	cholecystokinin	OB-rb	biologically-active long form leptin receptor
CIQTN4	complement-c1q tumor necrosis factor-related protein 4		
		PAI-1	plasminogen activator inhibitor-1
CNS	central nervous system	PDGFD	platelet derived growth factor D
CNTF	ciliary neurotrophic factor	PGRMC1	progesterone receptor membrane component 1

[2] The U.S. Department of Agriculture (USDA) prohibits discrimination in all its programs and activities on the basis of race, color, national origin, age, disability, and where applicable, sex, marital status, familial status, parental status, religion, sexual orientation, genetic information, political beliefs, reprisal, or because all or part of an individual's income is derived from any public assistance program. (Not all prohibited bases apply to all programs.) Persons with disabilities who require alternative means for communication of program information (Braille, large print, audiotape, etc.) should contact USDA's TARGET Center at (202) 720-2600 (voice and TDD). To file a complaint of discrimination, write to USDA, Director, Office of Civil Rights, 1400 Independence Avenue, S.W., Washington, D.C. 20250-9410, or call (800) 795-3272 (voice) or (202) 720-6382 (TDD). USDA is an equal opportunity provider and employer.

CRH	corticotrophin-releasing hormone	POMC	proopiomelanocortin
CTGF	connective tissue growth factor	PPARγ	proxisome proliferator activated receptor γ
CTRP4	complement-c1q tumor necrosis factor-related protein 4	PVN	paraventricular
EDNRB	endothelin receptor type B	RANTES	chemokine (c-c motif) ligand 5
EGFR	epidermal growth factor receptor	RBP	retinol binding protein
ESR1	estrogen receptor 1	RLN	relaxin
FFA	free fatty acids	RRC	Richard B. Russell Research Center
FSH	follicle-stimulating hormone	RTN	reticulon
GnRH	gonadotropin-releasing hormone	SQ-5	lung squamous carcinoma cell line 5
GNRHR2	gonadotropin-releasing hormone receptor 2	STAT-3	signal transducer and activator of transcription 3
GPR54	g protein coupled receptor 54	TGF	transforming growth factor
GT1-7	GT1-7 cells (immortalized hypothalamic cell line)	THR	thyroid hormone receptor
i.c.v.	intracerebroventricular	TLR	toll-like receptor
i.v.	intravenous	TNF	tumor necrosis factor
IFNG	interferon gamma	TNFα	tumor necrosis factor α
IGF	insulin-like growth factor	TSHR	thyroid-stimulating hormone receptor
IGF-IR	IGF-I receptor	USDA	United States Department of Agriculture
IGFBP	insulin-like growth factor binding protein	USMARC	U.S. Meat Animal Research Center
IL	interleukin	VEGFC	vascular endothelial growth factor C
INSR	insulin receptor		

7. References

Ahima, R. S. (2006). Adipose Tissue As an Endocrine Organ. *Obesity*, Vol.14, No.S8, (August 2006), pp. 242S-249S

Ahima, R. S.; Prabakaran, D.; Mantzoros, C.; Qu, D.; Lowell, B.; Maratos-Flier, E. & Flier, J. S. (1996). Role of Leptin in the Neuroendocrine Response to Fasting. *Nature*, Vol.382, No.6588, (July 1996), pp. 250-252

Ahima, R. S.; Dushay, J.; Flier, S. N.; Prabakaran, D. & Flier, J. S. (1997). Leptin Accelerates the Onset of Puberty in Normal Female Mice. *The Journal of Clinical Investigation*, Vol.99, No.3, (February 1997), pp. 391-395

Ahima, R. S.; Prabakaran, D. & Flier, J. S. (1998). Postnatal Leptin Surge and Regulation of Circadian Rhythm of Leptin by Feeding. Implications for Energy Homeostasis and Neuroendocrine Function. *The Journal of Clinical Investigation*, Vol.101, No.5, (March 1998), pp. 1020-1027

Ahmed, M. L.; Ong, K. K. L.; Morrell, D. J.; Cox, L.; Drayer, N.; Perry, L.; Preece, M. A. & Dunger, D. B. (1999). Longitudinal Study of Leptin Concentrations During Puberty: Sex Differences and Relationship to Changes in Body Composition. *The Journal of Clinical Endocrinology & Metabolism*, Vol.84, No.3, (March 1999), pp. 899-905

Amstalden, M.; Garcia, M. R.; Williams, S. W.; Stanko, R. L.; Nizielski, S. E.; Morrison, C. D.; Keisler, D. H. & Williams, G. L. (2000). Leptin Gene Expression, Circulating Leptin, and Luteinizing Hormone Pulsatility Are Acutely Responsive to Short-Term Fasting in Prepubertal Heifers: Relationships to Circulating Insulin and Insulin-Like Growth Factor I. *Biology of Reproduction*, Vol.63, No.1, (July 2000), pp. 127-133

Amstalden, M.; Garcia, M. R.; Stanko, R. L.; Nizielski, S. E.; Morrison, C. D.; Keisler, D. H. & Williams, G. L. (2002). Central Infusion of Recombinant Ovine Leptin Normalizes Plasma Insulin and Stimulates a Novel Hypersecretion of Luteinizing Hormone After Short-Term Fasting in Mature Beef Cows. *Biology of Reproduction*, Vol.66, No.5, (May 2002), pp. 1555-1561

Amstalden, M.; Zieba, D. A.; Edwards, J. F.; Harms, P. G.; Welsh, T. H., Jr.; Stanko, R. L. & Williams, G. L. (2003). Leptin Acts at the Bovine Adenohypophysis to Enhance Basal and Gonadotropin-Releasing Hormone-Mediated Release of Luteinizing Hormone: Differential Effects Are Dependent Upon Nutritional History. *Biology of Reproduction*, Vol.69, No.5, (November 2003), pp. 1539-1544

Armstrong, J. D. & Britt, J. H. (1987). Nutritionally-Induced Anestrus in Gilts: Metabolic and Endocrine Changes Associated With Cessation and Resumption of Estrous Cycles. *Journal of Animal Science*, Vol.65, No.2, (August 1987), pp. 508-523

Aydin, S.; Dag, E.; Ozkan, Y.; Erman, F.; Dagli, A. F.; Kilic, N.; Sahin, Í.; Karatas, F.; Yoldas, T.; Barim, A. O. & Kendir, Y. (2009). Nesfatin-1 and Ghrelin Levels in Serum and Saliva of Epileptic Patients: Hormonal Changes Can Have a Major Effect on Seizure Disorders. *Molecular and Cellular Biochemistry*, Vol.328, No.1, (August 2009), pp. 49-56

Backholer, K.; Smith, J. T.; Rao, A.; Pereira, A.; Iqbal, J.; Ogawa, S.; Li, Q. & Clarke, I. J. (2010a). Kisspeptin Cells in the Ewe Brain Respond to Leptin and Communicate With Neuropeptide Y and Proopiomelanocortin Cells. *Endocrinology*, Vol.151, No.5, (May 2010), pp. 2233-2243

Backholer, K.; Bowden, M.; Gamber, K.; Bjørbæk, C.; Iqbal, J. & Clarke, I. J. (2010b). Melanocortins Mimic the Effects of Leptin to Restore Reproductive Function in Lean Hypogonadotropic Ewes. *Neuroendocrinology*, Vol.91, No.1, (January 2010), pp. 27-40

Barash, I. A.; Cheung, C. C.; Weigle, D. S.; Ren, H.; Kabigting, E. B.; Kuijper, J. L.; Clifton, D. K. & Steiner, R. A. (1996). Leptin Is a Metabolic Signal to the Reproductive System. *Endocrinology*, Vol.137, No.7, (July 1996), pp. 3144-3147

Barb, C. R.; Kraeling, R. R.; Barrett, J. B.; Rampacek, G. B.; Campbell, R. M. & Mowles, T. F. (1991). Serum Glucose and Free Fatty Acids Modulate Growth Hormone and Luteinizing Hormone Secretion in the Pig. *Proceedings of the Society for Experimental Biology and Medicine*, Vol.198, No.1, (October 1991), pp. 636-642

Barb, C. R.; Kraeling, R. R. & Rampacek, G. B. (1995). Glucose and Free Fatty Acid Modulation of Growth Hormone and Luteinizing Hormone Secretion by Cultured Porcine Pituitary Cells. *Journal of Animal Science*, Vol.73, No.5, (May 1995), pp. 1416-1423

Barb, C. R.; Kraeling, R. R.; Rampacek, G. B. & Dove, C. R. (1997). Metabolic Changes During the Transition From the Fed to the Acute Feed-Deprived State in Prepuberal and Mature Gilts. *Journal of Animal Science*, Vol.75, No.3, (March 1997), pp. 781-789

Barb, C. R.; Barrett, J. B.; Kraeling, R. R. & Rampacek, G. B. (1999). Role of Leptin in Modulating Neuroendocrine Function: A Metabolic Link Between the Brain-Pituitary and Adipose Tissue. *Reproduction in Domestic Animals*, Vol.34, No.3-4, (August 1999), pp. 111-125

Barb, C. R.; Kraeling, R. R. & Rampacek, G. B. (2001a). Nutritional Regulators of the Hypothalamic-Pituitary Axis in Pigs. *Reproduction Supplement*, Vol.58, (2001), pp. 1-15

Barb, C. R.; Barrett, J. B.; Kraeling, R. R. & Rampacek, G. B. (2001b). Serum Leptin Concentrations, Luteinizing Hormone and Growth Hormone Secretion During Feed and Metabolic Fuel Restriction in the Prepuberal Gilt. *Domestic Animal Endocrinology*, Vol.20, No.1, (January 2001), pp. 47-63

Barb, C. R.; Barrett, J. B. & Kraeling, R. R. (2004). Role of Leptin in Modulating the Hypothalamic-Pituitary Axis and Luteinizing Hormone Secretion in the Prepuberal Gilt. *Domestic Animal Endocrinology*, Vol.26, No.3, (April 2004), pp. 201-214

Barb, C. R.; Kraeling, R. R.; Rampacek, G. B. & Hausman, G. J. (2006). The Role of Neuropeptide Y and Interaction With Leptin in Regulating Feed Intake and Luteinizing Hormone and Growth Hormone Secretion in the Pig. *Reproduction*, Vol.131, No.6, (June 2006), pp. 1127-1135

Barb, C. R.; Hausman, G. J.; Rekaya, R.; Lents, C. A.; Lkhagvadorj, S.; Qu, L.; Cai, W.; Couture, O. P.; Anderson, L. L.; Dekkers, J. C. M. & Tuggle, C. K. (2010a). Gene Expression in Hypothalamus, Liver, and Adipose Tissues and Food Intake Response to Melanocortin-4 Receptor Agonist in Pigs Expressing Melanocortin-4 Receptor Mutations. *Physiological Genomics*, Vol.41, No.3, (May 2010), pp. 254-268

Barb, C. R.; Hausman, G. J. & Kraeling, R. R. (2010b). Luteinizing Hormone Secretion As Influenced by Age and Estradiol in the Prepubertal Gilt. *Animal Reproduction Science*, Vol.122, No.3-4, (December 2010), pp. 324-327

Basu, U.; Romao, J. M. & Guan, L. L. (2012). Adipogenic Transcriptome Profiling Using High Throughput Technologies. *Journal of Genomics*, Vol.1, (2012), pp. 22-28

Bentsen, A. H.; Ansel, L.; Simonneaux, V.; Tena-Sempere, M.; Juul, A. & Mikkelsen, J. D. (2010). Maturation of Kisspeptinergic Neurons Coincides With Puberty Onset in Male Rats. *Peptides*, Vol.31, No.2, (February 2010), pp. 275-283

Blum, W. F.; Englaro, P.; Hanitsch, S.; Juul, A.; Hertel, N. T.; Müller, J.; Skakkebæk, N. E.; Heiman, M. L.; Birkett, M.; Attanasio, A. M.; Kiess, W. & Rascher, W. (1997). Plasma Leptin Levels in Healthy Children and Adolescents: Dependence on Body Mass Index, Body Fat Mass, Gender, Pubertal Stage, and Testosterone. *The Journal of Clinical Endocrinology & Metabolism*, Vol.82, No.9, (September 1997), pp. 2904-2910

Brailoiu, G. C.; Dun, S. L.; Brailoiu, E.; Inan, S.; Yang, J.; Chang, J. K. & Dun, N. J. (2007). Nesfatin-1: Distribution and Interaction With a G Protein-Coupled Receptor in the Rat Brain. *Endocrinology*, Vol.148, No.10, (October 2007), pp. 5088-5094

Bronson, F. H. (2001). Puberty in Female Mice Is Not Associated With Increases in Either Body Fat or Leptin. *Endocrinology*, Vol.142, No.11, (November 2001), pp. 4758-4761

Cameron, J. L.; Koerker, D. J. & Steiner, R. A. (1985). Metabolic Changes During Maturation of Male Monkeys: Possible Signals for Onset of Puberty. *American Journal of Physiology - Endocrinology and Metabolism*, Vol.249, No.4, (October 1985), p. E385-E391

Campfield, L. A.; Smith, F. J.; Guisez, Y.; Devos, R. & Burn, P. (1995). Recombinant Mouse OB Protein: Evidence for a Peripheral Signal Linking Adiposity and Central Neural Networks. *Science*, Vol.269, No.5223, (July 1995), pp. 546-549

Caraty, A.; Smith, J. T.; Lomet, D.; Ben Saïd, S.; Morrissey, A.; Cognie, J.; Doughton, B.; Baril, G.; Briant, C. & Clarke, I. J. (2007). Kisspeptin Synchronizes Preovulatory Surges in Cyclical Ewes and Causes Ovulation in Seasonally Acyclic Ewes. *Endocrinology*, Vol.148, No.11, (November 2007), pp. 5258-5267

Castellano, J. M.; Navarro, V. M.; Fernández-Fernández, R.; Nogueiras, R.; Tovar, S.; Roa, J.; Vazquez, M. J.; Vigo, E.; Casanueva, F. F.; Aguilar, E.; Pinilla, L.; Dieguez, C. & Tena-Sempere, M. (2005). Changes in Hypothalamic KiSS-1 System and Restoration of Pubertal Activation of the Reproductive Axis by Kisspeptin in Undernutrition. *Endocrinology*, Vol.146, No.9, (September 2005), pp. 3917-3925

Castellano, J. M.; Navarro, V. M.; Fernández-Fernández, R.; Roa, J.; Vigo, E.; Pineda, R.; Dieguez, C.; Aguilar, E.; Pinilla, L. & Tena-Sempere, M. (2006). Expression of Hypothalamic KiSS-1 System and Rescue of Defective Gonadotropic Responses by Kisspeptin in Streptozotocin-Induced Diabetic Male Rats. *Diabetes*, Vol.55, No.9, (September 2006), pp. 2602-2610

Castellano, J. M.; Bentsen, A. H.; Sánchez-Garrido, M. A.; Ruiz-Pino, F.; Romero, M.; Garcia-Galiano, D.; Aguilar, E.; Pinilla, L.; Diéguez, C.; Mikkelsen, J. D. & Tena-Sempere, M. (2011). Early Metabolic Programming of Puberty Onset: Impact of Changes in Postnatal Feeding and Rearing Conditions on the Timing of Puberty and Development of the Hypothalamic Kisspeptin System. *Endocrinology*, Vol.152, No.9, (September 2011), pp. 3396-3408

Cera, K. R.; Mahan, D. C. & Reinhart, G. A. (1989). Postweaning Swine Performance and Serum Profile Responses to Supplemental Medium-Chain Free Fatty Acids and Tallow. *Journal of Animal Science*, Vol.67, No.8, (August 1989), pp. 2048-2055

Chehab, F. F.; Mounzih, K.; Lu, R. & Lim, M. E. (1997). Early Onset of Reproductive Function in Normal Female Mice Treated With Leptin. *Science*, Vol.275, No.5296, (January 1997), pp. 88-90

Chen, X.; Cushman, S. W.; Pannell, L. K. & Hess, S. (2005). Quantitative Proteomic Analysis of the Secretory Proteins From Rat Adipose Cells Using a 2D Liquid Chromatography-MS/MS Approach. *Journal of Proteome Research*, Vol.4, No.2, (March 2005), pp. 570-577

Cheng, X.-B.; Wen, J.-P.; Yang, J.; Yang, Y.; Ning, G. & Li, X.-Y. (2011). GnRH Secretion Is Inhibited by Adiponectin Through Activation of AMP-Activated Protein Kinase and Extracellular Signal-Regulated Kinase. *Endocrine*, Vol.39, No.1, (February 2011), pp. 6-12

Cheung, C. C.; Thornton, J. E.; Nurani, S. D.; Clifton, D. K. & Steiner, R. A. (2001). A Reassessment of Leptin's Role in Triggering the Onset of Puberty in the Rat and Mouse. *Neuroendocrinology*, Vol.74, No.1, (July 2001), pp. 12-21

Combs, T. P.; Pajvani, U. B.; Berg, A. H.; Lin, Y.; Jelicks, L. A.; Laplante, M.; Nawrocki, A. R.; Rajala, M. W.; Parlow, A. F.; Cheeseboro, L.; Ding, Y.-Y.; Russell, R. G.; Lindemann, D.; Hartley, A.; Baker, G. R. C.; Obici, S.; Deshaies, Y.; Ludgate, M.; Rossetti, L. & Scherer, P. E. (2004). A Transgenic Mouse With a Deletion in the Collagenous Domain of Adiponectin Displays Elevated Circulating Adiponectin and Improved Insulin Sensitivity. *Endocrinology*, Vol.145, No.1, (January 2004), pp. 367-383

Constantin, S.; Caligioni, C. S.; Stojilkovic, S. & Wray, S. (2009). Kisspeptin-10 Facilitates a Plasma Membrane-Driven Calcium Oscillator in Gonadotropin-Releasing Hormone-1 Neurons. *Endocrinology*, Vol.150, No.3, (March 2009), pp. 1400-1412

Cravo, R. M.; Margatho, L. O.; Osborne-Lawrence, S.; Donato Jr, J.; Atkin, S.; Bookout, A. L.; Rovinsky, S.; Frazão, R.; Lee, C. E.; Gautron, L.; Zigman, J. M. & Elias, C. F. (2011). Characterization of Kiss1 Neurons Using Transgenic Mouse Models. *Neuroscience*, Vol.173, (January 2011), pp. 37-56

Czaja, K.; Lakomy, M.; Sienkiewicz, W.; Kaleczyc, J.; Pidsudko, Z.; Barb, C. R.; Rampacek, G. B. & Kraeling, R. R. (2002). Distribution of Neurons Containing Leptin Receptors in the Hypothalamus of the Pig. *Biochemical and Biophysical Research Communications*, Vol.298, No.3, (November 2002), pp. 333-337

Dyer, C. J.; Simmons, J. M.; Matteri, R. L. & Keisler, D. H. (1997). Leptin Receptor MRNA Is Expressed in Ewe Anterior Pituitary and Adipose Tissues and Is Differentially Expressed in Hypothalamic Regions of Well-Fed and Feed-Restricted Ewes. *Domestic Animal Endocrinology*, Vol.14, No.2, (March 1997), pp. 119-128

Estrada, K. M.; Clay, C. M.; Pompolo, S.; Smith, J. T. & Clarke, I. J. (2006). Elevated KiSS-1 Expression in the Arcuate Nucleus Prior to the Cyclic Preovulatory Gonadotrophin-Releasing Hormone/Lutenising Hormone Surge in the Ewe Suggests a Stimulatory Role for Kisspeptin in Oestrogen-Positive Feedback. *Journal of Neuroendocrinology*, Vol.18, No.10, (October 2006), pp. 806-809

Foo, K. S.; Brismar, H. & Broberger, C. (2008). Distribution and Neuropeptide Coexistence of Nucleobindin-2 MRNA/Nesfatin-Like Immunoreactivity in the Rat CNS. *Neuroscience*, Vol.156, No.3, (October 2008), pp. 563-579

Frisch, R. E. (1984). Body Fat, Puberty and Fertility. *Biol. Rev. Camb. Philos. Soc.*, Vol.59, No.2, (May 1984), pp. 161-188

Garcia, M. R.; Amstalden, M.; Williams, S. W.; Stanko, R. L.; Morrison, C. D.; Keisler, D. H.; Nizielski, S. E. & Williams, G. L. (2002). Serum Leptin and Its Adipose Gene Expression During Pubertal Development, the Estrous Cycle, and Different Seasons in Cattle. *Journal of Animal Science*, Vol.80, No.8, (August 2002), pp. 2158-2167

García-Galiano, D.; Navarro, V. M.; Roa, J.; Ruiz-Pino, F.; Sánchez-Garrido, M. A.; Pineda, R.; Castellano, J. M.; Romero, M.; Aguilar, E.; Gaytán, F.; Diéguez, C.; Pinilla, L. & Tena-Sempere, M. (2010). The Anorexigenic Neuropeptide, Nesfatin-1, Is Indispensable for Normal Puberty Onset in the Female Rat. *The Journal of Neuroscience*, Vol.30, No.23, (June 2010), pp. 7783-7792

García-Galiano, D.; Pineda, R.; Ilhan, T.; Castellano, J. M.; Ruiz-Pino, F.; Sánchez-Garrido, M. A.; Vazquez, M. J.; Sangiao-Alvarellos, S.; Romero-Ruiz, A.; Pinilla, L.; Diéguez, C.; Gaytán, F. & Tena-Sempere, M. (2012). Cellular Distribution, Regulated Expression, and Functional Role of the Anorexigenic Peptide, NUCB2/Nesfatin-1, in the Testis. *Endocrinology*, Vol.153, Published online before print February 14, 2012, doi: 10.1210/en.2011-2032 (Available from http://endo.endojournals.org/content/early/2012/02/08/en.2011-2032.abstract)

Garcia-Mayor, R. V.; Andrade, M. A.; Rios, M.; Lage, M.; Dieguez, C. & Casanueva, F. F. (1997). Serum Leptin Levels in Normal Children: Relationship to Age, Gender, Body Mass Index, Pituitary-Gonadal Hormones, and Pubertal Stage. *The Journal of Clinical Endocrinology & Metabolism*, Vol.82, No.9, (September 1997), pp. 2849-2855

Gil-Campos, M.; Cañete, R. & Gil, A. (2004). Adiponectin, the Missing Link in Insulin Resistance and Obesity. *Clinical Nutrition*, Vol.23, No.5, (October 2004), pp. 963-974

Gonzalez, R.; Tiwari, A. & Unniappan, S. (2009). Pancreatic Beta Cells Colocalize Insulin and Pronesfatin Immunoreactivity in Rodents. *Biochemical and Biophysical Research Communications*, Vol.381, No.4, (April 2009), pp. 643-648

Gonzalez, R.; Perry, R. L. S.; Gao, X.; Gaidhu, M. P.; Tsushima, R. G.; Ceddia, R. B. & Unniappan, S. (2011). Nutrient Responsive Nesfatin-1 Regulates Energy Balance and Induces Glucose-Stimulated Insulin Secretion in Rats. *Endocrinology*, Vol.152, No.10, (October 2011), pp. 3628-3637

Hausman, G. J. & Hausman, D. B. (2004). Ontogeny: Adipose Tissue, In: *Encyclopedia of Animal Science*, W.G. Pond & A.W. Bell, (Eds.), pp. 684-687, Marcel Dekker, Inc., ISBN 0-415-80286-5 [ei 1-4389-0932-1], New York, NY

Hausman, G. J.; Dodson, M. V.; Ajuwon, K.; Azain, M.; Barnes, K. M.; Guan, L. L.; Jiang, Z.; Poulos, S. P.; Sainz, R. D.; Smith, S.; Spurlock, M.; Novakofski, J.; Fernyhough, M. E. & Bergen, W. G. (2009). Board-Invited Review: The Biology and Regulation of Preadipocytes and Adipocytes in Meat Animals. Journal of Animal Science, Vol.87, No.4, (April 2009), pp. 1218-1246

Henry, B. A.; Goding, J. W.; Alexander, W. S.; Tilbrook, A. J.; Canny, B. J.; Dunshea, F.; Rao, A.; Mansell, A. & Clarke, I. J. (1999). Central Administration of Leptin to Ovariectomized Ewes Inhibits Food Intake Without Affecting the Secretion of Hormones From the Pituitary Gland: Evidence for a Dissociation of Effects on Appetite and Neuroendocrine Function. *Endocrinology*, Vol.140, No.3, (March 1999), pp. 1175-1182

Henry, B. A.; Goding, J. W.; Tilbrook, A. J.; Dunshea, F. R. & Clarke, I. J. (2001). Intracerebroventricular Infusion of Leptin Elevates the Secretion of Luteinising Hormone Without Affecting Food Intake in Long-Term Food-Restricted Sheep, but

Increases Growth Hormone Irrespective of Bodyweight. *The Journal of Endocrinology*, Vol.168, No.1, (January 2001), pp. 67-77

Herbison, A. E.; d'Anglemont de Tassigny, X.; Doran, J. & Colledge, W. H. (2010). Distribution and Postnatal Development of *Gpr54* Gene Expression in Mouse Brain and Gonadotropin-Releasing Hormone Neurons. *Endocrinology*, Vol.151, No.1, (January 2010), pp. 312-321

Irwig, M. S.; Fraley, G. S.; Smith, J. T.; Acohido, B. V.; Popa, S. M.; Cunningham, M. J.; Gottsch, M. L.; Clifton, D. K. & Steiner, R. A. (2004). Kisspeptin Activation of Gonadotropin Releasing Hormone Neurons and Regulation of KiSS-1 MRNA in the Male Rat. *Neuroendocrinology*, Vol.80, No.4, (2004), pp. 264-272

Islam, A.; Adamik, B.; Hawari, F. I.; Ma, G.; Rouhani, F. N.; Zhang, J. & Levine, S. J. (2006). Extracellular TNFR1 Release Requires the Calcium-Dependent Formation of a Nucleobindin 2-ARTS-1 Complex. *Journal of Biological Chemistry*, Vol.281, No.10, (March 2006), pp. 6860-6873

Iwasa, T.; Matsuzaki, T.; Murakami, M.; Fujisawa, S.; Kinouchi, R.; Gereltsetseg, G.; Kuwahara, A.; Yasui, T. & Irahara, M. (2010). Effects of Intrauterine Undernutrition on Hypothalamic *Kiss1* Expression and the Timing of Puberty in Female Rats. *The Journal of Physiology*, Vol.588, No.5, (March 2010), pp. 821-829

Kaplowitz, P. B. (2008). Link Between Body Fat and the Timing of Puberty. *Pediatrics*, Vol.121, No.Supplement 3, (February 2008), p. S208-S217

Kheterpal, I.; Ku, G.; Coleman, L.; Yu, G.; Ptitsyn, A. A.; Floyd, Z. E. & Gimble, J. M. (2011). Proteome of Human Subcutaneous Adipose Tissue Stromal Vascular Fraction Cells Versus Mature Adipocytes Based on DIGE. *Journal of Proteome Research*, Vol.10, No.4, (January 2011), pp. 1519-1527

Kohno, D.; Nakata, M.; Maejima, Y.; Shimizu, H.; Sedbazar, U.; Yoshida, N.; Dezaki, K.; Onaka, T.; Mori, M. & Yada, T. (2008). Nesfatin-1 Neurons in Paraventricular and Supraoptic Nuclei of the Rat Hypothalamus Coexpress Oxytocin and Vasopressin and Are Activated by Refeeding. *Endocrinology*, Vol.149, No.3, (March 2008), pp. 1295-1301

Kos, K.; Harte, A. L.; da Silva, N. F.; Tonchev, A.; Chaldakov, G.; James, S.; Snead, D. R.; Hoggart, B.; O'Hare, J. P.; McTernan, P. G. & Kumar, S. (2007). Adiponectin and Resistin in Human Cerebrospinal Fluid and Expression of Adiponectin Receptors in the Human Hypothalamus. *The Journal of Clinical Endocrinology & Metabolism*, Vol.92, No.3, (March 2007), pp. 1129-1136

Larsson, O.; Deeney, J. T.; Bränström, R.; Berggren, P.-O. & Corkey, B. E. (1996). Activation of the ATP-Sensitive K^+ Channel by Long Chain Acyl-CoA. *The Journal of Biological Chemistry*, Vol.271, No.18, (May 1996), pp. 10623-10626

Lehr, S.; Hartwig, S.; Lamers, D.; Famulla, S.; Müller, S.; Hanisch, F.-G.; Cuvelier, C.; Ruige, J.; Eckardt, K.; Ouwens, D. M.; Sell, H. & Eckel, J. (2012). Identification and Validation of Novel Adipokines Released From Primary Human Adipocytes. *Molecular & Cellular Proteomics*, Vol.11, No.1, (January 2012), p. M111.011734

Lents, C. A.; Heidorn, N. L.; Barb, C. R. & Ford, J. J. (2008). Central and Peripheral Administration of Kisspeptin Activates Gonadotropin but Not Somatotropin Secretion in Prepubertal Gilts. *Reproduction*, Vol.135, No.6, (March 2008), pp. 879-887

Levin, B. E.; Dunn-Meynell, A. A. & Routh, V. H. (1999). Brain Glucose Sensing and Body Energy Homeostasis: Role in Obesity and Diabetes. *AJP - Regulatory, Integrative and Comparative Physiology*, Vol.276, No.5, (May 1999), p. R1223-R1231

Li, Q.-C.; Wang, H.-Y.; Chen, X.; Guan, H.-Z. & Jiang, Z.-Y. (2010). Fasting Plasma Levels of Nesfatin-1 in Patients With Type 1 and Type 2 Diabetes Mellitus and the Nutrient-Related Fluctuation of Nesfatin-1 Level in Normal Humans. *Regulatory Peptides*, Vol.159, No.1-3, (January 2010), pp. 72-77

Lim, J.-M.; Sherling, D.; Teo, C. F.; Hausman, D. B.; Lin, D. & Wells, L. (2008). Defining the Regulated Secreted Proteome of Rodent Adipocytes Upon the Induction of Insulin Resistance. *Journal of Proteome Research*, Vol.7, No.3, (March 2008), pp. 1251-1263

Lin, J.; Barb, C. R.; Matteri, R. L.; Kraeling, R. R.; Chen, X.; Meinersmann, R. J. & Rampacek, G. B. (2000). Long Form Leptin Receptor MRNA Expression in the Brain, Pituitary, and Other Tissues in the Pig. *Domestic Animal Endocrinology*, Vol.19, No.1, (July 2000), pp. 53-61

Lin, J.; Barb, C. R.; Kraeling, R. R. & Rampacek, G. B. (2001). Developmental Changes in the Long Form Leptin Receptor and Related Neuropeptide Gene Expression in the Pig Brain. *Biology of Reproduction*, Vol.64, No.6, (June 2001), pp. 1614-1618

Lkhagvadorj, S.; Qu, L.; Cai, W.; Couture, O. P.; Barb, C. R.; Hausman, G. J.; Nettleton, D.; Anderson, L. L.; Dekkers, J. C. M. & Tuggle, C. K. (2009). Microarray Gene Expression Profiles of Fasting Induced Changes in Liver and Adipose Tissues of Pigs Expressing the Melanocortin-4 Receptor D298N Variant. *Physiological Genomics*, Vol.38, No.1, (June 2009), pp. 98-111

Lkhagvadorj, S.; Qu, L.; Cai, W.; Couture, O. P.; Barb, C. R.; Hausman, G. J.; Nettleton, D.; Anderson, L. L.; Dekkers, J. C. M. & Tuggle, C. K. (2010). Gene Expression Profiling of the Short-Term Adaptive Response to Acute Caloric Restriction in Liver and Adipose Tissues of Pigs Differing in Feed Efficiency. *AJP - Regulatory, Integrative and Comparative Physiology*, Vol.298, No.2, (February 2010), p. R494-R507

Loftus, T. M.; Jaworsky, D. E.; Frehywot, G. L.; Townsend, C. A.; Ronnett, G. V.; Lane, M. D. & Kuhajda, F. P. (2000). Reduced Food Intake and Body Weight in Mice Treated With Fatty Acid Synthase Inhibitors. *Science*, Vol.288, No.5475, (June 2000), pp. 2379-2381

Lu, M.; Tang, Q.; Olefsky, J. M.; Mellon, P. L. & Webster, N. J. G. (2008). Adiponectin Activates Adenosine Monophosphate-Activated Protein Kinase and Decreases Luteinizing Hormone Secretion in LβT2 Gonadotropes. *Molecular Endocrinology*, Vol.22, No.3, (March 2008), pp. 760-771

Luque, R. M.; Kineman, R. D. & Tena-Sempere, M. (2007). Regulation of Hypothalamic Expression of KiSS-1 and GPR54 Genes by Metabolic Factors: Analyses Using Mouse Models and a Cell Line. *Endocrinology*, Vol.148, No.10, (October 2007), pp. 4601-4611

Maciel, M. N.; Zieba, D. A.; Amstalden, M.; Keisler, D. H.; Neves, J. P. & Williams, G. L. (2004). Chronic Administration of Recombinant Ovine Leptin in Growing Beef Heifers:

Effects on Secretion of LH, Metabolic Hormones, and Timing of Puberty. *Journal of Animal Science*, Vol.82, No.10, (October 2004), pp. 2930-2936

Maejima, Y.; Sedbazar, U.; Suyama, S.; Kohno, D.; Onaka, T.; Takano, E.; Yoshida, N.; Koike, M.; Uchiyama, Y.; Fujiwara, K.; Yashiro, T.; Horvath, T. L.; Dietrich, M. O.; Tanaka, S.; Dezaki, K.; Oh-I, S.; Hashimoto, K.; Shimizu, H.; Nakata, M.; Mori, M. & Yada, T. (2009). Nesfatin-1-Regulated Oxytocinergic Signaling in the Paraventricular Nucleus Causes Anorexia Through a Leptin-Independent Melanocortin Pathway. *Cell Metabolism*, Vol.10, No.5, (November 2009), pp. 355-365

Matkovic, V.; Ilich, J. Z.; Skugor, M.; Badenhop, N. E.; Goel, P.; Clairmont, A.; Klisovic, D.; Nahhas, R. W. & Landoll, J. D. (1997). Leptin Is Inversely Related to Age at Menarche in Human Females. *The Journal of Clinical Endocrinology & Metabolism*, Vol.82, No.10, (October 1997), pp. 3239-3245

Messager, S.; Chatzidaki, E. E.; Ma, D.; Hendrick, A. G.; Zahn, D.; Dixon, J.; Thresher, R. R.; Malinge, I.; Lomet, D.; Carlton, M. B. L.; Colledge, W. H.; Caraty, A. & Aparicio, S. A. J. R. (2005). Kisspeptin Directly Stimulates Gonadotropin-Releasing Hormone Release Via G Protein-Coupled Receptor 54. *Proceedings of the National Academy of Sciences of the United States of America*, Vol.102, No.5, (February 2005), pp. 1761-1766

Miller, D. W.; Findlay, P. A.; Morrison, M. A.; Raver, N. & Adam, C. L. (2002). Seasonal and Dose-Dependent Effects of Intracerebroventricular Leptin on LH Secretion and Appetite in Sheep. *The Journal of Endocrinology*, Vol.175, No.2, (November 2002), pp. 395-404

Miller, J. C.; Gnaedinger, J. M. & Rapoport, S. I. (1987). Utilization of Plasma Fatty Acid in Rat Brain: Distribution of [^{14}C]Palmitate Between Oxidative and Synthetic Pathways. *Journal of Neurochemistry*, Vol.49, No.5, (November 1987), pp. 1507-1514

Morrison, C. D.; Daniel, J. A.; Holmberg, B. J.; Djiane, J.; Raver, N.; Gertler, A. & Keisler, D. H. (2001). Central Infusion of Leptin into Well-Fed and Undernourished Ewe Lambs: Effects on Feed Intake and Serum Concentrations of Growth Hormone and Luteinizing Hormone. *The Journal of Endocrinology*, Vol.168, No.2, (February 2001), pp. 317-324

Nakata, M.; Manaka, K.; Yamamoto, S.; Mori, M. & Yada, T. (2011). Nesfatin-1 Enhances Glucose-Induced Insulin Secretion by Promoting Ca^{2+} Influx Through L-Type Channels in Mouse Islet ß-Cells. *Endocrine Journal*, Vol.58, No.4, (April 2011), pp. 305-313

Navarro, V. M.; Castellano, J. M.; Fernández-Fernández, R.; Barreiro, M. L.; Roa, J.; Sanchez-Criado, J. E.; Aguilar, E.; Dieguez, C.; Pinilla, L. & Tena-Sempere, M. (2004a). Developmental and Hormonally Regulated Messenger Ribonucleic Acid Expression of KiSS-1 and Its Putative Receptor, GPR54, in Rat Hypothalamus and Potent Luteinizing Hormone-Releasing Activity of KiSS-1 Peptide. *Endocrinology*, Vol.145, No.10, (October 2004), pp. 4565-4574

Navarro, V. M.; Fernández-Fernández, R.; Castellano, J. M.; Roa, J.; Mayen, A.; Barreiro, M. L.; Gaytan, F.; Aguilar, E.; Pinilla, L.; Dieguez, C. & Tena-Sempere, M. (2004b). Advanced Vaginal Opening and Precocious Activation of the Reproductive Axis by KiSS-1 Peptide, the Endogenous Ligand of GPR54. *The Journal of Physiology*, Vol.561, No.2, (December 2004), pp. 379-386

Navarro, V. M.; Castellano, J. M.; Fernández-Fernández, R.; Tovar, S.; Roa, J.; Mayen, A.; Barreiro, M. L.; Casanueva, F. F.; Aguilar, E.; Dieguez, C.; Pinilla, L. & Tena-Sempere, M. (2005). Effects of KiSS-1 Peptide, the Natural Ligand of GPR54, on Follicle-Stimulating Hormone Secretion in the Rat. *Endocrinology*, Vol.146, No.4, (April 2005), pp. 1689-1697

Obici, S.; Feng, Z.; Morgan, K.; Stein, D.; Karkanias, G. & Rossetti, L. (2002). Central Administration of Oleic Acid Inhibits Glucose Production and Food Intake. *Diabetes*, Vol.51, No.2, (February 2002), pp. 271-275

Obici, S. (2009). Molecular Targets for Obesity Therapy in the Brain. *Endocrinology*, Vol.150, No.6, (June 2009), pp. 2512-2517

Ogiso, K.; Asakawa, A.; Amitani, H.; Nakahara, T.; Ushikai, M.; Haruta, I.; Koyama, K.-I.; Amitani, M.; Harada, T.; Yasuhara, D. & Inui, A. (2011). Plasma Nesfatin-1 Concentrations in Restricting-Type Anorexia Nervosa. *Peptides*, Vol.32, No.1, (January 2011), pp. 150-153

Oh-I, S.; Shimizu, H.; Satoh, T.; Okada, S.; Adachi, S.; Inoue, K.; Eguchi, H.; Yamamoto, M.; Imaki, T.; Hashimoto, K.; Tsuchiya, T.; Monden, T.; Horiguchi, K.; Yamada, M. & Mori, M. (2006). Identification of Nesfatin-1 As a Satiety Molecule in the Hypothalamus. *Nature*, Vol.443, No.7112, (October 2006), pp. 709-712

Pan, W.; Hsuchou, H. & Kastin, A. J. (2007). Nesfatin-1 Crosses the Blood-Brain Barrier Without Saturation. *Peptides*, Vol.28, No.11, (November 2007), pp. 2223-2228

Price, T. O.; Samson, W. K.; Niehoff, M. L. & Banks, W. A. (2007). Permeability of the Blood-Brain Barrier to a Novel Satiety Molecule Nesfatin-1. *Peptides*, Vol.28, No.12, (December 2007), pp. 2372-2381

Price, C. J.; Samson, W. K. & Ferguson, A. V. (2008). Nesfatin-1 Inhibits NPY Neurons in the Arcuate Nucleus. *Brain Research*, Vol.1230, (September 2008), pp. 99-106

Qian, H.; Barb, C. R.; Compton, M. M.; Hausman, G. J.; Azain, M. J.; Kraeling, R. R. & Baile, C. A. (1999). Leptin MRNA Expression and Serum Leptin Concentrations As Influenced by Age, Weight, and Estradiol in Pigs. *Domestic Animal Endocrinology*, Vol.16, No.2, (February 1999), pp. 135-143

Qiu, J.; Fang, Y.; Bosch, M. A.; Rønnekleiv, O. K. & Kelly, M. J. (2011). Guinea Pig Kisspeptin Neurons Are Depolarized by Leptin *Via* Activation of TRPC Channels. *Endocrinology*, Vol.152, No.4, (April 2011), pp. 1503-1514

Quennell, J. H.; Howell, C. S.; Roa, J.; Augustine, R. A.; Grattan, D. R. & Anderson, G. M. (2011). Leptin Deficiency and Diet-Induced Obesity Reduce Hypothalamic Kisspeptin Expression in Mice. *Endocrinology*, Vol.152, No.4, (April 2011), pp. 1541-1550

Ramanjaneya, M.; Chen, J.; Brown, J. E.; Tripathi, G.; Hallschmid, M.; Patel, S.; Kern, W.; Hillhouse, E. W.; Lehnert, H.; Tan, B. K. & Randeva, H. S. (2010). Identification of Nesfatin-1 in Human and Murine Adipose Tissue: A Novel Depot-Specific Adipokine With Increased Levels in Obesity. *Endocrinology*, Vol.151, No.7, (July 2010), pp. 3169-3180

Rapoport, S. (1996). *In Vivo* Labeling of Brain Phospholipids by Long-Chain Fatty Acids: Relation to Turnover and Function. *Lipids*, Vol.31, No.1, (March 1996), p. S97-S101

Redmond, J. S.; Baez-Sandoval, G. M.; Spell, K. M.; Spencer, T. E.; Lents, C. A.; Williams, G. L. & Amstalden, M. (2011). Developmental Changes in Hypothalamic *Kiss1* Expression During Activation of the Pulsatile Release of Luteinising Hormone in Maturing Ewe Lambs. *Journal of Neuroendocrinology*, Vol.23, No.9, (September 2011), pp. 815-822

Renes, J.; Rosenow, A. & Mariman, E. (2009). Novel Adipocyte Features Discovered by Adipoproteomics. *Adipobiology*, Vol.1, (2009), pp. 7-18

Roa, J.; García-Galiano, D.; Castellano, J. M.; Gaytan, F.; Pinilla, L. & Tena-Sempere, M. (2010). Metabolic Control of Puberty Onset: New Players, New Mechanisms. *Molecular and Cellular Endocrinology*, Vol.324, No.1-2, (August 2010), pp. 87-94

Rodriguez-Pacheco, F.; Martinez-Fuentes, A. J.; Tovar, S.; Pinilla, L.; Tena-Sempere, M.; Dieguez, C.; Castaño, J. P. & Malagon, M. M. (2007). Regulation of Pituitary Cell Function by Adiponectin. *Endocrinology*, Vol.148, No.1, (January 2007), pp. 401-410

Schäffler, A. & Schölmerich, J. (2010). Innate Immunity and Adipose Tissue Biology. *Trends in Immunology*, Vol.31, No.6, (June 2010), pp. 228-235

Shahab, M.; Mastronardi, C.; Seminara, S. B.; Crowley, W. F.; Ojeda, S. R. & Plant, T. M. (2005). Increased Hypothalamic GPR54 Signaling: A Potential Mechanism for Initiation of Puberty in Primates. *Proceedings of the National Academy of Sciences of the United States of America* , Vol.102, No.6, (February 2005), pp. 2129-2134

Shimizu, H.; Ohsaki, A.; Oh-I, S.; Okada, S. & Mori, M. (2009). A New Anorexigenic Protein, Nesfatin-1. *Peptides*, Vol.30, No.5, (May 2009), pp. 995-998

Smith, J. T.; Cunningham, M. J.; Rissman, E. F.; Clifton, D. K. & Steiner, R. A. (2005). Regulation of *Kiss1* Gene Expression in the Brain of the Female Mouse. *Endocrinology*, Vol.146, No.9, (September 2005), pp. 3686-3692

Smith, J. T.; Acohido, B. V.; Clifton, D. K. & Steiner, R. A. (2006). KiSS-1 Neurones Are Direct Targets for Leptin in the *Ob/Ob* Mouse. *Journal of Neuroendocrinology*, Vol.18, No.4, (April 2006), pp. 298-303

Smith, J. T.; Clay, C. M.; Caraty, A. & Clarke, I. J. (2007). KiSS-1 Messenger Ribonucleic Acid Expression in the Hypothalamus of the Ewe Is Regulated by Sex Steroids and Season. *Endocrinology*, Vol.148, No.3, (March 2007), pp. 1150-1157

Smith, J. T.; Li, Q.; Yap, K. S.; Shahab, M.; Roseweir, A. K.; Millar, R. P. & Clarke, I. J. (2011). Kisspeptin Is Essential for the Full Preovulatory LH Surge and Stimulates GnRH Release From the Isolated Ovine Median Eminence. *Endocrinology*, Vol.152, No.3, (March 2011), pp. 1001-1012

Stengel, A.; Goebel, M.; Yakubov, I.; Wang, L.; Witcher, D.; Coskun, T.; Taché, Y.; Sachs, G. & Lambrecht, N. W. G. (2009a). Identification and Characterization of Nesfatin-1 Immunoreactivity in Endocrine Cell Types of the Rat Gastric Oxyntic Mucosa. *Endocrinology*, Vol.150, No.1, (January 2009), pp. 232-238

Stengel, A.; Goebel, M.; Wang, L.; Rivier, J.; Kobelt, P.; Mönnikes, H.; Lambrecht, N. W. G. & Taché, Y. (2009b). Central Nesfatin-1 Reduces Dark-Phase Food Intake and Gastric Emptying in Rats: Differential Role of Corticotropin-Releasing Factor$_2$ Receptor. *Endocrinology*, Vol.150, No.11, (November 2009), pp. 4911-4919

Su, Y.; Zhang, J.; Tang, Y.; Bi, F. & Liu, J.-N. (2010). The Novel Function of Nesfatin-1: Anti-Hyperglycemia. *Biochemical and Biophysical Research Communications*, Vol.391, No.1, (January 2010), pp. 1039-1042

Tadross, J. A.; Patterson, M.; Wynne, K. J.; Patel, S.; Suzuki, K.; Ghatei, M. A. & Bloom, S. R. (2010). Nesfatin Suppresses Feeding and Stimulates the Hypothalamo-Pituitary-Gonadal Axis. *Endocrine Journal*, Vol.57 (Supplement 2), (2010), p. S442 (P3-1-3)

Tomikawa, J.; Homma, T.; Tajima, S.; Shibata, T.; Inamoto, Y.; Takase, K.; Inoue, N.; Ohkura, S.; Uenoyama, Y.; Maeda, K. & Tsukamura, H. (2010). Molecular Characterization and Estrogen Regulation of Hypothalamic *KISS1* Gene in the Pig. *Biology of Reproduction*, Vol.82, No.2, (February 2010), pp. 313-319

True, C.; Kirigiti, M.; Ciofi, P.; Grove, K. L. & Smith, M. S. (2011). Characterisation of Arcuate Nucleus Kisspeptin/Neurokinin B Neuronal Projections and Regulation During Lactation in the Rat. *Journal of Neuroendocrinology*, Vol.23, No.1, (January 2011), pp. 52-64

Wahab, F.; Ullah, F.; Chan, Y.-M.; Seminara, S. B. & Shahab, M. (2011). Decrease in Hypothalamic *Kiss1* and *Kiss1r* Expression: A Potential Mechanism for Fasting-Induced Suppression of the HPG Axis in the Adult Male Rhesus Monkey (*Macaca Mulatta*). *Hormone and Metabolic Research*, Vol.43, No.2, (February 2011), pp. 81-85

Wen, J.-P.; Lv, W.-S.; Yang, J.; Nie, A.-F.; Cheng, X.-B.; Yang, Y.; Ge, Y.; Li, X.-Y. & Ning, G. (2008). Globular Adiponectin Inhibits GnRH Secretion From GT1-7 Hypothalamic GnRH Neurons by Induction of Hyperpolarization of Membrane Potential. *Biochemical and Biophysical Research Communications*, Vol.371, No.4, (July 2008), pp. 756-761

Whisnant, C. S. & Harrell, R. J. (2002). Effect of Short-Term Feed Restriction and Refeeding on Serum Concentrations of Leptin, Luteinizing Hormone and Insulin in Ovariectomized Gilts. *Domestic Animal Endocrinology*, Vol.22, No.2, (April 2002), pp. 73-80

Woods, S. C.; Seeley, R. J.; Porte, D., Jr. & Schwartz, M. W. (1998). Signals That Regulate Food Intake and Energy Homeostasis. *Science*, Vol.280, No.5368, (May 1998), pp. 1378-1383

Xu, J.; Kirigiti, M. A.; Grove, K. L. & Smith, M. S. (2009). Regulation of Food Intake and Gonadotropin-Releasing Hormone/Luteinizing Hormone During Lactation: Role of Insulin and Leptin. *Endocrinology*, Vol.150, No.9, (September 2009), pp. 4231-4240

Yamada, S.; Uenoyama, Y.; Kinoshita, M.; Iwata, K.; Takase, K.; Matsui, H.; Adachi, S.; Inoue, K.; Maeda, K.-I. & Tsukamura, H. (2007). Inhibition of Metastin (Kisspeptin-54)-GPR54 Signaling in the Arcuate Nucleus-Median Eminence Region During Lactation in Rats. *Endocrinology*, Vol.148, No.5, (May 2007), pp. 2226-2232

Zegers, D.; Beckers, S.; Mertens, I. L.; Van Gaal, L. F. & Van Hul, W. (2011). Association Between Polymorphisms of the *Nesfatin* Gene, *NUCB2*, and Obesity in Men. *Molecular Genetics and Metabolism*, Vol.103, No.3, (July 2011), pp. 282-286

Zhang, A.-Q.; Li, X.-L.; Jiang, C.-Y.; Lin, L.; Shi, R.-H.; Chen, J.-D. & Oomura, Y. (2010). Expression of Nesfatin-1/NUCB2 in Rodent Digestive System. *World Journal of Gastroenterology*, Vol.16, No.14, (April 2010), pp. 1735-1741

Zhong, J.; Krawczyk, S. A.; Chaerkady, R.; Huang, H.; Goel, R.; Bader, J. S.; Wong, G. W.; Corkey, B. E. & Pandey, A. (2010). Temporal Profiling of the Secretome During Adipogenesis in Humans. *Journal of Proteome Research,* Vol.9, No.10, (August 2010), pp. 5228-5238

Zieba, D. A.; Amstalden, M.; Morton, S.; Maciel, M. N.; Keisler, D. H. & Williams, G. L. (2004). Regulatory Roles of Leptin at the Hypothalamic-Hypophyseal Axis Before and After Sexual Maturation in Cattle. *Biology of Reproduction,* Vol.71, No.3, (September 2004), pp. 804-812

Chapter 3

Endocannabinoids and Kisspeptins: Two Modulators in Fight for the Regulation of GnRH Activity

Rosaria Meccariello, Rosanna Chianese, Silvia Fasano and Riccardo Pierantoni

Additional information is available at the end of the chapter

http://dx.doi.org/10.5772/48443

1. Introduction

The master system in the control of reproductive functions is the communication into the hypothalamus-pituitary-gonadal axis (HPG), whose main actor is the hypothalamic gonadotropin releasing hormone (GnRH). Such a decapeptide triggers the release of pituitary gonadotropins [Follicular Stimulating Hormone (FSH) and Luteinizing Hormone (LH)] which in turn reach the gonads, induce the biosynthesis of steroids (mainly testosterone in males and estradiol/progesterone in females) and of other non steroidal substances (i.e. activin, follistastin, inhibin) modulating the gametogenesis in both sexes. In the last decades, a significant upsurge of studies aimed to define seveal actors and mechanisms supporting reproductive activity. Ultra short, short and long feedback in HPG communication finely modulate reproduction. Nevertheless, this picture is still puzzling and the complete knowledge of the full process has to be unravelled.

"*Only on the basis of an extensive comparative biology can authentic general biology emerge*" (Bern 1967). Besides the importance of evolutionary track in the research of adaptive phenomena, comparative approaches provide a deep insight into the physiological mechanism in building general models. At present, 25 GnRH molecular forms have been detected in metazoan, also in species lacking pituitary gland. Up to 15 molecular forms have been detected in vertebrates; fish, amphibians, reptiles, birds and also humans possess two GnRH molecular forms (GnRH1 and GnRH2, formerly known as mammalian GnRH and chicken 2 GnRH, respectively) as well as one GnRH receptor (GnRHR), at least. A third GnRH molecular form, GnRH3, is often detected in fish telencephalon and peripheral tissues (Pierantoni et al., 2002). In this respect, current hypothesis postulates that GnRH action progressively evolved from the control of simple basic functions in early metazoan to an indirect way to check gonadal activity in vertebrates, through a sophisticated network of finely tuned neurons (Chianese et al., 2011a; Kah et al., 2007; Kavanaugh et al., 2008; Pierantoni et al., 2002; White et al., 1998). Despite both GnRH1 and GnRH2 share the ability to trigger gonadotropin discharge (Pierantoni et al., 2002), the coexistence of multiple forms of GnRHs in the brain let to hypothesize the division of functional roles. In this respect, GnRH2 activity is also involved in processes other than gonadotropin discharge such as the control of sexual behaviour, or local action at gonadal level. Food intake and energy balance, stress and many other environmental cues deeply affect reproductive success *via* GnRH2. Hence, in such a complex scenario emerged: 1) the need to integrate and convey all information to GnRH neurons, the major hierarchical elements of the HPG and 2) the need to discover possible intermediary neuronal populations in this chain of events (Fernandez-Fernandez et al., 2006; Herbison & Pape, 2001).

Therefore, in this review, we focus on endocannabinoid (ECB) and kisspeptin systems, two modulators of GnRH activity. ECBs are lipidic mediators capable to inhibit the release of hypothalamic GnRH (Scorticati et al., 2004), affecting, as a consequence, both steroroidogenesis and gonadal functions (Wang et al., 2004). While ECBs exert such a negative effect upon GnRH release, kisspeptins, the product of *kiss* gene, positively affect GnRH release. Impairment of kisspeptin system causes idiopathic hypogonadotropic hypogonadism and affects puberty onset (de Roux et al., 2003; Seminara et al., 2003). Thus, at hypothalamic level ECBs and kisspeptin modulate GnRH circuitry in opposite manner. Similarly to GnRH, ECBs and kisspeptin exert a direct effect upon gonadic activity, affecting steroidogenesis, spermatogenesis, spermatozoa functions, follicular development and oocyte maturation, suggesting the existence of a possible local crosstalk among these systems. Thus, in the next paragraphs the activity of ECBs and kisspeptin along the HPG will be properly discussed.

2. New modulators of GnRH/gonadotropin activity at central level

2.1. Endocannabinoid system

The endocannabinoid system (ECS) is an ancient, evolutionarily conserved system, well-characterized in mammalian and non-mammalian vertebrates (Buznikov et al., 2010; Fasano et al., 2009; McPartland et al., 2006). Such a system comprises ECBs, several ECB receptors (CBs), many enzymatic machineries responsible for ECB degradation and biosynthesis and ECB transporters (EMT) (Pierantoni et al., 2009). A schematic representation of ECS components is depicted in Figure 1.

In general, ECBs are amides, esters and ethers of long-chain polyunsaturated fatty acid, isolated from brain, peripheral tissues and reproductive fluids (Devane et al., 1992; Sugiura et al., 1995; Schuel et al., 2002); they mimic the effects of the phytocannabinoid Δ^9-tetrahydrocannabinol (Δ^9-THC), the psychoactive constituent of marijuana plant, *Cannabis sativa*. The main ECBs are the N-arachidonoyl-ethanolamine (AEA, anandamide), the first ECB discovered in porcine brain (Devane et al., 1992), and 2-arachidonoylglycerol (2-AG) (Sugiura et al., 1995). ECBs have the ability to activate a wide range of CBs: the most studied are CB1 and CB2, classical seven transmembrane spanning G coupled receptors (Matsuda et al., 1990; Munro et al., 1993) widely distributed in both brain and peripheral tissues, gonads included (Galiegue et al., 1995, Shire et al., 1995, Brown et al., 2002). The orphan G coupled receptor GPR55 is currently accounted as the third CB (Lauckner et al., 2008). AEA, but not 2-AG, selectively acts as an intracellular ligand of the transient potential type1 vanilloid receptor (TRPV1) channel, a six transmembrane spanning receptor whose structure forms a ligand gated non selective cationic channel activated by capsaicin, one of red chilli pepper component (van der Stelt & Di Marzo, 2004, 2005). Lastly, direct nuclear action of ECBs has been postulated since many ECBs [for instance AEA, 2-AG, N-oleoyl-ethanolamine (OEA), N-palmitoyl-ethanolamine (PEA), noladin ether and virodhamine], the phytocannabinoid Δ^9-THC, CB agonists (HU210, WIN55121-2) as well as cannabinoid metabolites have the ability to activate also PPAR (peroxisome-proliferator-activated receptor) family of nuclear receptors (O'Sullivan, 2007; Sun & Bennett, 2007). In order to activate PPAR receptors, cytoplasmic-nuclear translocation of ECBs requires the fatty acid binding proteins (FABPs) as intracellular carriers (Kaczocha et al., 2012).

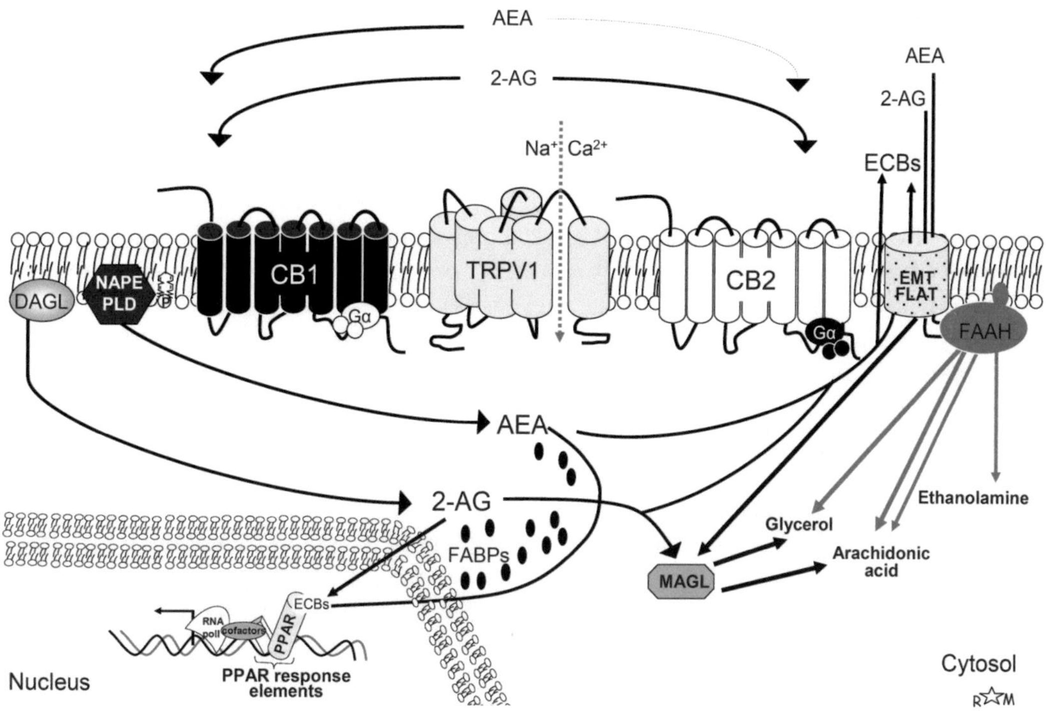

ECS comprises ECBs, CBs, ECB biosynthetic and hydrolizing enzymes, as well as membrane and intracellular carriers (See text for details). Figure modified from: Pierantoni et al., 2009.

Figure 1. Schematic representation of ECS components.

ECBs activity strongly depends on the balance between their biosynthetic and hydrolyzing pathways. AEA and 2-AG are usually released from membrane phospholipid precursors through the activation of N-acyl phosphatidylethanolamine phospholipase D (NAPE-PLD) and diacylglycerol lipase (DAGL), respectively (Bisogno et al., 2003; Okamoto et al., 2004).

Two fatty acid amide hydrolases (FAAH and FAAH-2) (Cravatt et al., 1996; Wei et al., 2006) as well as *N*-acylethanolamine-hydrolyzing acid amidase (NAAA) (Tsuboi et al., 2005; Ueda et al., 2010) release arachidonic acid and ethanolamine from AEA. Besides FAAH, 2-AG is cleaved into arachidonic acid and glycerol by a specific monoacylglycerol lipase (MAGL) (Dinh et al., 2002; Ho et al., 2002). Despite of their lipidic nature, data concerning the existence of a membrane carrier able to mediate ECBs transport is discussed. Recently, in neuronal cells a FAAH-like AEA transporter (FLAT) has been identified. Such a molecule is encoded by a splicing variant of *FAAH-1*, lacks the catalytic activity of FAAH but has the ability to bind AEA (Fu et al., 2011).

Nowadays, ECS elements have been identified in the central and peripheral nervous system as well as in gonads and gametes, demonstrating a deep involvement of the system in the control of reproductive functions, both at central and local level (Battista et al., 2012).

In marijuana smokers as well as in animal models, cannabinoids and ECBs interfere in the neuroendocrine control of reproductive function impairing GnRH and LH production, gonadic steroid production, spermatogenesis, ovulation, embryo development and implantation, as well as sexual behaviour (Murphy et al., 1998; Pagotto et al., 2006; Wang et al., 2006). In the brain, Δ^9-THC and ECBs are well known retrograde signals that act at presynaptic level in order to inhibit the release of specific neurotransmittes [i.e. γ-aminobutyric acid (GABA)]. Current opinion postulates that ECB mediated LH, but not FSH, inhibition is the result of hypothalamic ECB activity. In fact, ECBs are well known inhibitors of GnRH release (Scorticati et al., 2004) and GnRH transcription (Chianese et al., 2011b; Meccariello et al., 2008). By contrast, direct or indirect action of ECBs upon GnRH secreting neurons is still controversial and under investigation. ECBs inhibit several neuronal systems, positively involved in GnRH circuitry (i.e. norepinephrine and glutamate); by contrast, they activate well known inhibitors of GnRH activity [i.e. dopamine, endogenous opioid peptides and corticotrophin-releasing hormone (Murphy et al., 1998)]. Current hypothesis postulates that ECBs interfere in the well known regulation of GnRH neurons by long loop gonadal steroid feedback trough steroids receptor expressing afferents such as GABAergic neurons. For instance, there is a growing consensus that GABA can act through the GABAA receptor to exert both depolarizing and hyperpolarizing effects on GnRH neurons (Herbison & Moenter, 2011). In male mice, GnRH-secreting neurons tonically release 2-AG in presynaptic fissure, which in turn activates CB1 located on GABAergic afferents, in tight relationship with GnRH neurons. The activation of CB1 inhibits the spontaneous release of GABA (Figure 2). As a consequence, postsynaptic GABA receptors (GABAA and GABAB), located on GnRH-secreting neurons, are not activated and GnRH is not released (Farkas et al., 2010). ECB biosynthesis in GnRH secreting neurons might be induced by the activation of metabotropic glutamate receptor (mGluR) located on astrocytes. In fact, in female mice, a complementary hypothesis suggests that local GnRH-GABA circuits uses just the glia derived prostaglandins and/or ECBs in a steroid dependent fashion (Glanowska & Moenter, 2011). GnRH neurons interact with their afferent neurons using several mechanisms and these local circuits can be modified by both sex and steroid feedback. ECBs tone is certainly a key factor in ECBs activity. The inhibitory effect of AEA on GnRH-secreting neurons is reversed by estrogens (Scorticati et al., 2004), through the inhibition of astrocyte mGluR. Such a process inhibits prostaglandin mediated release of ECBs from GnRH secreting neurons (Glanowska & Moenter, 2011). Alternatively, estradiol might directly prevent the ECB mediated inhibition of GABA neurons (Glanowska & Moenter, 2011). In the brain, functional relationships between CB1 and FAAH emerged, since they have a quite overlapping localization (Egertovà et al., 1998). Since estradiol modulates the transcription of FAAH hydrolase, whose promoter contains an ERE element (Waleh et al., 2002), it is not excluded that estradiol might reverse the adverse activity of AEA on GnRH neurons, by means of FAAH upregulation and AEA degradation.

Conversely, it is not excluded that neuronal systems other than GABAergic, as for example kisspeptin neurons described in the next paragraphs, might modulate GnRH-secreting neurons activity *via* ECBs in an estradiol dependent fashion. A model for proposed circuits and possible mechanisms of GnRH neurons activity in males and females are, respectively, reported in Figures 2 and 3. The use of CB1 knockout mice ($CB1^{-/-}$) also contributed to elucidate the mechanism of ECB mediated LH inhibition. AEA decreases both LH and prolactin (PRL) in $CB1^{-/-}$ mice whereas 2-AG is able to suppress LH in wild-type, but not in $CB1^{-/-}$ mice (Olàh et al., 2008). Thus, receptors other than CB1 might be involved in such a signalling. In such a context, the main candidate is TRPV1 (Olàh et al., 2008), whose expression has been reported in the hypothalamus but not in pituitary gland.

The basal crosstalk between ECS and GnRH is evolutionarily conserved, since it has been described also in lower vertebrates (Chianese et al., 2008, 2011b; Cottone et al., 2008, Meccariello et al., 2008). In both amphibians and teleost fish, CB1 was detected in the forebrain, the encephalic macro-area containing the anterior preoptic area, the encephalic region mainly involved in GnRH activity and in the control of gonadotropin discharge (Cottone et al., 2003, 2005; Lam et al., 2006; Migliarini et al., 2006; Meccariello et al., 2008; Valenti et al., 2005). Besides an involvement in food intake, also in lower vertebrates ECS negatively modulates neuroendocrine machinery and reproduction. In fish forebrain, CB1 colocalizes with GnRH3, the GnRH molecular form mainly detected in the telencephalon of fish (Cottone et al., 2008). A CB1 mediated self modulation of GnRH secreting neurons emerged in the anuran amphibian *Rana esculenta* (Meccariello et al., 2008). In male frogs, GnRH1 and CB1 share the localization inside the basal telencephalon and septum (Cottone et al., 2008; Meccariello et al., 2008); most GnRH1 secreting neurons are close to CB1 expressing neurons whereas a subpopulation of GnRH1 secreting neurons - in the approximate order of 20% - coexpresses CB1 (Meccariello et al., 2008). Such a neuroanatomical observation finds a possible functional explanation at molecular level. In fact, mRNA and protein profiles of CB1 and GnRH1 are opposite in frog diencephalon during the annual sexual cycle (Chianese et al., 2008; Meccariello et al., 2008). Treatments of male diencephalons with buserelin, a long acting GnRH analogue, inhibit *GnRH1* transcription and upregulate *CB1* transcription; conversely, AEA treatments downregulate *GnRH1* expression. In this respect, GnRH secreting neurons might produce ECBs in order to properly suppress GnRH secreting activity (ultrashort feedback). This saga is becoming more intricate since in this amphibian a second GnRH molecular form - GnRH2, with a suggested hypophisiotropic role (Pierantoni et al., 2002) - and three GnRHRs (GnRHR1,

GnRHR2, GnRHR3) have been cloned (Chianese et al., 2011b). In different periods of the annual reproductive cycle, AEA also inhibits *GnRH2* expression and upregulates the expression of *GnRHR1, GnRHR2,* but not of *GnRHR3* (Chianese et al., 2011b). Also immortalized neuronal cell lines (GT1) are both target and source of ECBs; *in vitro* they have the ability to produce and secrete ECBs (2-AG and AEA), to uptake and degrade ECBs, and possess CBs (both CB1 and CB2); the activation of CBs inhibits the pulsatile release of GnRH (Gammon et al., 2005). Nevertheless, such observations did not found any confirmation *in vivo,* although GnRH secreting neurons are close to cannabinergic fibres and scantly express CB1 (Gammon et al., 2005). By contrast, micro-array analysis revealed CB2 expression in a subpopulation of GnRH secreting neurons (Todman et al., 2005).

ECS interferes in GnRH circuitry also modulating the activity of neuronal populations that usually converge environmental, stressors, metabolic and photoperiodic cues at different levels of HPG. Stress and food intake, well-known processes under ECBs control (Pagotto et al., 2006), interfere in GnRH secretion. It is interesting to include in this scenario the gonadotropin-inhibitory hormone (GnIH). GnIH belongs to the super-family of RFamide neuropeptides, but its role in the control of gonadotropin secretion is negative, thus proposing the existence of a balance between stimulatory and inhibitory systems in the control of reproduction. Interestingly, this concept does not represent a rule; in fact, in male Syrian hamster, the mammalian ortholog of avian GnIH, the RFRP-3, works on the gonadotropic axis as a stimulator, inducing LH, FSH and testosterone secretion, *via* GnRH neurons activation. Furthermore, this effect might not only vary across species, but also include sex-specific differences in the same species, due to the loss of RFRP-3 mediated stimulation in females (Ancel et al., 2012).

Besides the effect in the hypothalamus, still controversial is the direct activity of ECBs on the pituitary. ECB binding sites, as well as the expression of CBs, biosynthetic and hydrolyzing enzymes have been reported in pituitary *pars distalis* and in pituitary cell cultures (Gonzales et al., 1999, 2000; Lynn & Herkenham, 1994; Murphy et al., 1998; Wenger et al., 1999).

Nevertheless, the localization of CBs in the gonadotropes is confirmed in amphibians and mammals, but not in humans (Cesa et al., 2002; Wenger et al., 1999; Yasuo et al., 2010a). For instance, in rats, AEA exhibits differential effects on the *in vitro* secretion of LH, and pituitary hormones other than gonadotropins [i.e. PRL, corticotrophin (ACTH) and growth hormone (GH)] (Wenger et al., 2000). In a sex steroid dependent fashion, rats express *CB1* in pituitary gland. In females, CB1 expression and AEA content depende on the phase of the ovarian cycle and, in general, pituitary AEA content is opposite to that observed in the hypothalamus (Gonzales et al., 2000). Recently, ECBs have been included among tuberalins, the messengers supposed to be secreted from the *pars tuberalis* - a brain area located between the median eminence, the pituitary portal vessels and the pituitary *pars distalis* - to target the pituitary *pars distalis* (Yasuo et al., 2010b). In both hamsters and humans, *pars tuberalis* produces high levels of 2-AG and low levels of other ECBs (AEA, PEA and OEA), while the pituitary *pars distalis* possesses CB1 (Yasuo et al., 2010a, 2010b). Such a crosstalk might be involved in gonadal response to photoperiodic changes.

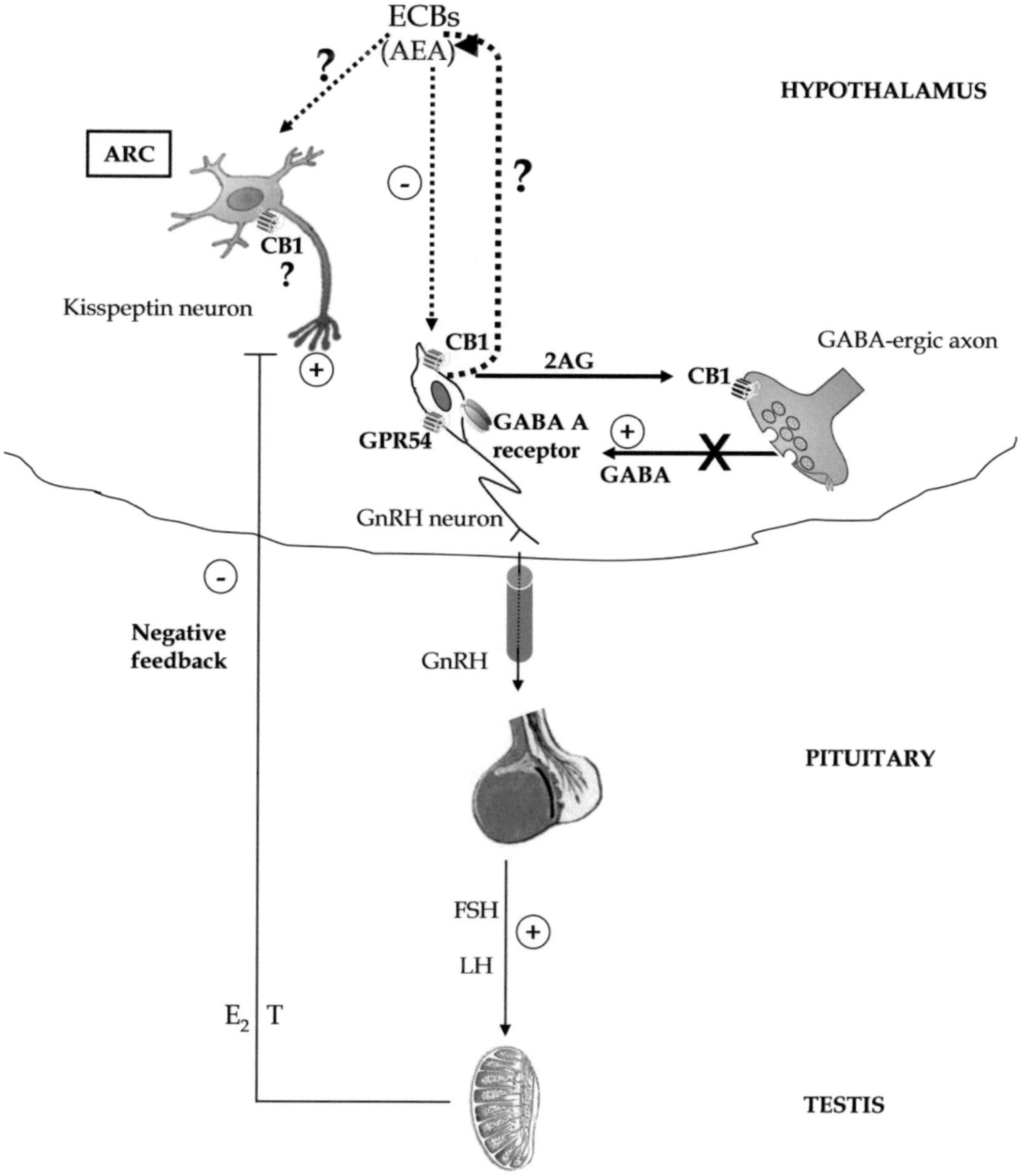

GnRH neuron, through GPR54 receptor, directly receives ARC kisspeptin input and conveys it to pituitary and testis. Gonadal steroids inhibit GnRH secretion through ARC kisspeptin neurons. 2-AG synthesized from GnRH neuron - by means of the CB1 activation - blocks GABA release toward GnRH neuron. ECBs directly act upon GnRH neuron since it express CB1; possibly, ECBs may have a further action on kisspeptin neuron. Anyway, an autocrine regulation of GnRH neuron - through ECBs - may exist.

Figure 2. Model for possible regulatory network along the male HPG.

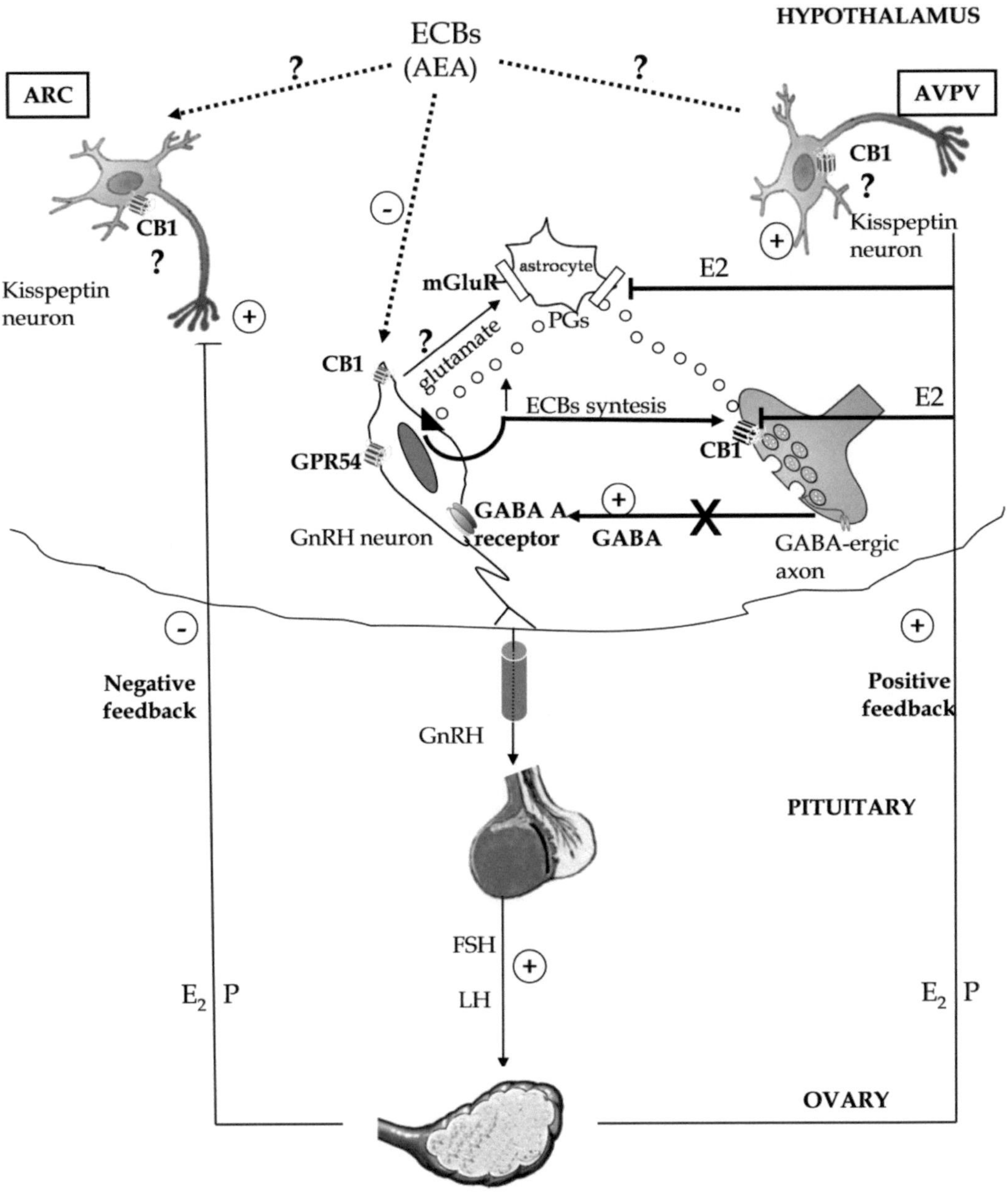

Gonadal steroids exert both inhibitory and stimulatory effects on GnRH neurons, through ARC and AVPV kisspeptin neurons, respectively. While CB1 expression and so ECBs action on GnRH neuron are sure, it remains doubtful the mediation of kisspeptin neurons in the inhibitory regulation of GnRH neuron from ECBs. GnRH neuron is able to produce ECBs; these, in turn, bind CB1 on the GABA-ergic afferent, thus to inhibit GABA release. A possible alternative mechanism for this regulation supposes possible glutamate release from GnRH neuron. Glutamate - through metabotropic glutamate receptor (mGluR) activation - stimulates astrocytes to produce prostaglandins (PGs). These in turn can stimulate GnRH neuron to produce ECBs or regulate CB1 trafficking on GABA-ergic axon. Estradiol blocks this circuit inhibiting mGluR or CB1 activity.

Figure 3. Model for possible regulatory network along the female HPG.

2.2. Kisspeptin system

Kisspeptins belong to the family of RFamide peptides, encoded by the *kiss1* gene, originally detected as a metastasis-suppressor gene in several malignancies (Lee et al., 1996). Kiss name just derives from its role as a suppressor sequence (ss); the letters "Ki" were added after in homage to the location of its discovery, Hershey, Pennsylvania, home of the famous "Hershey Chocolate Kiss". The major kisspeptin product - known as kisspeptin-54 - is a 54 amino acid peptide (Ohtaki et al., 2001); for its instability, it is proteolitically cleaved into shorter peptides (kisspeptin-10, -13 and -14) (Kotani et al., 2001). In 2001, four independent groups showed that all kisspeptin forms bind and activate with similar affinity the orphan G protein-coupled membrane receptor, GPR54 (Clements et al., 2001; Kotani et al., 2001; Muir et al., 2001; Ohtaki et al., 2001).

Hypogonadotropic hypogonadism has been described in mice lacking a functional *kiss* gene or in human and mice with mutations/targeted deletions of *GPR54* genes (Oakley et al., 2009).

Multiple and intricate are the molecular pathways activated by the kisspeptin/GPR54 system to exert its functions in a cell specific way. Starting from G-protein $G_{q/11}$ stimulation, kisspeptins induce phospholipase C (PLC) activation and intracellular calcium mobilization; kisspeptins are also able to induce a strong, sustained stimulation of phosphorylation of the MAP kinases extracellular signal regulated kinases ERK1 and ERK2 and a weak stimulation of p38 MAPK phosphorylation, whereas no activation was observed for stress-activated protein kinase/c-Jun NH2-terminal kinase (SAPK/JNK) (Castaño et al., 2009 and references therein).

The "reproductive" facet of kisspeptins got its disclosure in 2003 when mutations in *kiss1* or *GPR54* genes were associated with idiopathic hypogonadotropic hypogonadism and impaired pubertal maturation (de Roux et al., 2003; Seminara et al., 2003).

Since, the demonstration that kisspeptins are able to stimulate LH and, to a lesser extent, FSH secretion in several species (Roa et al., 2009 and references therein). However, a more consistent hypogonadotropic phenotype characterizes *GPR54* knock-out (KO) mice, compared to *kiss*-KO, suggesting the existence of other possible endogenous ligands for the receptor.

By contrast, GPR54 seems to be the only receptor responsible for the effects of kisspeptins (Lapatto et al., 2007). The main experimental evidences supporting the involvement of kisspeptin in the control of GnRH secreting neuron activity and gonadotropin discharge are summarized in Table 1. The activation of GnRH neurons appears under the control of a kisspeptin tone, but also involves an increase of the kisspeptin neuron projections to GnRH neurons (Roa et al., 2008). Accordingly, in rodents, the detection of kisspeptin-immunoreactive fibres around GnRH neuron cell bodies only starts from postnatal day 25 onwards, and the number of kisspeptin fibres increases at puberty (Clarkson & Herbison, 2006), suggesting that GnRH neurons become more sensitive to kisspeptin just before the onset of puberty. Surprisingly, at least in rodents, electrophysiological studies have demonstrated that a subset of GnRH neurons - responsive to group I metabotropic glutamate receptor agonists - is insensitive to kisspeptins (Dumalska et al., 2008).

In rodents, two major kisspeptin neuronal populations are located at the arcuate nucleus (ARC) and the preoptic area (POA) or the anteroventral periventricular nucleus (AVPV) of the hypothalamus (Mikkelsen et al., 2009). Although in these encephalic districts the kisspeptin-immunoreactive neuron distribution is highly similar in both male and female, the number of cell bodies detected in the AVPV shows a substantial sexual dimorphism being higher in female than in male, at least in rodents (Clarkson & Herbison, 2006). In contrast, in sheep and primates, hypothalamic kisspeptin neurons are especially located in the ARC/infundibular region (Estrada et al., 2006). In this neuro-anatomical picture, although GPR54 and kisspeptin immunoreactivities are rather overlapping, there are some examples of receptor-ligand mismatch. In particular, the ARC is rich in kisspeptin fibres and devoid of GPR54 (Herbison et al., 2010). Over again, the existence of unidentified receptors or ligands appears an intriguing interpretation of this phenomenon.

Key aspect of kisspeptin populations is the high degree of anatomical heterogeneity that may underlie a functional discernable network in the control of GnRH secretion. In this view, in the ARC - but not in the POA/AVPV - kisspeptin neurons co-localize two other neuropeptides, neurokinin B (NKB) and dynorphin (DYN), in several species analyzed to date. For convenience, these cells have been termed KNDy (*K*isspeptin, *N*eurokinin B, *D*ynorphin) (Cheng et al., 2010). They constitute a central node in the control of GnRH secretion, given also the recent observation that genetic inactivation of *TAC3* or *TACR3*, which encode NKB peptide and its receptor, respectively, causes hypogonadotropic hypogonadism (Topaloglu et al., 2009). KNDy cells establish an interconnected network, through extensive reciprocal connections, which might serve to promote auto-regulatory mechanisms; in addition, they have a suggested dual peptidergic as well as glutamatergic phenotype (Lehman et al., 2010a). Conversely, in the AVPV kisspeptin neurons co-localize galanin, a neuropeptide involved in female reproductive functions (Vida et al., 2009), and tyrosine hydroxylase, a marker for dopaminergic neurons (Kauffman et al., 2007). Starting from ARC and AVPV nuclei, both trans-synaptic (indirect) and direct kisspeptin appositions respectively reach GnRH neurons (Clarkson & Herbison, 2006). Evidence for potential inputs at GnRH terminals in the median eminence has also been reported (Lehman et al., 2010a). Anyway, the presence of GPR54 at GnRH nerve terminal level has yet to be demonstrated.

Most work has emphasized the ability of kisspeptin neurons to mediate gonadal steroid feedback on GnRH release. Indistinctly from the specific kisspeptin population observed, all neurons co-localize estradiol (ER), progesterone (PR) and androgen (AR) receptors; particular attention concerns ER, since the greatest percentage of both ARC and AVPV kisspeptin neurons expresses the isoform ERα, in comparison with GnRH neurons that express the isoform ß (Lehman et al., 2010b and references therein). In female, throughout most of the cycle, GnRH/LH secretion is under a negative feedback from ovarian steroids, with estradiol that controls pulse amplitude and progesterone pulse frequency. The feedback becomes positive at the end of the follicular phase to sustain pre-ovulatory GnRH/LH surge and the ovulation (Karsch, 1987). This sexually dimorphic event - only females of most species exhibit it – specifically depends on ERα and occurs *via* a classical mechanism involving transcriptional regulation of gene expression. Of important note, AVPV kisspeptin neurons mediate this positive feedback triggering ovulation; in this respect, kisspeptin signalling might have potential therapeutic roles in the control of ovulation (Clarkson & Herbison, 2009). On the other hand, ARC KNDy neurons convey to GnRH neurons the estrogen negative feedback, at least in rodents, sheep and primates (Roa et al., 2008). Differently, in ewes, KNDy neurons alone govern both inhibitory and stimulatory estrogen effects on GnRH secretion, leaving open the question of how the same sub-population of neurons is able to discern these inputs; a possible explanation could lie in DYN that has the well known ability to mediate the inhibitory feedback of progesterone on GnRH secretion (Goodman et al., 2004). Although some aspects of ARC KNDy neurons have been elucidated, their physiology and their ability to integrate inputs in the control of reproduction are still partially unknown. The use of experimental approach such as cell ablation, that consists in the complete elimination of a whole cell type, can result in quite different phenotypes from complementary gene KO approach. This is the case of kisspeptin/GPR54 neuron ablation (Mayer & Boehm, 2011). The major upsetting observations coming from this study concern the loss of effect of kisspeptin/GPR54 ablation on the timing of puberty onset in female mice, suggesting a regulatory circuit upstream GnRH pulse, independent from kisspeptin signalling. Despite the formation of smaller ovaries, these animals are fertile and, even if GPR54 neuron ablation notably reduces the number of GnRH neurons to almost 10%, this limited percentage seems to be sufficient for a normal reproductive development. Only in the case of acute kisspeptin neuron ablation, animals show acyclicity and infertility, suggesting an essential role for kisspeptin neurons themselves, but not for kisspeptin signalling in ovulatory cyclicity (Mayer & Boehm, 2011).

Reproductive success strongly depends on energy balance, environmental and stressor cues (Bouret et al., 2004). In this perspective, ARC KNDy neurons have been suggested to convey metabolic and stressor information on HPG by means of the expression of glucocorticoid and leptin receptor - where leptin is a hormone secreted by white adipose tissue in proportion to the amount of body energy stores (Bouret et al., 2004, Kinsey-Jones et al., 2009). Conditions of hypoleptinemia have been linked to decreased hypothalamic expression of *kiss1* mRNA and to the inhibition of reproductive functions (Smith et al., 2006). Since GnRH neurons do not directly respond to nutritional conditions (Louis et al., 2011), current hypothesis is that kisspeptin neurons represent intermediate obligate pathways to transmit leptin actions to GnRH neurons that do not express leptin receptor (Castellano et al., 2009, Smith et al., 2006, Tena-Sempere, 2010).

Thus, not only kisspeptins represent a new well consolidated class of modulators of GnRH neuron activity, but also there is an intricate network of regulators that operate up-stream kisspeptin neurons making the study of their physiology much more complicate. Therefore, it is interesting to include in this scenario also the GnIH; it is remarkable that GnIH - through its ability to induce an increase of *kiss1* expression in the the ARC - could act up-stream and not always opposite to kisspeptin neurons, thus to completely upset the idea of the balance kisspeptin/GnIH conceived to date (Ancel et al., 2012).

Evidence	*Reference*
- *Hypothalamus*	
GnRH antagonists completely abrogate kisspeptin releasing effects on LH and FSH	Matsui et al., 2004; Navarro et al., 2005a; Navarro et al., 2005b
GnRH neurons in the rat forebrain express *GPR54* gene	Irwig et al., 2004
Kisspeptin induces *c-fos* expression in rodent GnRH neurons	Irwig et al., 2004
Kisspeptin induces long-lasting depolarization responses of GnRH neurons	Han et al., 2005
Kisspeptin loses its stimulatory effect upon LH secretion in GnRH-deficient *hpg* mice	Roa et al., 2009
- *Hypothalamus cell lines*	
GT1-7 cell lines - parentally related to GnRH neurons - express *GPR54* and respond to kisspeptin stimulation	Quaynor et al., 2007
- *Pituitary*	
Kiss1 and *GPR54* expression is differentially regulated by steroids	Richard et al., 2008
- *Pituitary cell lines*	
GPR54 is expressed in fractions of ovine pituitary cells enriched for gonadotropes, somatotropes and lactotropes	Smith et al., 2008b
Gonadotrope and somatotrope functions are regulated by kisspeptins in nonhuman primate pituitary	Luque et al., 2011
Kisspeptin inhibits LH expression in eel	Pasquier et al., 2011

This table provides a list of references in which the involvement of kisspeptins in the control of GnRH neuron activity as well as of gonadotropin discharge has been demonstrated.

Table 1. Experimental evidences supporting the mechanisms of action of kisspeptins.

As puberty, physiological conditions as pregnancy, lactation and aging suppose a strong contribution of kisspeptins in the regulation of gonadotropin secretion.

During pregnancy, in particular, hypothalamic *kiss1* expression increases and global state of hyper-responsiveness to kisspeptin, probably due to elevated levels of estradiol and progesterone, emerges. Moreover, circulating levels of kisspeptin - mainly derived from the placenta - dramatically increase, suggesting a possible involvement of this signalling in the regulation of trophoblast invasion during the first trimester (Horikoshi et al., 2003). Instead, the suckling stimulus during lactation might be responsible for the suppression of *kiss1* expression in the ARC and so for LH reduction (Yamada et al., 2007). Lastly, aging causes a high degree of reproductive system disruption, most obviously in females; this defect mainly concerns AVPV nucleus. Of note, during menopause, kisspeptin neurons are subjected to a high degree of hypertrophy (Downs & Wise, 2009).

Besides mammals, some important evidences concerning kisspeptin system have also been obtained in non-mammalian species. Recent advances have let to the identification of multiple isoforms of both *kiss* and *GPR54* in non-mammalian vertebrates, contrarily to mammals where only one gene coding for both the ligand and the receptor is present. This complication has been suggested as a consequence of genome duplication events (Tena-Sempere et al., 2012; Um et al., 2010). In this light, fish have two forms of kisspeptin (*kiss1* and *kiss2*) and GPR54 (*GPR54-1* and *GPR54-2*), whereas in amphibians a second round of gene duplication may have contributed to the generation of subtypes for both ligand and receptor (*kiss1a, -1b, -2; GPR54-1a, -1b, -2*) (Tena-Sempere et al., 2012; Um et al., 2010). As previously suggested for GnRH, the presence of two kisspeptin systems might indicate a diversity of roles. Accordingly, zebrafish possess two independent kisspeptin systems, with kiss2 mostly involved in the control of reproductive functions, through interactions with GnRH neurons, whereas kiss1 is supposed to be implicated in the perception of environmental and metabolic signals (Servili et al., 2011). A possible relationship between food intake and kisspeptin signalling has been proposed in Senegalese sole, as well; this function has been attributed to kiss2, being the only isoform found in this specie, in contrast to the evident situation in most fish (Mechaly et al., 2011).

Lower vertebrates, as in particular fish models, strongly respond to environmental conditions, mostly thermal and light cues. In tilapia brain, GPR54 co-localizes with neurons expressing GnRH1, GnRH2 and GnRH3, suggesting an involvement of kisspeptin system in the regulation of GnRH system expression as in mammals (Parhar et al., 2004). Higher levels of *GPR54* expression in the brain have been discovered in mature than in immature animals, thus to hypothesize a link between gonadal development and encephalic *GPR54* expression (Parhar et al., 2004). Similarly to mammals, *kiss1* gene has been identified in two distinct neuronal populations that exhibited a differential response to steroid milieu (Kanda et al., 2008). Furthermore, in fish, light has been shown to have a strong impact on kisspeptin system; in particular, long day - a typical permissive light condition - induces an increase in kisspeptin neuron number, supporting a role for this system in the mediation of light response and reproduction. Such a mediation has been evaluated in mammals, as well. In particular, *kiss1* mRNA and protein expression in ARC of Syrian hamsters decreases in short day condition, in correlation with decreased reproductive activity (Revel et al., 2006). Taken together these findings assign to kisspeptins an important role in the photoperiodic control of reproduction, processes under control of melatonin signals, whose actions on GnRH neurons are not direct. Currently, another wedge has been added to the picture, just in Syrian hamster with the demonstration that RFRP-3 is able to reactivate the reproductive axis blocked under photoinhibitory short-day conditions, thus suggesting that RFRP-3 could be the missing link between melatonin and kisspeptins (Ancel et al., 2012). In sheep, reproductive function is activated by short-day and inhibited by long-day photoperiods; during the breeding season, ARC shows an increase of *Kiss1* and a decrease of *RFRP* expression. Furthermore, the number of kisspeptin fibres onto GnRH neurons increases in comparison to that of RFRP, thus suggesting that these two peptides act in concert, with opposing effects, to regulate GnRH neuron activity (Smith et al., 2008a).

In goldfish, *in vivo* administration of kisspeptin induces LH release, indicating a conserved role from fish to mammals (Li et al., 2009). Anyway, the physiology of kisspeptin system seems to be rather controversial even among piscine species. This is the case of the eel, *Anguilla anguilla*, where kisspeptin - through a direct activity on the pituitary has an inhibitory - and not a stimulatory - effect on *LHβ* expression; this effect is also specific, since no action on other pituitary glycoprotein hormone subunits has been shown (Pasquier et al., 2011).

In amphibian model, the presence of three isoforms for both ligand and receptor makes the evaluation of possible physiological roles for each component likely complex. As in fish, in amphibian all isoforms of kisspeptin and GPR54 are highly expressed in the brain, notably in the hypothalamus, allowing to hypothesize a conserved neuroendocrine and neuromodulatory role in the control of puberty onset and reproduction. Moreover, the expression of *GPR54-1a* and *-2* in the pituitary would support a direct neuroendocrine action at pituitary level (Lee et al., 2009). In *Rana catesbeiana*, in particular, GPR54 is primarily expressed in the hypothalamus and pituitary, and weakly expressed in the testis. Of note, neither a faint signal has been detected in other peripheral tissues, such as heart, spleen, liver, supporting an exclusive role for kisspeptin system in the control of central functions (Moon et al., 2009).

Peripheral administration of kisspeptin also stimulates LH as well as GH and PRL secretion (Kadokawa et al., 2008; Yang et al., 2010). Therefore, an additional target of kisspeptin might be outside the blood-brain barrier (Matsui et al., 2004) and some evidences suggest autocrine/paracrine actions of kisspeptins at the pituitary level. Hence, indicative results as the presence of a functional kisspeptin receptor in the pituitary, combined with the finding that kisspeptin is released in hypophyseal portal blood, reinforce the idea that kisspeptin could be able of a dual action at both the hypothalamus and pituitary level. In support of this hypothesis, both *kiss* and *GPR54* are expressed in the pituitary of several species investigated to date (Richard et al., 2009); GPR54 has also been detected in ovine cellular fractions enriched of gonadotropes, somatotropes and lactotropes (Smith et al., 2008b). Once again, this duality suggested in many species is not the rule, since in a sheep model of hypothalamo-pituitary disconnection, kisspeptin loses its stimulatory action on LH secretion, thus assuming an exclusive effect upstream of the pituitary (Smith et al. 2008b). Anyway, this debate is still open and surely warrants further investigations.

3. Gonadic action of GnRH molecular forms

3.1. GnRH molecular forms and GnRHRs expression and activity in male and female gonads

An intriguing question is the synthesis of GnRH at gonadal level. Despite in hypophysectomised animals GnRH agonist administration induces steroidogenesis and GnRH like molecules have been detected in the main circulation of elasmobranches, in tetrapods the peptide has never been detected in plasma (King et al., 1992). Extra brain synthesis and function of GnRH - expecially GnRH2 - and GnRHRs (both mRNA and protein) have been detected in vertebrate gonads, humans included, endometrium, placenta, and endometrial cancer cells (Pierantoni et al., 2002; Ramakrishnappa et al., 2005; Singh et al., 2007; Wu et al., 2009).

In males, GnRH involvement in paracrine Sertoli/Leydig cell communication has been postulated in both mammals and lower vertebrates (Pierantoni et al., 2002; Sharpe 1986). In rodent and human testis, the main source of testicular GnRH are Sertoli cells, as well as spermatogenetic cells whereas GnRHR has been mainly located in interstitial Leydig cells (Bahk et al., 1995). Thus, GnRH likely acts as paracrine mediator for steroidogenesis and spermatogenesis progression. GnRH involvement in sperm release has also been reported since GnRH agonist/antagonist, induces/suppresses the spermiation in amphibians and lampreys (Deragon & Sower 1994; Pierantoni et al., 1984a, 1984b). Despite the presence of a functional GnRHR in spermatozoa is questionable, GnRH involvement in sperm function at fertilization has also been proposed, since GnRH antagonists inhibit *in vivo* and *in vitro* fertilization in rodents (Morales et al., 2002a). Most information concerning the local activity of GnRH derived from studies carried out in lower vertebrates, where, as in humans, GnRH2 is the main form detected at peripheral level (Pierantoni et al., 2002; White et al., 1998). However, it is not excluded that the existence of multiple forms of GnRH might be linked to the development of specific functions. For instance, in the amphibian, *Rana esculenta,* we have just cloned and characterized two GnRH molecular forms (GnRH1 and GnRH2) and three GnRHRs, with a specific expression pattern in testis, a specific testicular localization and probably, a specific function during the spermatogenesis (Chianese et al., unpublished). In the frog *Rana esculenta,* GnRH cooperates with estradiol in order to gain spermatogonial proliferation in a mechanism involving the protooncogene *c-fos* (Cobellis et al., 2002). During the frog annual sexual cycle, FOS protein appeared inside the cytoplasm of spermatogonia before the proliferative period, whereas it appeared inside the nucleus as soon as spermatogonia proliferation resumes (Cobellis et al., 2002). Estradiol, produced by Leydig cells, induces the transcription of *c-fos* inside the spermatogonia and the protein is stored in cytoplasmic compartment (Cobellis et al., 2002); then, at the end of the winter stasis, GnRH, produced by Sertoli cells, induces FOS activity by means of FOS protein traslocation from cytoplasmic to nuclear compartment (Cobellis et a., 2003) with a consequent increase of spermatogonial mitotic index. The involvement of *c-fos* as well as of estradiol in spermatogonial proliferation has recently been confirmed also in cell lines (He et al., 2008; Sirianni et al., 2008). However, GnRH role in spermatogonial proliferation is an evolutionarily conserved mechanism since it has been demonstrated also in bivalve mollusc (Treen et al., 2012).

As for testis, also in the ovary of mammalian and non-mammalian vertebrates GnRH binding sites as well as at least one GnRH molecular form and one GnRHR have been detected (Pierantoni et al., 2002). Besides testis, in the ovary GnRH activity highly depends on the state of maturation (Guilgur et al., 2009; Pierantoni et al., 2002; Uzbekova et al., 2002; Wu et al., 2009). In lamprey, GnRH induces both steroidogenesis and ovulation, whereas in teleost fish different GnRH molecular forms differentially modulate both meiosis resumption and steroidogenesis (Nabissi et al. 2000; Pati & Habibi, 2000). In rodents,

GnRHR expression rate and localization change during the reproductive cycle, with high expression levels observed in granulosa cells of atretic follicles as well as in mural granulosa cells of Graffian and preovulatory follicles (Bauer-Dantoin & Jameson, 1995; Kogo et al., 1995). Thus, GnRH seems to have a direct role in follicular atresia, a well known phenomenon of cell death. In *in vitro* cultures, GnRH inhibits DNA synthesis (Saragueta et al., 1997) or induces apoptosis in rat granulosa cells (Billig et al., 1994). Studies have shown the evidence for GnRH-induced remodelling of the extra cellular matrix by inducing structural luteolysis in superovulated rats through stimulation of specific matrix metalloproteinase (Goto et al., 1999). In human ovary, GnRH acts as an autocrine modulator of granulosa cells and has the ability to inhibit progesterone biosynthesis (Peng et al, 1994). Lastly, in addition to endocrine regulation, GnRH is also known to act in an autocrine and paracrine manner in order to suppress cell proliferation and to activate apoptosis in the endometrium and endometrial cancer cells through several mechanisms (Wu et al., 2009). In human ovary cell lines, such a mechanism involves GnRH2 and not GnRH1, and opens question of a functional GnRHR2 in humans (Leung et al., 2003). Hypothesis of remnant *GnRHR2* genes in human, mouse and rat genomes is reported in literature (Pawson et al., 2003); at present, it remains unknown whether or not GnRHR2 is expressed as a full-length, properly processed and functional transcript in humans.

However, both GnRH1 and GnRH2 exhibit regulatory roles in tissue remodelling during embryo implantation and placentation, which suggests that these hormones may have important roles in embryo implantation and early pregnancy (Wu et al., 2009).

3.2. Are ECBs and kisspeptin putative local modulators of GnRH/gonadotropin activity?

As for GnRH, also ECBs and kisspeptin biosynthesis and activity have been reported at gonadal levels, thus opening new questions in their possible local crosstalk. Besides the well known suppression of LH in both marijuana smokers and animal model, events due to hypothalamic GnRH suppression, ECBs deeply affect male and female reproductive functions (Wang et al., 2006; Wenger et al., 2001) and they have been detected in reproductive fluids (Schuel et al., 2002; Wang et al., 2006). In males, ECS modulates the progression of spermatogenesis, spermatozoa functions and the activity of testicular somatic cells in mammalian, non-mammalian vertebrates as well as in invertebrates. (Battista et al., 2012; Cacciola et al 2008; Cobellis et al., 2006; Cottone et al., 2008; Grimaldi et al., 2009; Maccarrone et al., 2003, 2005; Pierantoni et al., 2009, Schuel et al., 1991; Wang et al., 2006). In females, ECBs represent fertility signals in folliculogenesis, follicle maturation, oocyte maturation and ovulation (El-Talatini et al., 2009). Then, ECBs and CBs drive embryo transport, survival, implantation, development and growth, placentation and labour (Battista et al., 2012). Consistently, marijuana smokers exhibit several reproductive dysfunctions such as decreased LH levels in both sexes, decreased testosterone level, decreased sperm quality (oligospermia), sperm abnormality and block of acrosome reaction in males, whereas menstrual cycle disorders, reduced birth rates, preterm birth, low foetal birth weight have been described in women (Bari et al., 2011; Wang et al., 2006).

As for kisspeptin concerns, at present, the physiological significance of kisspeptin signalling at gonadal level is under investigation. Besides hypothalamic kisspeptin signalling is critical for puberty onset (Mayer & Boehm, 2011), human and rodent gonads express both *GPR54* and *kiss1* genes (Funes et al., 2003; Terao et al., 2004). With respect to GnRH and ECS, in rat ovary, in particular, *kiss1* mRNA expression shows a fluctuation dependent on the phase of the cycle, with a strong increase before ovulation and a dramatic decrease when ovary is at an immature state (Roa et al., 2007). Also in zebrafish females, *GPR54* expression follows the ovarian development with a decline of expression going toward the reproductive maturity; conversely, an increase of *kiss1* expression coincides with the appearance of mature oocytes (Biran et al., 2008; Filby et al., 2008).

At 7 weeks of age, *GPR54* KO mice display a reduced size of the internal and external reproductive organs with hypoplasia of seminiferous tubules, interstitial Leydig cells, uterine horns and mammary glands; these results let to hypothesize an involvement of GPR54 in cell proliferation and differentiation that are properly necessary for gonadal development (Funes et al., 2003). Interestingly, in zebrafish male, high levels of both ligand and receptor expression have been observed during the first stages of spermatogenesis, when testis is mainly populated by type A spermatogonia to decrease after puberty (Biran et al., 2008; Filby et al., 2008). Kisspeptin expression is modulated by estradiol (Clarkson & Herbison, 2009) and estradiol cooperates with GnRH in order to induce proliferation of spermatogonia (Cobellis et al., 2003), thus raising the possibility of kisspeptin involvement in such a process. The presence of CB2 protein in mouse differentiating spermatogonia (Grimaldi et al., 2009) makes such an item an interesting issue for future investigations.

In disagreement with the general idea that kisspeptin signalling might have a positive impact on reproductive functions, also at a local level, a degenerative effect of kisspeptin administration on maturing rat testes has been reported (Ramzan & Qureshi, 2011). In particular, LH and testosterone suppression and severe degeneration of spermatogenesis in prepubertal testes in a dose-dependent manner have been reported. Such a disruption consists in: Sertoli cells impairment, meiosis inhibition concomitantly to increased spermatogonial proliferation. Already at low doses of kisspeptins, seminiferous tubules show intraepithelial vacuolizations that could be the cause of their massive degeneration, germ cells undergo necrosis, round and elongated spermatids have abnormal acrosome and the interstitial compartment is enlarged. Anyway, testicular degeneration observed after kisspeptin treatment has been suggested to be centrally mediated, and specifically due to an acute hyper-stimulation of the HPG axis (Thompson et al., 2009).

Worth mentioning, the negative effect of kisspeptin on testosterone secretion just reported in rats is in total disagreement with many other evidences provided in both rodents and humans where kisspeptin administration increases testosterone levels (Dhillo et al., 2005; Patterson et al., 2006). Such a point might represent a key switch in autocrine-paracrine communications in Leydig-Sertoli cells - germ cells circuitry involving also GnRH and ECS. AEA administration suppresses testosterone levels (Wenger et al., 2001). Such an issue is surely a consequence of hypothalamic GnRH inhibition, but it is not excluded a direct action at testicular level. Leydig cells are the main source of testicular steroids and express both *GnRHR* and *CB1* (Bahk et al., 1995; Wenger et al 2001); Sertoli cells are the suggested source of GnRH and, in a FSH dependent fashion, modulate ECB tone and aromatase activity (Bahk et al., 1995; Rossi et al., 2007); germ cells are a suggested source of ECBs and have the ability to respond to ECBs and GnRH (Grimaldi et al., 2009). In such a story, the localization of kisspeptin/GPR54 inside the testis, to our knowledge, is completely lacking.

Really interesting might be the sequential activation of ECS, kisspeptin and GnRH in the diachronic process of epididymal sperm motility acquisition, post-ejaculatory events (capacitation and hyperactivation), and the capacity to recognize and to bind to the oocyte investments and egg plasma membrane. Mammalian spermatozoa acquire the ability to swim during their transit from the testis to the oviduct under the control of several external and intracellular factors. In vertebrates, spermatozoa possess a complete ECS and, at least in humans, evidence of kisspeptin system activity has been provided (Pinto et al., 2012; Wang et al., 2006). ECBs, *via* CB1, operate into the epididymis to regulate sperm motility acquisition and to prevent premature acrosome reaction (Cobellis et al., 2010; Ricci et al., 2007; Wang et al., 2006). To date, in species with external fertilization ECBs control the number of motile spermatozoa keeping sperm motility quiescent until their release in aquatic environment (Cobellis et al., 2006). *In vitro*, kisspeptin stimulates an irregular flagellar beating that is typical of a hyperactivation state, a condition critical for fertilization (Pinto et al., 2012). Then, it is intriguing to note that CB1, but not kisspeptin, controls the zona pellucida induced acrosome reaction (Wang et al., 2006) and GnRH increases sperm-zona pellucida binding in humans (Morales et al., 2002b).

4. Closing remarks

Astonishing progress has been accomplished the understanding of how intricate is the scenario that sustains the functionality of the reproductive axis. However, numerous new regulators are still emerging thus suggesting that many other key aspects have to be unravelled. A deep involvement of ECS and kisspeptin system in the modulation of GnRH activity clearly emerged at hypothalamic level. Nevertheless, a functional crosstalk between kisspeptin system, ECS and GnRH has never been investigated so far, neither in the brain nor in male and female gonads. At central level, ECBs and kisspeptins have opposite effects upon GnRH secreting neurons and glutamatergic glial cell surrounding GnRH neurons. In this respect, the balance between AEA and kisspeptin tone might represent a cooperative switch on/off signal for the activity of HPG axis. This aspect becomes more intriguing whether related to the existence of a complicate and multifunctional hypothalamic/gonadal GnRH system in non- mammalian vertebrates and humans.

Most work has attempted to rapidly decipher molecular mechanisms that control kisspeptin, ECBs and GnRH activity at peripheral level, but at moment many aspects of this debate are far from being fully elucidated and warrant further investigation.

Thus, altogether, the putative crosstalk among ECS, kisspeptin system and GnRH might provide a deep insight into the complex field of reproductive biology, opening the avenue to novel therapeutic approaches able to cure and prevent human infertility.

Author details

Rosaria Meccariello*
Dipartimento di Studi delle Istituzioni e dei Sistemi Territoriali, Università di Napoli Parthenope, Napoli, Italy

Rosanna Chianese, Silvia Fasano and Riccardo Pierantoni
Dipartimento di Medicina Sperimentale sez "F. Bottazzi", Seconda Università di Napoli, Napoli, Italy

Acknowledgement

Financial support by Italian Ministry of the University (COFIN 2008/BXCKKX to R.P) and Sorveglianza Sanitaria ex Esposti Mesoteliomi.

Abbreviations

AEA, anandamide; 2-AG, 2-arachidonoylglycerol; AR, androgen receptor; ARC, arcuate nucleus; AVPV, anteroventral periventricular nucleus; CBs, ECB receptors; ER, estradiol receptor; DAGL, diacylglycerol lipase; Δ^9-THC, Δ^9-tetrahydrocannabinol; DYN, dynorphin; ECBs, endocannabinoids; ECS, endocannabinoid system; EMT, ECB transporters; FABPs, fatty acid binding proteins; FAAH, fatty acid amide hydrolase; FLAT, FAAH-like AEA transporter; FSH, follicular Stimulating Hormone; GH, growth hormone; GnIH; gonadotropin-inhibitory hormone; GnRH, gonadotropin releasing hormone; HPG, hypothalamus-pituitary-gonadal axis; KNDy, *K*isspeptin, *N*eurokinin B, *D*ynorphin cells; LH, Luteinizing Hormone; MAGL, monoacylglycerol lipase; NAAA, *N*-acylethanolamine-hydrolyzing acid amidase; NAPE-PLD, N-acyl phosphatidylethanolamine phospholipase D; NKB, neurokinin B; POA, preoptic area; PPAR, peroxisome-proliferator-activated receptor; PR, progesterone receptor; PRL, prolactin; RFRP-3, RFamide-related peptide.

5. References

Ancel, C., Bentsen, AH., Sebert, ME., Tena-Sempere, M., Mikkelsen, JD., & Simmoneaux, V. (2012). Stimulatory effect of RFRP-3 on the gonadotrophic axis in the male Syrian Hamster: the exception proves the rule. *Endocrinol*, 153, 1352-1363.

Bahk, JY., Hyun, JS., Chung, SH., Lee, H., Kim, MO., Lee, BH., & Choi, WS. (1995). Stage specific identification of the expression of GnRH mRNA and localization of the GnRH receptor in mature rat and adult human testis. *J Urol*, 154, 1958-1961.

Bari, M., Battista, N., Pirazzi, V., & Maccarrone, M. (2011). The manifold actions of endocannabinoids on female and male reproductive events. *Front Biosci*, 16, 498-516.

Battista, N., Meccariello, R., Cobellis, G., Fasano, S., Di Tommaso, M., Pirazzi, V., Konje, JC., Pierantoni, R., & Maccarrone, M. (2012). The role of endocannabinoids in gonadal

* Corresponding Author

function and fertility along the evolutionary axis. *Mol Cell Endocrinol* [Epub ahead of print].

Bauer-Dantoin, AC., & Jameson, JL. (1995). Gonadotropin-releasing hormone receptor messenger ribonucleic acid expression in the ovary during the rat estrous cycle. *Endocrinol*, 136, 4432-4438.

Bern, HA. (1967). Hormones and endocrine glands in fishes. Studies on fish endocrinology reveal major physiologic and evolutionary problems. *Science*, 158, 455-462.

Billig, H., Furuta, I., & Hsueh, AJ. (1994). Gonadotropin-releasing hormone directly induces apoptotic cell death in the rat ovary: biochemical and in situ detection of deoxyribonucleic acid fragmentation in granulosa cells. *Endocrinol*, 134, 245-252.

Biran, J., Ben-Dor, S., & Levavi-Sivan, B. (2008). Molecular identification and functional characterization of the kisspeptin/kisspeptin receptor system in lower vertebrates. *Biol Reprod*, 79, 776-786.

Bisogno, T., Howell, F., Williams, G., Minassi, A., Cascio, MG., Ligresti, A., Matias, I., Schiano-Moriello, A., Paul, P., Williams, EJ., Gangadharan, U., Hobbs, C., Di Marzo, V., & Doherty, P. (2003). Cloning of the first sn1-DAG lipases points to the spatial and temporal regulation of endocannabinoid signaling in the brain. *J Cell Biol*, 63, 463-468.

Bouret, SG., Draper, SJ., & Simerly, RB. (2004). Trophic action of leptin on hypothalamic neurons that regulate feeding. *Science*, 304, 108-110.

Brown, SM., Wager-Miller, J., & Mackie, K. (2002). Cloning and molecular characterization of the rat CB2 cannabinoid receptor. *Biochim Biophys Acta*, 1576, 255-264.

Buznikov, GA., Nikitina, LA., Bezuglov, VV., Francisco, ME., Boysen, G., Obispo-Peak, IN., Peterson, RE., Weiss, ER., Schuel, H., Temple, BR., Morrow, AL., & Lauder, JM. (2010). A putative 'pre-nervous' endocannabinoid system in early echinoderm development. *Dev Neurosci*, 32, 1-18.

Cacciola, G., Chioccarelli, T., Mackie, K., Meccariello, R., Ledent, C., Fasano, S., Pierantoni, R., & Cobellis, G. (2008). Expression of type-1 cannabinoid receptor during rat postnatal testicular development: Possible Involvement in adult Leydig cell differentiation. *Biol Reprod*, 79, 758-765.

Castaño, JP., Martínez-Fuentes, AJ., Gutiérrez-Pascual, E., Vaudry, H., Tena-Sempere, M., & Malagón, MM. (2009). Intracellular signalling pathways activated by kisspeptins through GPR54: do multiple signals underlie function diversity? *Peptides*, 30, 10-15.

Castellano, JM., Roa, J., Luque, RM., Dieguez, C., Aguilar, E., Pinilla, L., & Tena-Sempere, M. (2009). KiSS-1/kisspeptins and the metabolic control of reproduction: physiologic roles and putative physiopathological implications. *Peptides*, 30, 139-145.

Cesa, R., Guastalla, A., Cottone, E., Mackie, K., Beltramo, M., & Franzoni, MF. (2002). Relationships between CB1 cannabinoid receptors and pituitary endocrine cells in Xenopus laevis: an immunohistochemical study. *Gen Comp Endocrinol*, 25, 17-24.

Cheng, G., Coolen, LM., Padmanabhan, V., Goodman, RL., & Lehman, MN. (2010). The Kisspeptin/Neurokinin B/Dynorphin (KNDy) cell population of the arcuate nucleus: sex differences and effects of prenatal testosterone in sheep. *Endocrinol*, 151, 301-311.

Chianese, R., Cobellis, G., Pierantoni, R., Fasano, S., & Meccariello, R. (2008). Non mammalian vertebrate models and the endocannabinoid system: relationships with gonadotropin-releasing hormone. *Mol Cell Endocrinol,* 286, S46-51.

Chianese, R., Chioccarelli, T., Cacciola, G., Ciaramella, V., Fasano, S., Pierantoni, R., Meccariello, R., & Cobellis G. (2011a). The contribution of lower vertebrate animal models in human reproduction research. *Gen Comp Endocrinol,* 171, 17-27.

Chianese, R., Ciaramella, V., Fasano, S., Pierantoni, R., & Meccariello, R. (2011b). Anandamide modulates the expression of *GnRH-II* and *GnRHRs* in frog, *Rana esculenta,* diencephalon. *Gen Comp Endocrinol,* 173, 389-395.

Clarkson, J., & Herbison, AE. (2006). Postnatal development of kisspeptin neurons in mouse hypothalamus; sexual dimorphism and projections to gonadotropin-releasing hormone neurons. *Endocrinol,* 147, 5817-5825.

Clarkson, J., & Herbison, AE. (2009). Oestrogen, kisspeptin, GPR54 and the pre-ovulatory luteinising hormone surge. *J Neuroendocrinol,* 21, 305-311.

Clements, MK., McDonald, TP., Wang, R., Xie, G., O'Dowd, BF., George, SR., Austin, CP., & Liu, Q. (2001). FMRFamide-related neuropeptides are agonists of the orphan G-protein-coupled receptor GPR54. *Biochem Biophys Res Commun,* 284, 1189-1193.

Cobellis, G., Meccariello, R., Finga, G., Pierantoni, R., & Fasano, S. (2002). Cytoplasmic and nuclear Fos protein forms regulate resumption of spermatogenesis in the frog, *Rana esculenta. Endocrinol,* 143, 163-170.

Cobellis, G., Meccariello, R., Minucci, S., Palmiero, C., Pierantoni, R., & Fasano, S. (2003). Cytoplasmic versus nuclear localization of Fos-related proteins in the frog, *Rana esculenta,* testis: *in vivo* and direct *in vitro* effect of a gonadotropin-releasing hormone agonist. *Biol Reprod,* 68, 954-960.

Cobellis, G., Cacciola, G., Scarpa, D., Meccariello, R., Chianese, R., Franzoni, MF., Mackie, K., Pierantoni, R., & Fasano, S. (2006). Endocannabinoid system in frog and rodent testis: type-1 cannabinoid receptor and fatty acid amide hydrolase activity in male germ cells. *Biol Reprod,* 75, 82-89.

Cobellis, G., Ricci, G., Cacciola, G., Orlando, P., Petrosino, S., Cascio, MG., Bisogno, T., De Petrocellis, L., Chioccarelli, T., Altucci, L., Fasano, S., Meccariello, R., Pierantoni, R., Ledent, C., & Di Marzo, V. (2010). A gradient of 2-arachidonoylglycerol regulates mouse epididymal sperm cell start-up. *Biol Reprod,* 82, 451-458.

Cottone, E., Salio, C., Conrath, M., & Franzoni, MF. (2003). Xenopus laevis CB1 cannabinoid receptor: molecular cloning and mRNA distribution in the central nervous system. *J Comp Neurol,* 464, 487-496.

Cottone, E., Forno, S., Campantico, E., Guastalla, A., Viltono, L., Mackie, K., & Franzoni, MF. (2005). Expression and distribution of CB1 cannabinoid receptors in the central nervous system of the African cichlid fish Pelvicachromis pulcher. *J Comp Neurol,* 485, 293-303.

Cottone, E., Guastalla, A., Mackie, K., & Franzoni, MF. (2008). Endocannabinoids affect the reproductive functions in teleosts and amphibians. *Mol Cell Endocrinol,* 286, S41-S45.

Cravatt, BF., Giang, DK., Mayfield, SP., Boger, DL., Lerner, RA., & Gilula, NB. (1996). Molecular characterization of an enzyme that degrades neuromodulatory fatty-acid amides. *Nature,* 384, 83-87.

Deragon, KL., & Sower, SA. (1994). Effects of lamprey gonadotropin-releasing hormone-III on steroidogenesis and spermiation in male sea lampreys. *Gen Comp Endocrinol*, 95, 363-367.

de Roux, N., Genin, E., Carel, JC., Matsuda, F., Chaussain, JL., & Milgrom, E. (2003). Hypogonadotropic hypogonadism due to loss of function of the Kiss1-derived peptide receptor GPR54. *Proc Natl Acad Sci USA*, 100, 10972-10976.

Devane, WA., Hanus, L., Breuer, A., Pertwee, RG., Stevenson, LA., Griffin, G., Gibson, D., Mandelbaum, A., Etinger, A., & Mechoulam, R. (1992). Isolation and structure of a brain constituent that binds to the cannabinoid receptor. *Science*, 258, 1946-1949.

Dhillo, W.S., Chaudhri, O.B., Patterson, M., Thompson, E.L., Murphy, K.G., Badman, M.K., McGowan, B.M., Amber, V., Patel, S., Ghatei, M.A., & Bloom S.R. (2005). Kisspeptin-54 stimulates the hypothalamic-pituitary gonadal axis in human males. *J Clin Endocrinol Metab*, 90, 6609-6615.

Dinh, TP., Freund, TF., & Piomelli, D. (2002). A role for monoglyceride lipase in 2-arachidonoylglycerol inactivation. *Chem Phys Lipids*, 121, 149-158.

Downs, JL., & Wise, PM. (2009). The role of the brain in female reproductive aging. *Mol Cell endocrinol*, 299, 32-38.

Dumalska, I., Wu, M., Morozova, E., Liu, R., van den Pol, A., & Alreja, M. (2008). Excitatory effects of the puberty-initiating peptide kisspeptin and group I metabotropic glutamate receptor agonists differentiate two distinct subpopulations of gonadotropin-releasing hormone neurons. *J Neurosci*, 28, 8003-8013.

Egertová, M., Giang, DK., Cravatt, BF., & Elphick, MR. (1998). A new perspective on cannabinoid signalling: complementary localization of fatty acid amide hydrolase and the CB1 receptor in rat brain. *Proc Biol Sci*, 265, 2081-2085.

El-Talatini, MR., Taylor, AH., Elson, JC., Brown, L., Davidson, AC., & Konje, JC. (2009). Localisation and function of the endocannabinoid system in the human ovary. *PLoS One*, 4, e4579.

Estrada, KM., Clay, CM., Pompolo, S., Smith, JT., & Clarke, IJ. (2006). Elevated Kiss-1 expression in the arcuate nucleus prior to the cyclic preovulatory gonadotrophin-releasing hormone/luteinising hormone surge in the ewe suggests a stimulatory role for kisspeptin in oestrogen-positive feedback. *J Neuroendocrinol*, 18, 806-809.

Farkas, I., Kalló, I., Deli, L., Vida, B., Hrabovszky, E., Fekete, C., Moenter, SM., Watanabe, M., & Liposits, Z. (2010). Retrograde endocannabinoid signaling reduces GABAergic synaptic transmission to Gonadotropin-Releasing Hormone neurons. *Endocrinol*, 151, 5818-5829

Fasano, S., Meccariello, R., Cobellis, G., Chianese, R., Cacciola, G., Chioccarelli, T., & Pierantoni, R. (2009). The Endocannabinoid System: An Ancient Signaling Involved in the Control of Male Fertility. *Ann NY Acad Sci*, 1163, 112-124.

Fernandez-Fernandez, R., Martini, AC., Navarro, VM., Castellano, JM., Dieguez, C., Aguilar, E., Pinilla, L., & Tena-Sempere, M. (2006). Novel signals for the integration of energy balance and reproduction. *Mol Cell Endocrinol*, 254-255, 127-132.

Filby, AL., van Aerle, R., Duitman, JW., & Tyler, CR. (2008). The Kisspeptin/gonadotropin-releasing hormone pathway and molecular signaling of puberty in fish. *Biol Reprod*, 78, 278-289.

Fu, J., Bottegoni, G., Sasso, O., Bertorelli, R., Rocchia, W., Masetti, M., Guijarro, A., Lodola, A., Armirotti, A., Garau, G., Bandiera, T., Reggiani, A., Mor, M., Cavalli, A., & Pomelli, D. (2011). A catalytically silent FAAH-1 variant drives anandamide transport in neurons. *Nat Neurosci*, 15, 64-69.

Funes, S., Hedrick, JA., Vassleva, G., Markowitz, L., Abbondanzo, S., Golovko, A., Yang, S., Monsma, FJ., & Gustafson EL. (2003). The KISS-1 receptor GPR54 is essential for the development of the murine reproductive system. *Biochem Biophys Res Commun*, 312, 1357-1363.

Gammon, CM., Freeman, GM. Jr., Xie, W., Petersen, SL., & Wetsel, WC. (2005). Regulation of gonadotropin-releasing hormone secretion by cannabinoids. *Endocrinol*, 146, 4491-4499.

Galiegue, S., Mary, S., Marchand, J., Dussossoy, D., Carriere, D., Carayon, P., Bouaboula, M., Shire, D., Le Fur, G., & Casellas, P. (1995). Expression of central and peripheral cannabinoid receptors in human immune tissues and leukocyte subpopulations. *Eur J Biochem*, 232, 54-61.

Glanowska, KM., & Moenter, SM. (2011). Endocannabinoids and prostaglandins both contribute to GnRH neuron-GABAergic afferent local feedback circuits. *J Neurophysiol*, 106, 3073-3081.

González, S., Manzanares, J., Berrendero, F., Wenger, T., Corchero, J., Bisogno, T., Romero, J., Fuentes, JA., Di Marzo, V., Ramos, JA., & Fernández-Ruiz, J. (1999). Identification of endocannabinoids and cannabinoid CB(1) receptor mRNA in the pituitary gland. *Neuroendocrinol*, 70, 137-145.

González, S., Bisogno, T., Wenger, T., Manzanares, J., Milone, A., Berrendero, F., Di Marzo, V., Ramos, JA., & Fernández-Ruiz, JJ. (2000). Sex steroid influence on cannabinoid CB(1) receptor mRNA and endocannabinoid levels in the anterior pituitary gland. *Biochem Biophys Res Commun*, 270, 260-266.

Goodman, RL., Coolen, LM., Anderson, GM., Hardy, SL., Valent, M., Connors, JM., Fitzgerald, ME., & Lehman, MN. (2004). Evidence that dynorphin plays a major role in mediating progesterone negative feedback on gonadotropin-releasing hormone neurons in sheep. *Endocrinol*, 145, 2959-2967.

Goto, T., Endo, T., Henmi, H., Kitajima, Y., Kiya, T., Nishikawa, A., Manase, K., Sato, H., & Kudo, R. (1999). Gonadotropin-releasing hormone agonist has the ability to induce increased matrix metalloproteinase (MMP)-2 and membrane type 1-MMP expression in corpora lutea, and structural luteolysis in rats. *J Endocrinol*, 161, 393-402.

Grimaldi, P., Orlando, P., Di Sena, S., Lolicato, F., Petrosino, S., Bisogno, T., Geremia, R., De Petrocellis, L., & Di Marzo, V. (2009). The endocannabinoid system and pivotal role of the CB2 receptor in mouse spermatogenesis. *Proc Natl Acad Sci USA*, 106, 11131-11136.

Guilgur, LG., Strüssmann, CA., & Somoza, GM. (2009). mRNA expression of GnRH variants and receptors in the brain, pituitary and ovaries of pejerrey (Odontesthes bonariensis) in relation to the reproductive status. *Fish Physiol Biochem*, 35, 157-166.

Han, SK., Gottsch, ML., Lee, KJ., Popa, SM., Smith, JT., Jakawich, SK. (2005). Activation of gonadotropin-releasing hormone neurons by kisspeptin as a neuroendocrine switch for the onset of puberty. *J Neurosci*, 25, 11349-11356.

He, Z., Jiang, J., Kokkinaki, M., Golestaneh, N., Hofmann, MC., & Dym, M. (2008). Gdnf upregulates c-Fos transcription via the Ras/Erk1/2 pathway to promote mouse spermatogonial stem cell proliferation. *Stem Cells*, 26, 266-278.

Herbison, AE., & Pape, JR. (2001). New evidence for estrogen receptors in gonadotropin-releasing hormone neurons. *Front Neuroendocrinol*, 22, 292-308.

Herbison, AE., d'Anglemont de Tassigny, X., Doran, J., & Colledge, WH. (2010). Distribution and postnatal development of Gpr54 gene expression in mouse brain and gonadotropin-releasing hormone neurons. *Endocrinol*, 151, 312-321.

Herbison, AE., & Moenter, SM. (2011). Depolarising and hyperpolarising actions of GABA(A) receptor activation on gonadotrophin-releasing hormone neurones: towards an emerging consensus. *J Neuroendocrinol*, 23, 557-569.

Ho, SY., Delgado, L., & Storch, J. (2002). Monoacylglycerol metabolism in human intestinal Caco-2 cells: evidence for metabolic compartmentation and hydrolysis. *J Biol Chem*, 277, 1816-1823.

Horikoshi, Y., Matsumoto, H., Takatsu, Y., Ohtaki, T., Kitada, C., Usuki, S., & Fujino, M. (2003). Dramatic elevation of plasma metastin concentrations in human pregnancy: metastin as a novel placenta-derived hormone in humans. *J Clin Endocrinol Metab*, 88, 914-919.

Irwig, MS., Fraley, GS., Smith, JT., Acohido, BV., Popa, SM., Cunningham, MJ., Gottsch, ML., Clifton, DK., & Steiner, RA. (2004). Kisspeptin activation of gonadotropin releasing hormone neurons and regulation of KISS-1 mRNA in the male rat. *Neuroendocrinol*, 80, 264-272.

Kaczocha, M., Vivieca, S., Sun, J., Glaser, ST., & Deutsch, DG. (2012). Fatty acid-binding proteins transport N-acylethanolamines to nuclear receptors and are targets of endocannabinoid transport inhibitors. *J Biol Chem*, 287, 3415-3424.

Kadokawa, H., Suzuki, S., & Hashizume, T. (2008). Kisspeptin-10 stimulates the secretion of growth hormone and prolactin directly from cultured bovine anterior pituitary cells. *Anim Reprod Sci*, 105, 404-408.

Kah, O., Lethimonier, C., Somoza, G., Guilgur, LG., Vaillant, C., Lareyre, JJ. (2007). GnRH and GnRH receptors in metazoa: a historical, comparative, and evolutive perspectives. *Gen Comp Endocrinol*, 153, 346-364.

Kanda, S., Akazome, Y., Matsunaga, T., Yamamoto, N., Yamada, S., Tsukamura, H., Maeda, K., & Oka, Y. (2008). Identification of Kiss-1 product kisspeptin and steroid-sensitive sexually-dimorphic kisspeptin neurons in medaka (Oryzias latipes). Endocrinol, 149, 2467-2476.

Karsch, FJ. (1987). Central actions of ovarian steroids in the feedback regulation of pulsatile secretion of luteinizing hormone. *Annu Rev Physiol*, 49, 365-382.

Kauffman, AS., Gottsch, ML., Roa, J., Byquist, AC., Crown, A., Clifton, DK., Hoffman, GE., Steiner, RA., & Tena-Sempere, M. (2007). Sexual differentiation of Kiss1 gene expression in the brain of the rat. *Endocrinol*, 148, 1774-1783.

Kavanaugh, SI., Nozaki, M., & Sower, SA. (2008). Origins of gonadotropin-releasing hormone (GnRH) in vertebrates: identification of a novel GnRH in a basal vertebrate, the sea lamprey. *Endocrinol*, 149, 3860-3869.

King, JA., Steneveld, AA., Millar, RP., Fasano, S., Romano, G., Spagnuolo, A., Zanetti, L., & Pierantoni, R. (1992). Gonadotropin-releasing hormone in elasmobranch (electric ray, *Torpedo marmorata*) brain and plasma: chromatographic and immunological evidence for chicken GnRH-II and novel molecular forms. *Peptides*, 13, 27-35.

Kinsey-Jones, JS., Li, XF., Knox, AM., Wilkinson, ES., Zhu, XL., Chaudhary, AA., Millian, SR., Lightman, SL., & O'Byrne, KT. (2009). Down-regulation of hypothalamic kisspeptin and its receptor, Kiss1r, mRNA expression is associated with stress-induces suppression of luteinising hormone secretion in the female rat. *J Neuroendocrinol* 209, 21, 20-29.

Kogo, H., Kudo, A., Park, MK., Mori, T., & Kawashima, S. (1995). In situ detection of gonadotropin-releasing hormone (GnRH) receptor mRNA expression in the rat ovarian follicles. *J Exp Zool*, 272, 62-68.

Kotani, M., Detheux, M., Vandenbogaerde, A., Communi, D., vanderwinden, JM., Le Poul, E., Brezillon, S., Tyldesley, R., Suarez-Huerta, N., Vandeput, F., Blanpain, C., Schiffmann, SN., Vassart, G., & Parmentier, M. (2001). The metastasis suppressor gene KISS-1 encodes kisspeptins, the natural ligands of the orphan G protein-coupled receptor GPR54. *J Biol Chem*, 276, 34631-34636.

Lam, CS., Rastegar, S., & Strähle, U. (2006). Distribution of cannabinoid receptor 1 in the CNS of zebrafish. *Neurosci*, 138, 83-95.

Lapatto, R., Pallais, JC., Zhang, D., Chan, YM., Mahan, A., Cerrato, F., Le, WW., Hoffman, GE., & Seminara, SB. (2007). Kiss1-/- mice exhibit more variable hypogonadism than Gpr54-/- mice. *Endocrinol*, 148, 4927-4936.

Lauckner, JE., Jensen, JB., Chen, HY., Lu, HC., Hille, B., & Mackie, K. (2008). GPR55 is a cannabinoid receptor that increases intracellular calcium and inhibits M current. *Proc Natl Acad Sci USA*, 105, 2699-2704.

Lee, JH., Miele, ME., Hicks, DJ., Phillips, KK., Trent, JM., Weissman, BE., & Welch, DR. (1996). Kiss-1, a novel human malingnant melanoma metastasis-suppressor gene. *J Natl Cancer Inst*, 88, 1731-1737.

Lee, YR., Tsunekawa, K., Moon, MJ., Um, HN., Hwang, JI., Osugi, T., Otaki, N., Sunakawa, Y., Kim, K., Vaudry, H., Kwon, HB., Seong, JY., & Tsutsui, K. (2009). Molecular evolution of multiple forms of kisspeptins and GPR54 receptors in vertebrates. *Endocrinol*, 150, 2837-2846.

Lehman, MN., Coolen, LM., & Goodman, RL. (2010a). Minireview: Kisspeptin/Neurokinin B/Dynorphin (KNDy) cells of the arcuate nucleus: a central node in the control of gonadotropin-releasing hormone secretion. *Endocrinol*, 151, 3479-3489.

Lehman, MN., Merkley, CM., Coolen, LM., & Goodman, RL. (2010b). Anatomy of the kisspeptin neural network in mammals. *Brain Res*, 1364, 90-102.

Leung, PC., Cheng, CK., & Zhu, XM. (2003). Multi-factorial role of GnRH-I and GnRH-II in the human ovary. *Mol Cell Endocrinol*, 202, 145-153.

Li, S., Zhang, Y., Liu, Y., Huang, X., Huang, W., Lu, D., Zhu, P., Shi, Y., Cheng, CH., Liu, X., & Lin, H. (2009). Structural and functional multiplicity of the kisspeptin/GPR54 system in goldfish (Carassius auratus). *J Endocrinol*, 201, 407-418.

Louis, GW., Greenwald-Yarnell, M., Phillips, R., Coolen, LM., Lehman, MN., & Myers, MG Jr. (2011). Molecular mapping of the neural pathways linking leptin to the neuroendocrine reproductive axis. *Endocrinol*, 152, 2302-2310.

Luque, RM., Córdoba-Chacón, J., Gahete, MD., Navarro, VM., Tena-Sempere, M., Kineman, RD., & Castaño JP. (2011). Kisspeptin regulates gonadotroph and somatotroph function in nonhuman primate pituitary via common and distinct signaling mechanisms. *Endocrinol*, 152, 957-966.

Lynn, AB., & Herkenham, M. (1994). Localization of cannabinoid receptors and nonsaturable high-density cannabinoid binding sites in peripheral tissues of the rat: implications for receptor-mediated immune modulation by cannabinoids. *J Pharmacol Exp Ther*, 268, 1612-1623.

Maccarrone, M., Cecconi, S., Rossi, G., Battista, N., Pauselli, R., & Finazzi-Agrò, A. (2003). Anandamide activity and degradation are regulated by early postnatal aging and follicle-stimulating hormone in mouse Sertoli cells. *Endocrinol*, 144, 20-28.

Maccarrone, M., Barboni, B., Paradisi, A., Bernabò, N., Gasperi, V., Pistilli, MG., Fezza, F., Lucidi, P., & Mattioli, M. (2005). Characterization of the endocannabinoid system in boar spermatozoa and implications for sperm capacitation and acrosome reaction. *J Cell Sci*, 118, 4393-4404.

Matsuda, LA., Lolait, SJ., Brownstein, MJ., Young, AC., & Bonner, TI. (1990). Structure of a cannabinoid receptor and functional expression of the cloned cDNA. *Nature*, 346, 561-564.

Matsui, H., Takatsu, Y., Kumano, S., Matsumoto, H., & Ohtaki, T. (2004). Peripheral administration of metastin induces marked gonadotropin release and ovulation in the rat. *Biochem Biophys Res Commun*, 320, 383-388.

Mayer, C., & Boehm, U. (2011). Female reproductive maturation in the absence of kisspeptin/GPR54 signaling. *Nat Neurosci*, 14, 704-710.

McPartland, JM., Matias, I., Di Marzo, V., & Glass, M. (2006). Evolutionary origins of the endocannabinoid system. *Gene*, 370, 64-74.

Meccariello, R., Franzoni, MF., Chianese, R., Cottone, E., Scarpa, D., Donna, D., Cobellis, G., Guastalla, A., Pierantoni, R., & Fasano, S. (2008). Interplay between the endocannabinoid system and GnRH-I in the forebrain of the anuran amphibian *Rana esculenta*. Endocrinol, 149, 2149-2158.

Mechaly, AS., Vinas, J., & Piferrer, F. (2011). Gene structure analysis of kisspeptin-2 (*kiss2*) in the Senegalese sole (*Solea senegalensis*): characterization of two splice variants of *kiss2*, and novel evidence for metabolic regulation of kisspeptin signaling in non-mammalian species. *Mol Cell Endocrinol*, 339, 14-24.

Migliarini, B., Marucci, G., Ghelfi, F., & Carnevali, O. (2006). Endocannabinoid system in Xenopus laevis development: CB1 receptor dynamics. *FEBS Lett*, 580, 1941-1945.

Mikkelsen, JD., & Simonneaux, V. (2009). The neuroanatomy of the kisspeptin system in the mammalian brain. *Peptides*, 30, 26-33.

Moon, JS., Lee, YR., Oh, DY., Hwang, JI., Lee, JY., Kim, JI., Vaudry, H., Kwon, HB., & Seong, JY. (2009). Molecular cloning of the bullfrog kisspeptin receptor GPR54 with high sensitivity to Xenopus kisspeptin. *Peptides*, 30, 171-179.

Morales, P., Pasten, C., & Pizzarro, E. (2002a). Inhibition of *in vivo* and *in vivo* fertilization in rodents by gonadotropin-releasing hormone antagonist. *Biol Reprod*, 67, 1360-1365.

Morales, P., Pizarro, E., Kong, M., & Pasten, C. (2002b). Sperm binding to the human zona pellucida and calcium influx in response to GnRH. *Andrologia*, 34, 301-307.

Muir, AI., Chamberlain, L., Elshourbagy, NA., Michalovich, D., Moore, DJ., Calamari, A., Szekeres, PG., Sarau, HM., Chambers, JK., Murdock, P., Steplewski, K., Shabon, U., Miller, JE., Middleton, SE., Darker, JG, Larminie, CG., Wilson, S., Bergsma, DJ., Emson, P., Faull, R., Philpott, KL., & Harrison, DC. (2001). AXOR12, a novel human G protein-coupled receptor, activated by the peptide Kiss-1. *J Biol Chem*, 276, 28969-28975.

Munro, S., Thomas, KL., & Abu-Shaar, M. (1993). Molecular characterization of a peripheral receptor for cannabinoids. *Nature*, 365, 61-65.

Murphy, LL., Muñoz, RM., Adrian, BA., & Villanúa, MA. (1998). Function of cannabinoid receptors in the neuroendocrine regulation of hormone secretion. *Neurobiol Dis*, 5, 432-446.

Nabissi, M., Soverchia, L., Polzonetti-Magni, AM., & Habibi, HR. (2000). Differential splicing of three gonadotropin-releasing hormone transcript in the ovary of the sea bream Sparus aurata. *Biol Reprod*, 62, 1329-1334.

Navarro, VM., Castellano, JM., Fernandez-Fernandez, R., Tovar, S., Roa, J., Majen, A., Barreiro, ML., Casanueva, FF., Aguilar, E., Dieguez, C., Pinilla, L., Tena-Sempere, M. (2005a). Effects of Kiss-1 peptide, the natural ligand of GPR54, on follicle-stimulating hormone secretion in the rat. *Endocrinol*. 146, 1689-1697.

Navarro, VM., Castellano, JM., Fernández-Fernández, R., Tovar, S., Roa, J., Mayen, A., Nogueiras, R., Vazquez, MJ., Barreiro, ML., Magni, P., Aguilar, E., Dieguez, C., Pinilla, L., Tena-Sempere, M. (2005b). Characterization of the potent luteinizing hormone-releasing activity of Kiss-1 peptide, the natural ligand of GPR54. Endocrinol, 146, 156-163.

Oakley, AE., Clifton, DK., Steiner, RA. (2009). Kisspeptin signalin in the brain. *Endocr Rev*, 30, 713-743.

Ohtaki, T., Shintani, Y., Honda, S., Matsumoto, H., Hori, A., Kanehashi, K., Terao, Y., Kumano, S., Takatsu, Y., Masuda, Y., Ishibashi, Y., Watanabe, T., Asada, M., Yamada, T., Suenaga, M., Kitada, C., Usuki, S., Kurokawa, T., Onda, H., Nishimura, O., & Fujino, M. (2001). Metastasis suppressor gene KISS-1 encodes peptide ligand of a G protein-coupled receptor. *Nature*, 411, 613-617.

Okamoto, Y., Morishita, J., Tsuboi, K., Tonai, T., & Ueda, N. (2004). Molecular characterization of a phospholipase D generating anandamide and its congeners. *J Biol Chem*, 279, 5298-5305.

Oláh, M., Milloh, H., & Wenger, T. (2008). The role of endocannabinoids in the regulation of luteinizing hormone and prolactin release. Differences between the effects of AEA and 2AG. *Mol Cell Endocrinol*, 286, S36-40.

O'Sullivan, S.E. (2007). Cannabinoids go nuclear: evidence for activation of peroxisome proliferator-activated receptors. *Br J Pharmacol*, 152, 576-582.

Pagotto, U., Marsicano, G., Cota, D., Lutz, B., & Pasquali, R. (2006). The emerging role of the endocannabinoid system in endocrine regulation and energy balance. *Endocrine Rev*, 27, 73-100.

Parhar, IS., Ogawa, S., & Sakuma, Y. (2004). Laser-captured single digoxigenin-labeled neurons of gonadotropin-releasing hormone types reveal a novel G protein-coupled receptor (GPR54) during maturation in cichlid fish. *Endocrinol*, 145, 3613-3618.

Pasquier, J., Lafont, A-G., Leprince, J., Vaudry, H., Rousseau, K., & Dufour, S. (2011). First evidence for a direct inhibitory effect of kisspeptins on LH expression in the eel, *Anguilla anguilla*. *Gen Comp Endocrinol*, 173, 216-225.

Pati, D., & Habibi, HR. (2000). Direct action of GnRH variants on goldfish oocyte meiosis and follicular steroidogenesis. *Mol Cell Endocrinol*, 160, 75-88.

Patterson, M., Murphy, K.G., Thompson, E.L., Patel, S., Ghatei, M.A., & Bloom, S.R. (2006). Administration of kisspeptin-54 into discrete regions of the hypothalamus potently increases plasma luteinising hormone and testosterone in male adult rats. *J Neuroendocrinol* 2006, 18, 349-354.

Pawson, AJ., Morgan, K., Maudsley, SR., & Millar, RP. (2003). Type II gonadotrophin-releasing hormone (GnRH-II) in reproductive biology. *Reprod*, 126, 271-278.

Peng, C., Fan, NC., Ligier, M., Väänänen, J., & Leung, PC. (1994). Expression and regulation of gonadotropin-releasing hormone (GnRH) and GnRH receptor messenger ribonucleic acids in human granulosa-luteal cells. *Endocrinol*, 135, 1740-1746.

Pierantoni, R., Fasano, S., Di Matteo, L., Minucci, S., Varriale, B., & Chieffi, G. (1984a). Stimulatory effect of a GnRH agonist (buserelin) in *in vitro* and *in vivo* testosterone production by the frog (*Rana esculenta*) testis. *Mol Cell Endocrinol*, 38, 215-219.

Pierantoni, R., Iela, L., d'Istria, M., Fasano, S., Rastogi, RK., & Delrio, G. (1984b). Seasonal testosterone profile and testicular responsiveness to pituitary factors and gonadotrophin releasing hormone during two different phases of the sexual cycle of the frog (*Rana esculenta*). *J Endocrinol*, 102, 387-392.

Pierantoni, R., Cobellis, G., Meccariello, R., & Fasano, S. (2002). Evolutionary aspects of cellular communication in the vertebrate hypothalamo-hypophysio-gonadal axis. *Int Rev Cytol*, 218, 69-141.

Pierantoni, R., Cobellis, G., Meccariello, R., Cacciola, G., Chianese, R., Chioccarelli, T., & Fasano, S. (2009). CB1 Activity in Male Reproduction: Mammalian and Nonmammalian Animal Models. *Vitam Horm*, 81, 367-387.

Pinto, FM., Cejudo-Román, A., Ravina, CG., Fernández-Sánchez, M., Martín-Lozano, D., Illanes, M., Tena-Sempere, M., & Candenas, ML. (2012). Characterization of the kisspeptin system in human spermatozoa. *Int J Androl*, 35, 63-73.

Quaynor, S., Hu, L., Leung, PK., Feng, H., Mores, N., Krsmanovic, LZ., & Catt, KJ. (2007). Expression of a functional g protein-coupled receptor 54-kisspeptin autoregulatory system in hypothalamic gonadotropin-releasing hormone neurons. *Mol Endocrinol*, 21, 3062-3070.

Ramakrishnappa, N., Rajamahendran, R., Lin, YM., & Leung, PC. (2005). GnRH in non-hypothalamic reproductive tissues. *Anim Reprod Sci*, 88, 95-113.

Ramzan, F., & Qureshi, IZ. (2011). Intraperitoneal kisspeptin-10 administration induces dose-dependent degenerative changes in maturing rat testes. *Life Sci*, 88, 246-256.

Revel, FG., Saboureau, M., Masson-Pévet, M., Pévet, P., Mikkelsen, JD., & Simonneaux V. (2006). Kisspeptin mediates the photoperiodic control of reproduction in hamsters. *Curr Biol*, 16, 1730-1735.

Ricci, G., Cacciola, G., Altucci, L., Meccariello, R., Pierantoni, R., Fasano, S., & Cobellis, G. (2007). Endocannabinoid control of sperm motility: the role of epididymus. *Gen Comp Endocrinol*, 153, 320-322.

Richard, N., Galmiche, G., Corvaiser, S., Caraty, A., & Kottler, ML. (2008). Kiss-1 and GPR54 genes are co-expressed in rat gonadotrophs and differentially regulated in vivo by oestradiol and gonadotrophin-releasing hormone. *J Neuroendocrinol*, 20, 381-393.

Richard, N., Corvaiser, S., Camacho, E., & Kottler, ML. (2009). Kiss-1 and GPR54 at the pituitary level: overview and recent insights. *Peptides*, 30, 123-129.

Roa, J., & Tena-Sempere M. (2007). Kiss-1 system and reproduction: comparative aspects and roles in the control of female gonadotropic axis in mammals. *Gene Comp Endocrinol*, 153, 132-140.

Roa, J., Aguilar, E., Dieguez, C., Pinilla, L., & Tena-Sempere, M. (2008). New frontiers in kisspeptins/GPR54 physiology as fundamental gatekeepers of reproductive function. *Front Neuroendocrinol*, 29, 48-69.

Roa, J., Castellano, JM., Navarro, VM., Handelsman, DJ., Pinilla, L., & Tena-Sempere, M. (2009). Kisspeptins and the control of gonadotropin secretion in male and female rodents. *Peptides*, 30, 57-66.

Rossi, G., Gasperi, V., Paro, R., Barsacchi, D., Cecconi, S., & Maccarrone, M. (2007). Follicle-stimulating hormone activates fatty acid amide hydrolase by protein kinase A and aromatase-dependent pathways in mouse primary Sertoli cells. *Endocrinol*, 148, 1431-1439.

Sarагüeta, PE., Lanuza, GM., & Barañao, JL. (1997). Inhibitory effect of gonadotrophin-releasing hormone (GnRH) on rat granulosa cell deoxyribonucleic acid synthesis. *Mol Reprod Dev*, 47, 170-174.

Schuel, H., Chang, MC., Berkery, D., Schuel, R., Zimmerman, AM., & Zimmerman S. (1991). Cannabinoids inhibit fertilization in sea urchins by reducing the fertilizing capacity of sperm. *Pharmacol Biochem Behav*, 40, 609-15.

Schuel, H., Burkman, LJ., Lippes, J., Crickard, K., Forester, E., Piomelli, D., & Giuffrida, A. (2002). N-Acylethanolamines in human reproductive fluids. *Chem Phys Lipids*, 121, 211-227.

Scorticati, C., Fernandez-Solari, J., De Laurentiis, A., Mohn, C., Prestifilippo, JP., Lasaga, M., Seìlicovich, A., Billi, S., Franchi, A., McCann, S., & Rettori, V. (2004). The inhibitory effect of anandamide on luteinizing hormone-releasing hormone secretion is reversed by oestrogen. *Proc Natl Acad Sci USA*, 32, 11891-11896.

Seminara, SB., Messager, S., Chatzidaki, EE., Thresher, RR., Acierno, JS. Jr, Shagoury, JK., Bo-Abbas, Y., Kuohung, W., Schwinof, KM., Hendrick, AG., Zahn, D., Dixon, J., Kaiser, UB., Slaugenhaupt, SA., Gusella, JF., O'Rahilly, S., Carlton, MB., Crowley, WF. Jr, Aparicio, SA., & Colledge, WH. (2003). The GPR54 gene as a regulator of puberty. *N Engl J Med*, 349, 1614-1627.

Servili, A., Le Page, Y., Leprince, J., Caraty, A., Escobar, S., Parhar, IS., Seong, JY., Vaudry, H., & Kah, O. (2011). Organization of two independent kisspeptin systems derived from evolutionary-ancient kiss genes in the brain of zebrafish. *Endocrinol*, 152, 1527-1540.

Sharpe, RM. (1986). Paracrine control of the testis. *Clin Endocrinol Metab*, 15, 185-207.

Shire, D., Carillon, C., Kaghad, M., Calandra, B., Rinaldi-Carmona, M., Le Fur, G., Caput, D., & Ferrara, P. (1995). An ammino-terminal variant of the central cannabinoid receptor resulting from alternative splicing. *J Biol Chem*, 270, 3726-3731.

Singh, P., Krishna, A., Sridaran, R. (2007). Localization of gonadotrophin-releasing hormone I, bradykinin and their receptors in the ovaries of non-mammalian vertebrates. *Reprod*, 133, 969-981.

Sirianni, R., Chimento, A., Ruggiero, C., De Luca, A., Lappano, R., Andò, S., Maggiolini, M., Pezzi, V. (2008). The novel estrogen receptor, G protein-coupled receptor 30, mediates the proliferative effects induced by 17beta-estradiol on mouse spermatogonial GC-1 cell line. *Endocrinol*, 149, 5043-5051.

Smith, JT., Acohido, BV., Clifton, DK., & Steiner, RA. (2006). Kiss-1 neurons are direct target for leptin in the ob/ob mouse. *J Neuroendocrinol*, 18, 298-303.

Smith, JT., Coolen, LM., Kriegsfeld, LJ., Sari, IP., Jaafarzadehshirazi, MR., Maltby, M., Bateman, K., Goodman, RL., Tilbrook, AJ., Ubuka, T., Bentley, GE., Clarke, IJ., & Lehman, MN. (2008a). Variation in kisspeptin and RFamide-related peptide (RFRP) expression and terminal connections to gonadotropin-releasing hormone neurons in the brain: a novel medium for seasonal breeding in the sheep. *Endocrinol*, 149, 5770-5782.

Smith, JT., Rao, A., Pereira, A., Caraty, A., Millar RP., & Clarke, IJ. (2008b). Kisspeptin is present in ovine hypophysial portal blood does not increase during the preovulatory luteinizing hormone surge: evidence that gonadotropes are not direct targets of kisspeptin in vivo. *Endocrinol*, 149, 1951-1959.

Sugiura, T., Kondo, S., Sukagawa, A., Nakane, S., Shinoda, A., Itoh, K., Yamashita, A., & Waku, K. (1995). 2-Arachidonoylglycerol: a possible endogenous cannabinoid receptor ligand in brain. *Biochem Res Commun*, 215, 89-97.

Sun, Y., & Bennett, A. (2007). Cannabinoids: A New Group of Agonists of PPARs. *PPAR Res.* Vol 2007;ARTICLE ID:23513.

Tena-Sempere M. (2010). Kisspeptin signalling in the brain: recent developments and future challenges. *Mol Cell Endocrinol*, 314, 164-169.

Tena-Sempere, M., Felip, A., Gomez, A., Zanuy, S., & Carillo, M. (2012). Comparative insights of the kisspeptin/kisspeptin receptor system: lessons from non-mammalian vertebrates. *Gen Comp Endocrinol*, 175, 234-243.

Terao, Y., Kumano, S., Takatsu, Y., Hattori, M., Nishimura, A., Ohtaki, T., & Shintani Y. (2004). Expression of KISS-1, a metastasis suppressor gene, in trophoblast giant cells of the rat placenta. *Biochim Biophys Acta*, 1678, 102-110.

Thompson, EL., Amber, V., Stamp, GW., Patterson, M., Curtis, AE., Cooke, JH., Appleby, GF., Dhillo, WS., Ghatei, MA., Bloom, SR., & Murphy, KG. (2009). Kisspeptin-54 at high doses acutely induces testicular degeneration in adult male rats via central mechanisms. *Br J Pharmacol*, 156, 609-625.

Todman, MG., Han, SK., & Herbison, AE. (2005). Profiling neurotransmitter receptor expression in mouse gonadotropin-releasing hormone neurons using green fluorescent protein-promoter transgenics and microarrays. *Neurosci*, 132, 703-712.

Topaloglu, AK., Reimann, F., Guclu, M., Yalin, AS., Kotan, LD., Porter, KM., Serin, A., Mungan, NO., Cook, JR., Ozbek, MN., Imamoglu, S., Akalin, NS., Yuksel, B., O'Rahilly, S., & Semple, RK. (2009). TAC3 and TACR3 mutations in familial hypogonadotropic hypogonadism reveal a key role for Neurokinin B in the central control of reproduction. *Nat Gen*, 41, 354-358.

Treen, N., Itoh, N., Miura, H., Kikuchi, I., Ueda, T., Takahashi, KG., Ubuka, T., Yamamoto, K., Sharp, PJ., Tsutsui, K., & Osada, M. (2012). Mollusc gonadotropin-releasing hormone directly regulates gonadal functions: A primitive endocrine system controlling reproduction. *Gen Comp Endocrinol* [Epub ahead of print].

Tsuboi, K., Sun, YX., Okamoto, Y., Araki, N., Tonai, T., & Ueda, N. (2005). Molecular characterization of N-acylethanolamine-hydrolyzing acid amidase, a novel member of the choloylglycine hydrolase family with structural and functional similarity to acid ceramidase. *J Biol Chem*, 280, 11082-11092.

Ueda, N., Tsuboi, K., & Uyama, T. (2010). Enzymological studies on the biosynthesis of N-acylethanolamines. *Biochim Biophys Acta*, 1801, 1274-1285.

Um, HN., Han, JM., Hwang, JI., Hong, SI., Vaudry, H., & Seong, JY. (2010). Molecular coevolution of kisspeptins and their receptors from fish to mammals. *Ann N Y Acad Sci*, 1200, 67-74.

Uzbekova, S., Lareyre, JJ., Madigou, T., Davail, B., Jalabert, B., & Breton, B. (2002). Expression of prepro-GnRH and GnRH receptor messengers in rainbow trout ovary depends on the stage of ovarian follicular development. *Mol Reprod Dev*, 62, 47-56.

Valenti, M., Cottone, E., Martinez, R., De Pedro, N., Rubio, M., Viveros, MP., Franzoni, MF., Delgrado, MJ., & Di Marzo, V. (2005). The endocannabinoid system in the brain of Carassius auratus and its possible role in the control of food intake. *J Neurochem*, 95, 662-672.

van der Stelt, M., & Di Marzo, V. (2004). Endovanilloids. Putative endogenous ligands of transient receptor potential vanilloid 1 channels. *Eur J Biochem*, 271, 1827-1834.

van der Stelt, M., & Di Marzo, V. (2005). Anandamide as an intracellular messenger regulating ion channel activity. *Prostaglandins Other Lipid Mediat*, 77, 111-122.

Vida, B., Hrabovsky, E., Caraty, A., Ciofi, P., Coen, CW., Liposits, Z., & Kallo, Dr I. (2009). Gender differences in the co-localisation of neuropeptides with kisspeptin in the hypothalamic neurons of the mouse brain. In Annual Meeting of the Society of Neuroscience. Vol Ed, Chicago, IL. pp. Poster 865.9.

Waleh, NS., Cravatt, BF., Apte-Deshpande, A., Terao, A., & Kilduff, TS. (2002). Transcriptional regulation of the mouse fatty acid amide hydrolase gene. *Gene*, 291, 203-210.

Wang, H., Dey, SK., & Maccarrone, M. (2006). Jekyll and Hyde: two faces of cannabinoid signalling in male and female fertility. *Endocr Rev*, 27, 427-448.

Wei, BQ., Mikkelsen, TS., McKinney, MK., Lander, ES., & Cravatt, BF. (2006). A second fatty acid amide hydrolase with variable distribution among placental mammals. *J Biol Chem*, 281, 36569-36578.

Wenger, T., Fernández-Ruiz, JJ., & Ramos, JA. (1999). Immunocytochemical demonstration of CB1 cannabinoid receptors in the anterior lobe of the pituitary gland. *J Neuroendocrinol*,11, 873-878.

Wenger, T., Jamali, KA., Juaneda, C., Bascsy, E., & Tramu, G. (2000). The endogenous cannabinoid, anandamide regulates anterior pituitary secretion in vitro. *Addiction Biol*, 5, 59-64.

Wenger, T., Ledent, C., Csernus, V., & Gerendai, I. (2001). The central cannabinoid receptor inactivation suppresses endocrine reproductive functions. *Biochem Biophys Res Commun*, 284, 363-368.

White, RB., Eisen, JA., Kasten, TL., & Fernald, RD. (1998). Second gene for gonadotropin-releasing hormone in humans. *Proc Natl Acad Sci USA*, 95, 305-309.

Wu, HM., Wang, HS., Huang, HY., Soong, YK., MacCalman, CD., & Leung, PC. (2009). GnRH signaling in intrauterine tissues. *Reprod*, 137, 769-777.

Yamada, S., Uenoyama, Y., Kinoshita, M., Iwata, K., Takase, K., Matsui, H., Adachi, S., Inoue, K., Maeda, KI., & Tsukamura, H. (2007). Inhibition of metastin (kisspeptin-54)-GPR54 signaling in the arcuate nucleus-median eminence region during lactation in rats. *Endocrinol*, 148, 2226-2232.

Yang, B., Jiang, Q., Chan, T., Ko, WK., & Wong, AO. (2010). Goldfish kisspeptin: molecular cloning, tissue distribution of transcript expression, and stimulatory effects on prolactin, growth hormone and luteinizing hormone secretion and gene expression via direct actions at the pituitary level. *Gen Comp Endocrinol*, 165, 60-71.

Yasuo, S., Unfried, C., Kettner, M., Geisslinger, G., & Korf, HW. (2010a). Localization of an endocannabinoid system in the hypophysial pars tuberalis and pars distalis of man. *Cell Tissue Res*, 342, 273-281.

Yasuo, S., Koch, M., Schmidt, H., Ziebell, S., Bojunga, J., Geisslinger, G., & Korf, HW. (2010b). An endocannabinoid system is localized to the hypophysial pars tuberalis of Syrian hamsters and responds to photoperiodic changes. *Cell Tissue Res*, 40, 127-136.

Chapter 4

Influence of Neuropeptide – Glutamic Acid-Isoleucine (NEI) on LH Regulation

María Ester Celis

Additional information is available at the end of the chapter

http://dx.doi.org/10.5772/48672

1. Introduction

Neuropeptide- glutamic acid isoleucine (NEI) is a peptide related to reproduction. Although it also has an important function on behavior [2-6], we will focus here on the relationship between NEI and LH.

NEI is derived from the precursor pre- prohormone named pp melanin-concentrating hormone (pp-MCH). This precursor also gives rise to melanin concentrating hormone (MCH) and to neuropeptide-glycine-glutamic acid (NGE) [7-9].

Some studies have suggested a role of NGE at the level of the hypothalamus. For instance, NGE increases the number of neurofilaments and the production of synaptophysin in rat neurons within 18 days of development [10-12].

Immunoreactivity and mRNA expression of both MCH and NEI have been observed in certain regions of the central nervous system. The first region is the diencephalon including the rostralmedial part of the zona incerta, later refer to as the incerto-hypothalamic area (Ihy) by Sita et al. [13]; the three subdivisions (anterior, tuberal and posterior) of the lateral hypothalamus (LHA); the area between the dorsomedial and ventromedial nuclei of the hypothalamus, which Swanson [14] designated as the internuclear area, the anterior periventricular nucleus; and the dorso medial aspects of the tuberomammillary complex. The second region includes the olfatory tubercle, located in the basal forebrain. The third region includes the paramedian pontine reticular formation in the pons [7]. It is important to note that the highest concentration of MCH/NEI ir cells is found in the Ihy and the LHA. We found nearly all the cells in these two regions were immureactive for both MCH and NEI (mean +-S.E.M, 96 +-3%) (Fig.1 and 2)

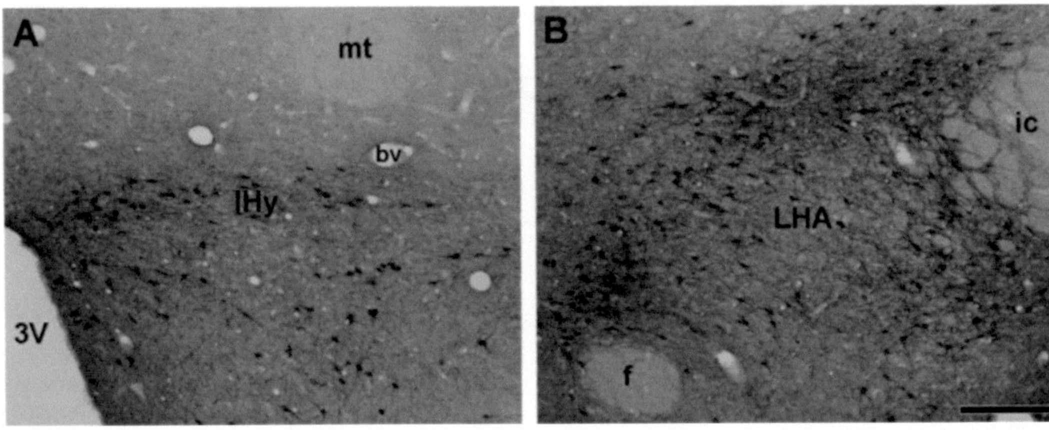

Figure 1. Diencephalic distribution of NEI-immunoreactivity-containing cells. Brightfield photomicrographs of immunoperoxidase material stained for NEI-ir. (A) NEI-ir-containing cells in the incerto-hypothalamic area. (B) NEI-ircontaining cells in the lateral hypothalamic area. Abbreviations: mt, mammilothalamic tract; bv, blood vessels; IHy, incerto hypothalamic area; 3v, third ventricle; ic, internal capsule; LHA, lateral hypothalamic area; f, fornix. Bar = 200 mm. - Reproduced from Bittencourt and Celis, 2008, with permission from Peptides (29:1441-50).

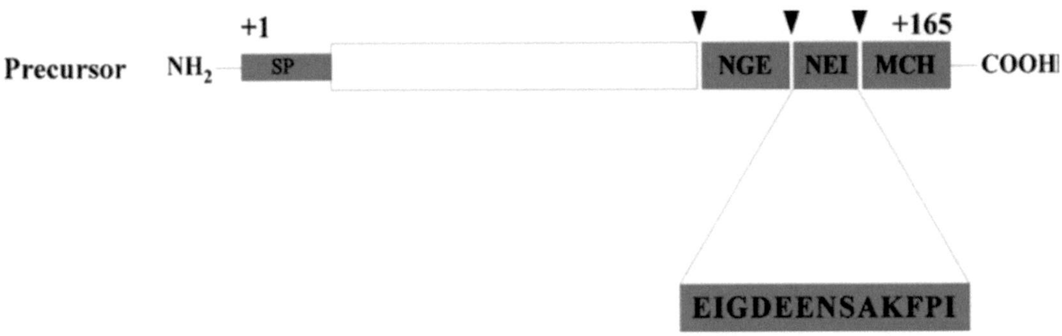

Figure 2. Deduced structure of rat prepro-MCH. The relative positions of the amino (NH2) terminal signal peptide (SP), and the putative MCH, NEI and NGE sequences at the carboxy (COOH) terminus are indicated. The amino acids sequence of NEI is expanded below it. The putative proteolitic processing sites are marked with arrowheads. - Reproduced from Bittencourt and Celis, 2008, with permission from Peptides (29:1441-50).

Peptides such as NGE, NEI and MCH are highly conserved among vertebrates, being abundant and widely distributed in the brain, suggesting that they could be performing important physiological functions. NEI is a 13 aminoacid peptide and has an extensive distribution in the central nervous system (CNS), acting as a neurotransmitter or neuromodulator [15-17]. Neurotranmitter NEI induces grooming behavior, locomotor activity, and stimulates sexual receptivity in female rats [1-6]. NEI injections can modify the levels of noradrenaline and dopamine in specific areas of the brain [4], and earlier studies demonstrated that MCH injection into the preoptic area or median eminence induces luteinizing hormone (LH) secretion. Subsequent studies have shown that modified circulating hormonal levels might modulate ppMCH neurons [18] It has been reported that treatment with 17β-estradiol increases MCH and NEI immunoreactivity throughout the entire diencephalon of ovariectomized cynomologous monkeys [18]. Similar effects were observed in ovariectomized rats receiving no gonadal estradiol treatment [19]. Levels of ppMCH mRNA are only increased in the medial zone incerta (ZI) [15], which houses the A13 group, a collection of dopaminergic neurons that have been previously demonstrated to play a stimulating role in gonadotropin release [20].

More recently, various studies have explored the potential mechanisms by which MCH induces LH secretion [21-27]. Surprisingly, few have examined the role played by NEI in this process.

2. Ovarian steroids effects

Viale et al (1999) proposed a central role of the MCH/NEI neuronal system in the regulation of reproductive functions in rats [18]. In fact, the MCH/NEI system of immunoreactive fibers and terminals that is encountered in hypothalamic areas such as the medial preoptic area (MPOA), is well known to be involved in the control of pre-ovulatory LH surge. These authors studied the effects of the treatment with estrogen on the immunoreactivity of NEI and MCH in OVX animals, using the non-human primate (*M. Fasscicularis*). A slight increase of MCH-IR after 30 days post treatment with estrogen, along with a concurrent significant rise in NEI-IR was observed. A three-fold increase in MCH and NEI –Ir was seen at 72 h post estrogen treatment, compared with the amount of both peptides-ir at 48h post treatment. These facts suggest the possible involvement of these peptides in the regulation of the pre-ovulatory mid- cycle LH surge in primates [19].

The MCH receptors are classified into five subtypes: MC1-R to MC5-R [28]. MCH stimulates gonadotropin-releasing hormone (GnRH) release from hypothalamic explants, and it is interesting to note that MCH affects the release of LH [23] in the female rat. When MCH was injected bilaterally into the rostral preoptic area (rPOA) or medial preoptic area (mPOA) of estrogen-primed ovariectomized rats, LH release was stimulated. Two MCH receptors are involved in the MCH effect. The stimulatory action of MCH in the rPOA was inhibited by administration of antagonists for either MC-1 R or MC-5R, indicating that both ones, MC-1R and MC-5 are involved in the central control of GnRH release by MCH [19-27].

3. The effect of neuropeptide EI on LH regulation

For this study we used male and female rats, aged 10-14 weeks which were bred in our laboratory and maintained with food and water ad libitum, with a cycle of 14h/ light/10h dark and a temperature controlled environment (22±2ºC). The animal procedures were consistent with the standards established by the National Institutes of Health Guide for the Care and Use of Laboratory Animals (1996) and the AmericanVeterinarian Guidelines of Eutanasia.

The first evidence, on the effects of NEI on LH regulation was provided by Attademo et al [1], using male and ovariectomized rats treated with estrogen benzoate (10 ug) and low doses of progesterone (40ug). These animals revealed the following: when male rats were treated with intraventricular injections of NEI (1ug/1ul), the peptide induced an increase of serum LH concentration throughout the entire period studied (10-90 min). At 90 min the serum LH slightly decreased, possibly signaling initiation of the recovery of normal LH serum levels. Control rats injected with artificial cerebrospinal fluid showed practically no changes on serum LH concentrations (Fig. 3). It was also possible to see the NEI effect on ovariectomized female rats treated with estrogen plus progesterone, by using a low dose of progesterone to permit the visualization of modifications in the LH surge. Again, the neuropeptide increased LH release compared with control animals (Fig.4)

The fact that the effect of NEI may be mediated by the noradrenergic system must be taken into consideration. The peptide is known to modify DA and NA in the nucleus accumbens and caudate putamen during grooming behavior and locomotion activity [4]. As NEI behaves similarly to α-MSH, it is important to note that there is some relation between MCH-NEI and α-MSH, indicating that all three peptides are associated in a complex inter-relationship [1].

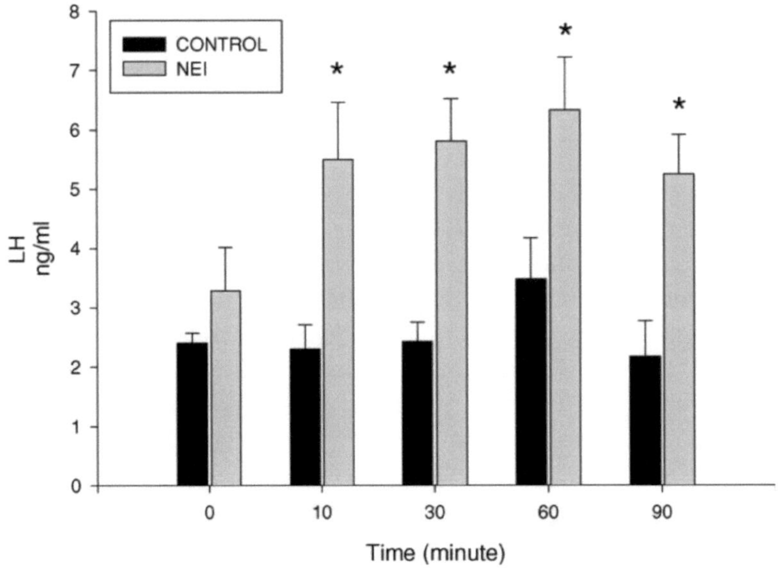

Figure 3. Effect of icv administration of NEI or ACSF (controls) on plasma LH concentration in male rats. Blood samples were collected at 0 (before NEI or ACSF injection), 10, 30, 60 and 90 min post-injection. Bars represent the mean ± S.E.M. $*P < 0.05$ compared to controls. - Reproduced from Attademo et al, 2004, with permission from Peptides.

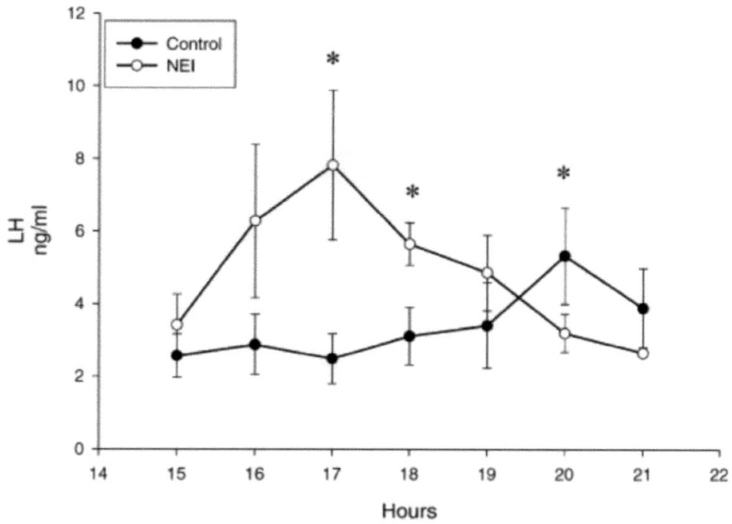

Figure 4. Time course of LH release in CHR-OVX-EB-progesterone treated female rats in the presence (◦) or absence (•) of NEI. CHR-OVX rats were subcutaneously injected with 10 ug EB and 3 days later with 40 ug progesterone at 13:00 h. On the same day of the progesterone injection, the animals were injected icv 1 ug/ul of NEI or ASCF (controls) at 12:00 and 14:00 h. Blood samples were obtained between 15:00 and 21:00 h via the jugular vein, and the plasma levels of LH were measured. The plotted values represent the mean ± S.E.M. ($n = 6$). $*P < 0.05$ compared to controls. - Reproduced from Attademo et al, 2004, with permission from Peptides.

4. Distribution of NEI immunoreactivity

In this study, we described the anatomical substrate underlying the NEI effect of inducing LH secretion, using techniques of double and triple label immunohitochemistry, as well as dual label immunofluorescence. A group of female rats were perfused on day 15 postovariectomy; a second group received10 μg of estradiol benzoate and were perfused two days later and a third group received 10 μg of estradiol benzoate and two days later 40 μg of progesterone and were perfused 5 h after treatment. To mimic the manipulation of the animals, we used a fourth group of ovariectomized rats treated with sesame oil, and also used female intact rats at proestrus and diestrus [28].

Using these techniques, we were able to obtain the following results:

NEI-ir neurons were observed in the medial ZI, in the perifornix at the tuberal hypothalamic level and in the lateral hypothalamus. Fibers were distributed throughout the forebrain, including areas related to reproductive control and LH secretion. We observed a dense number of NEI-ir fibers in the medial septal nucleus, the diagonal band of Broca, the environs of OVLT, the preoptic area and in the internal layer of the median eminence (Fig. 5).

All fibers seen in these areas show varicosities and terminal-like structures. NEI and terminal-like structures were in close apposition with portal blood vessels and GnRH neurons expressing Fos (Fig. 6 A and B)

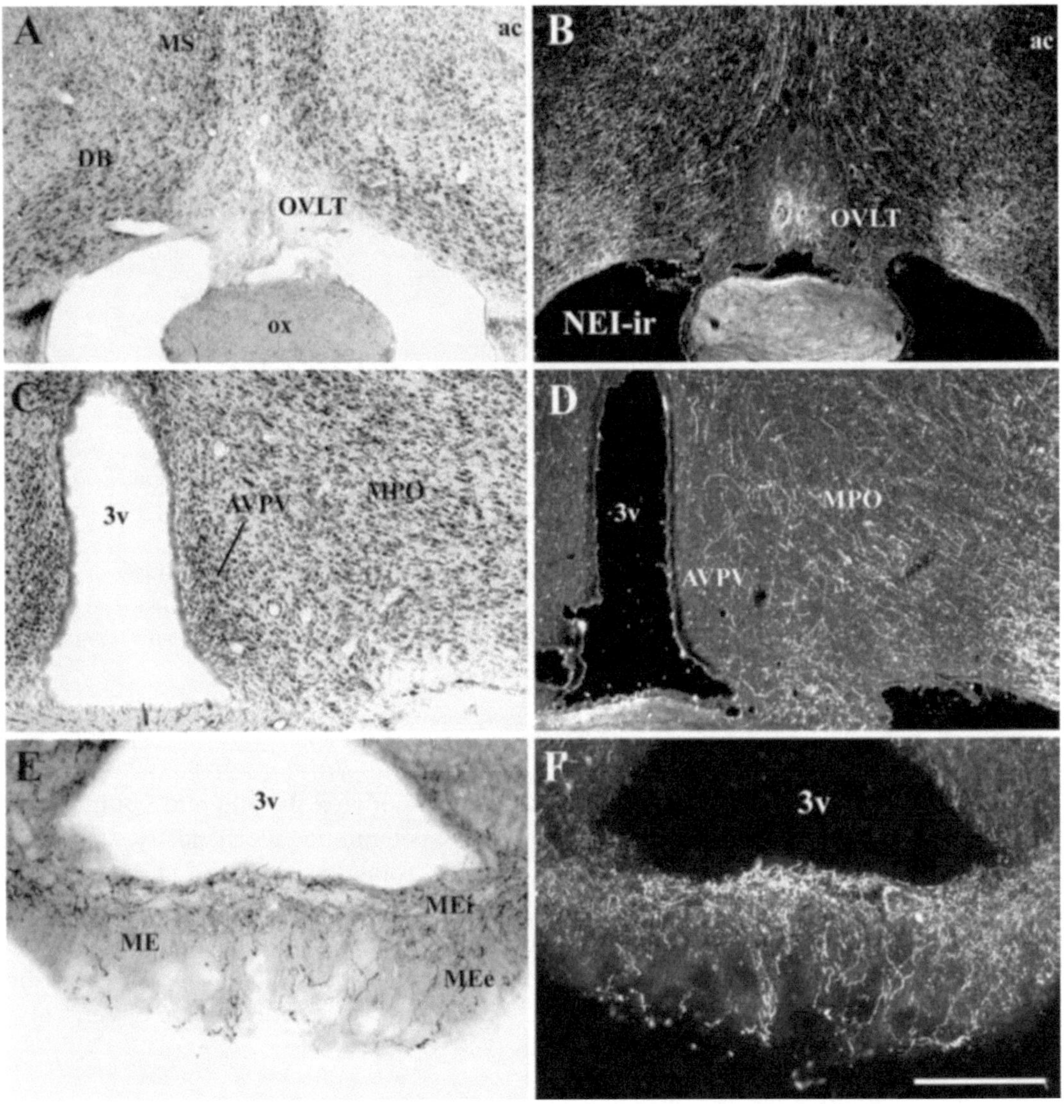

Figure 5. Distribution of NEI-ir fibers in forebrain areas related to reproduction. Bright-field photomicrographs of reference sections with thionine staining showing the OVLT (**A**) and AVPV (**C**). Dark-field photomicrographs showing the distribution of NEI-ir fibers in the environs of the OVLT (**B**) and in the AVPV (**D**). **E** Bright-field photomicrograph showing the distribution of NEI-ir fibers in the median eminence (ME). **F** Dark-field photomicrograph of the same section showing the distribution of NEIir fibers in the ME. MEi = Internal layer of the median eminence; MEe = external layer of the median eminence; ox = optic chiasm; 3v = third ventricle; ac = anterior commissure; DB = nucleus of the diagonal band; MPO = medial preoptic nucleus; MS = medial septal nucleus. Scale bar: 400 μm (**A–D**), 200 μm (**E** , **F**). - Reproduced from Attademo et al, 2006, with permission from Neuroendocrinology.

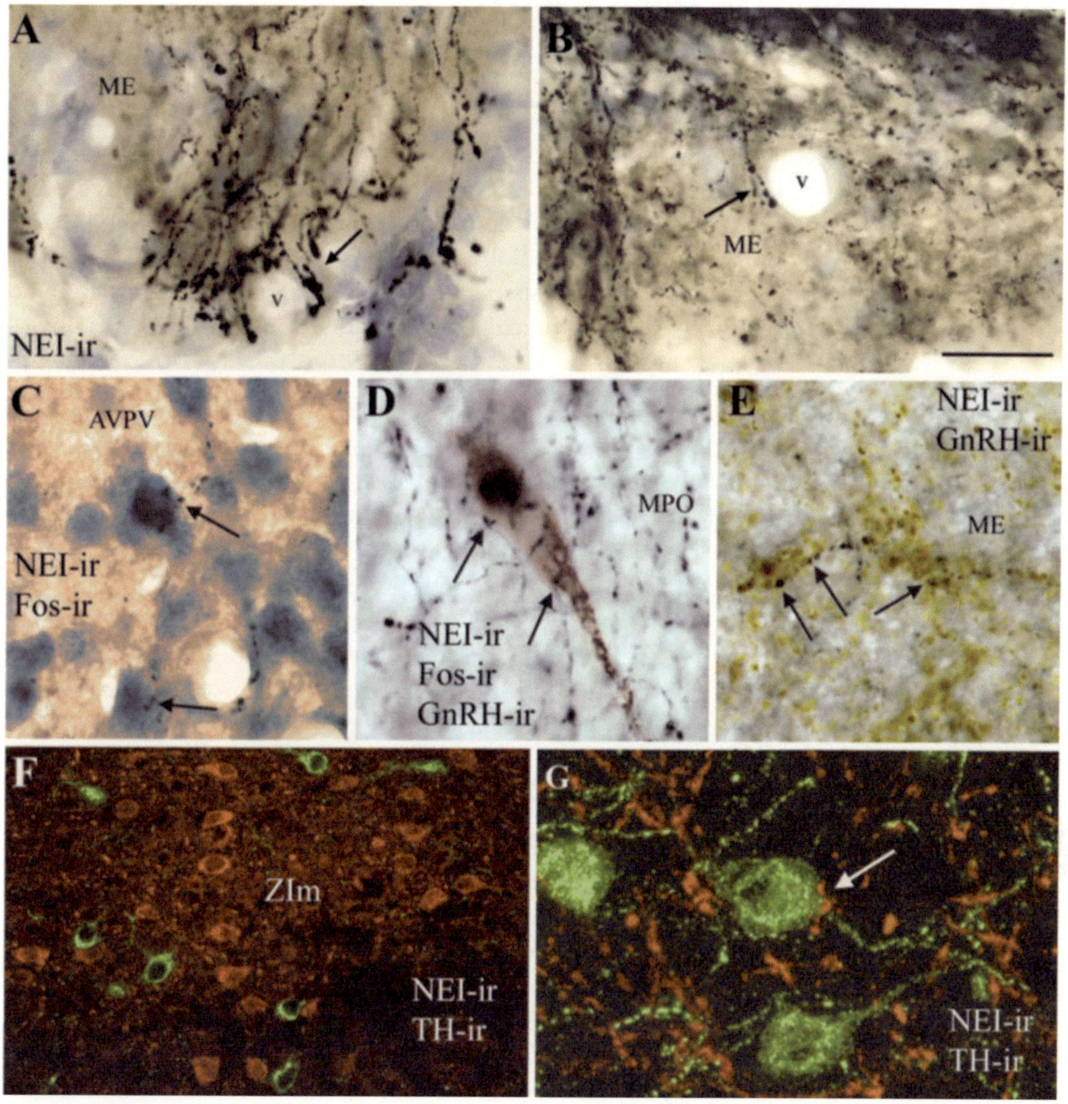

Figure 6. Alternative pathways for NEI induction of LH secretion. **A** , **B** Bright-field photomicrographs showing NEI-ir varicosities and terminal-like structures in the median eminence (ME). Note the close proximity to blood vessels (arrows). **C** Bright-field photomicrograph showing NEI-ir varicosities in close apposition with AVPV neurons expressing Fos (Fos-ir) in the afternoon of the proestrus day (arrows). **D** Bright-field photomicrograph showing NEI-ir fibers in close apposition with GnRH-ir neurons expressing Fos in the afternoon of the proestrus day (arrows). **E** Bright-field photomicrograph showing NEI-ir varicosities (in black) in close apposition with GnRH-ir fibers (in light brown) in the ME. **F** Fluorescence photomicrograph showing the close association between NEI-ir (in green, AlexaFluor 488) and TH-immunoreactive (TH-ir, in red, AlexaFluor 594) neurons in the medial zona incerta (ZIm). **G** Fluorescence photomicrograph showing TH-ir fibers in close apposition with NEI-ir neurons in the ZIm (arrow). v = Blood vessel; MPO = medial preoptic nucleus. Scale bar: 50 μm (**A–E** , **G**); 100 μm (**F**). - Reproduced from Attademo et al, 2006, with permission from Neuroendocrinology.

5. NEI-ir fibers innervate GnRH and AVPV neurons expresing fos

We observed an increased expression of Fos immunoreactivity in the anteroventral periventricular nucleus (AVPV) neurons of rats perfused during the afternoon of the day of proestrus, as well as in ovariectomized rats treated with estradiol benzoate plus progesterone, as described by others [30, 31]. Close to a 10% of the AVPV neurons expressing Fos receive NEI fibers in close apposition. Very little Fos immunoreactivity was observed in rats perfused in the afternoon of the diestrus day, for either of the following conditions: ovariectomized treated with estradiol benzoate or ovariectomized treated with sesame oil. In addition, all groups, showed a sparse distribution of Fos immunoreactivity in the medial zone incerta and in the LHA, whereas co-localization of NEI fibers with any of these cells was not observed (Fig. 6 D).

It has been reported that Fos protein is expressed in a portion of GnRH neurons that are active in the afternoon of the proestrus day, as well as in the GnRH neurons of ovariectomized rats treated with estradiol benzoate plus progesterone [31-33]. Based on these results, we investigated the pattern of NEI innervations in areas that expressed GnRH neurons in these animals. Most of the neurons expressing Fos were found to be in the vicinity of the organum vasculosum of the lamina terminalis (OVLT) and of the preoptic area. NEI fibers were also found in the median eminence, and NEI and GnRH varicosities presented similar distribution, thus revealing close apposition between them. Immediately before and during LH surge (on the afternoon of the proestrus day or following treatment with estrogen plus progesterone), only a portion of the GnRH neurons expressed Fos [30,31,33,34-36].

AVPV, is a nucleus that also expresses Fos in the afternoon of the proestrus day and has been widely implicated in the control of reproduction [32], with Fos expression indicating neuronal response [36]. However, in rats perfused on the diestrus day or in ovariectomized rats receiving estradiol benzoate or sesame oil, we did not find Fos expression in GnRH neurons. The pattern of distribution of NEI-ir and GnRH ir in the median eminence, showed NEI fibers to be denser in the internal layer than in the external one. Nevertheless, in the external layer, NEI and GnRH varicosities presented similar distributions, revealing an apparent close apposition between them. In the present study, we labeled distinctive cell compartments by using dual and triple-label immunohistochemistry which revealed NEI-ir fibers to be innervating the Fos-positive neurons in the AVPV, as well as the GnRH neurons positive for Fos immunoreactivity. In these experiments we labeled distinct cell compartments (cytoplasm, nuclei and terminals) using various antisera, all raised in rabbit. In the control tests, the second or third antisera were omitted, and no reaction was evident. This indicates that the observed labeling of cell bodies, fibers or both was not the result of cross-reactivity of the secondary antibody. In addition, evaluation of the data under light microscopy at a high magnification revealed only a suggestion of synaptic contact (Fig 6 A-B).

6. NEI innervation of GnRH neurons

Our results indicated that NEI fibers were in close apposition with GnRH neurons expressing Fos in the afternoon of the proestrus day. Since Fos protein expression in GnRH neurons increases in parallel with rises in the plasma LH levels [27, 31, 32], it can be assumed that these neurons project to the median eminence and induce LH secretion during proestrus. Therefore, we can suggest that NEI (through projections to a subset of GnRH neurons) modulated GnRH activity and, consequently, LH surges.

The role that NEI plays in GnRH secretion has not been investigated. However, NEI varicosities in some parts of the median eminence display a pattern of distribution similar to that of GnRH, revealing a possible effect on the modulation of GnRH secretion directly at the terminals. This may represent one of the mechanisms by which intracerebroventricular administration of NEI causes an increase in LH secretion (Fig. 6 E)

Experiments using in vitro preparations or intracerebroventricular injections have shown that various neurotransmitters can regulate gonadotropin release [38-40]. One such neurotransmitters is the cocaine- and amphetamine- regulated transcript (CART) peptide, which has been shown to increase the GnRH pulse amplitude in cycling female rats and to decrease GnRH pulse intervals in prepubertal rats [41-43]. These effects can be achieved through direct CART innervation of the GnRH neurons [39, 40]. Interestingly, in the medial ZI and lateral hypothalamus, MCH/NEI neurons coexpress CART [44, 46]. In the present study, we did not explore the origins of NEI innervation of GnRH neurons or areas related to reproductive behavior. However, it is intriguing that the number of NEI-ir neurons in ovariectomized rats was increased only in the medial ZI, a brain region that projects to the AVPV and GnRH- containing areas [47,48], as well as to the circumventricular organs, probably including the median eminence [44, 45]. This result is in agreement with those of other studies in which ppMCH mRNA expression was found to be greater in the medial ZI of untreated ovariectomized rats than in that of ovariectomized rats primed with estradiol benzoate or estradiol benzoate plus progesterone.

7. In vitro studies

Taken into account the above results, we decided to investigate whether NEI could act directly at the pituitary level by modulating hormone secretion. With this purpose the effects of NEI were studied in pituitary cell cultures from female rats on the release of several pituitary hormones (GH, LH and prolactin). Furthermore, the ability of NEI to activate pituitary cells was evaluated by electron microscopy and immunocitochemistry [49], and finally, the ability of NEI to potentiate GnRH-induced LH release was tested. The study of the effects of physiological stimuli involved in the regulation of pituitary hormone secretion was facilitated by the availability of a system consisting of a suspension of single dispersed pituitary cells, in which the cell functions were essentially the same as in situ [50]. For this study we used female rats in order to obtain a primary culture. The results were as follows:

NEI induced a fast release of LH in the culture cell media. In addition, there were differences in the LH levels obtained for the various time periods of hormonal stimuli assayed, which were closely associated with the doses applied. The lowest dose of NEI (100x 10^{-8}M) induced a significant increase of LH secretion after 2h of stimulus, achieving maximum response after 4h of NEI treatment. At this time, the LH levels almost reached a five-fold increase over controls and then maintained these values (Fig.7). In spite of NEI being effective in stimulating LH secretion, none of the assayed doses were capable of significantly promoting FSH secretion from gonadotrophs. In addition, no significant increases were observed on prolactin or GH secretion, at doses ranging from 100x10^{-8} to 400x10^{-8} M NEI in primary cell cultures, thus confirming the specificity of NEI stimuli on LH secretion (Table 1). To determine whether or not NEI was able to synergize with GnRH in stimulating LH release, pituitary cells were simultaneously incubated with GnRH (0.1 or 1x10^{-9}M) and different concentrations of NEI (1, 10 or 100x10^{-8}M) for 3 h and then the media was collected and tested for LH by RIA (Fig. 8). Although NEI at the dose of 10x10^{-8}M had no effect on LH secretion, GnRH 1x10^{-9}M plus NEI 10x10^{-8}M induced a slight but significant increase in LH concentrations (16%; $p< 0.01$). A combined treatment with the highest doses of both NEI and GnRH significantly stimulated the secretory response, which was more effective than that observed with the same dose of GnRH alone [49] (Fig.8).

When pituitary cells from female rats were cultured, different types of secretory cells were observed (Fig. 9). These were identifiable by their ultra structural characteristics, essentially by the profile of the secretory granules, which constituted a distinctive feature. The most frequent populations observed were lactotroph and somatotroph cells, which were in close contact with gonadotrph cells. In the control group, the lactotroph and somatotroph cells have numerous polymorphic and round mature secretory granules respectively. These also had high electron densities and were stored in the cytoplasm. The gonadotroph were

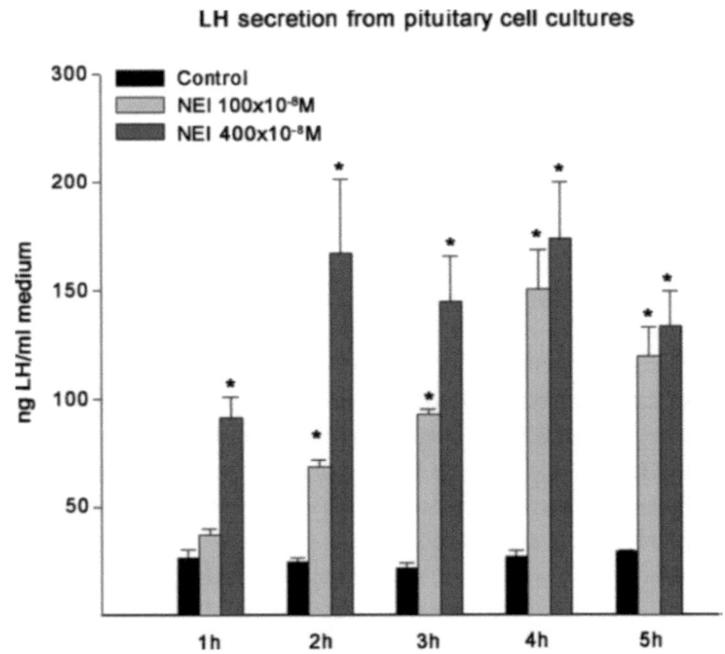

Figure 7. Time-course study of the effects of NEI on LH secretion in the culture media. The cell cultures were treated with NEI 100 or 400 x 10^{-8} M for 1–5 h, in serum free conditions. The data are represented as mean ± S.E.M. of three independent experiments. Data were evaluated by the ANOVA–Fisher test; *$p < 0.01$ vs Control group. – Reproduced from De Paul et al, 2009, with permission from Peptides.

	Time exposition	Control Mean ± S.E.M.	NEI 100 × 10^{-8} M Mean ± S.E.M.	NEI 400 × 10^{-8} M
FSH secretion	1 h	32.41 ± 4.93	38.16 ± 1.05	38.1 ± 3.30
	2 h	32.24 ± 3.22	38.46 ± 1.70	31.92 ± 5.59
	3 h	28.83 ± 3.15	36.23 ± 1.82	24.65 ± 1.35
	4 h	25.80 ± 2.22	29.53 ± 2.09	19.88 ± 1.36
	5 h	28.30 ± 3.18	28.91 ± 3.15	22.35 ± 1.30
PRL secretion	1 h	839.42 ± 47.96	998.65 ± 42.09	926.64 ± 96.40
	2 h	1079.81 ± 56.38	1204.50 ± 93.25	951.60 ± 69.38
	3 h	1182.30 ± 92.82	1338.38 ± 141.05	936.41 ± 27.40
	4 h	1567.68 ± 95.27	1703.32 ± 26.56	1373.41 ± 157.41
	5 h	1537.53 ± 66.10	1736.56 ± 129.94	130.88 ± 56.86
GH secretion	1 h	395.20 ± 56.05	309.13 ± 36.45	502.79 ± 26.09
	2 h	485.51 ± 49.54	426.75 ± 42.88	533.82 ± 36.48
	3 h	522.03 ± 70.54	585.64 ± 37.47	508.72 ± 49.67
	4 h	740.07 ± 96.60	729.82 ± 76.28	618.08 ± 71.91
	5 h	730.90 ± 38.26	897.58 ± 72.80	676.75 ± 66.53

Table 1. Time-course study of the effects of NEI on FSH, PRL and GH secretion accumulated in the culture media (ng/ml of culture medium). Pituitary cells were treated with NEI 100 or 400×10^{-8}M for 1–5 h. The data are shown as the mean ±S.E.M. of three independent experiments and were evaluated by the ANOVA–Fisher test.

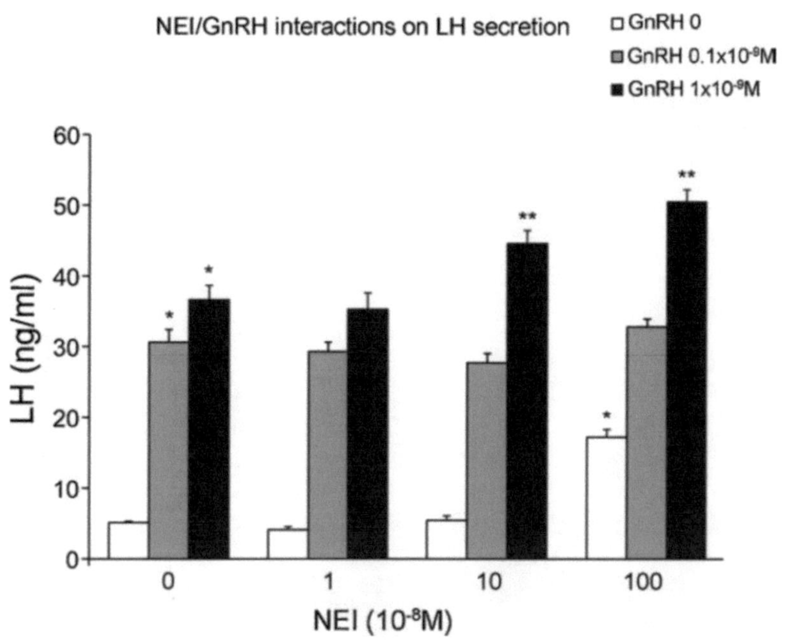

Figure 8. NEI and GnRH combined treatments on LH secretion. The presence of 10 and 100 x 10^{-8} M NEI in the culture media for 3 h promoted a significant increase in LH release stimulated by GnRH 1 x10^{-9} M. Data are shown as the mean ± S.E.M. of three independent experiments. ANOVA–Fisher test; *$p < 0.01$ vs control group; **$p < 0.01$ vs GnRH 1 x 10^{-9} M. – Reproduced from De Paul et al, 2009, with permission from Peptides.

characterized by a conspicuous accumulation of round secretory granules of two different sizes and by electron densities in the cytoplasm. The most abundant granules were about 150nm in diameter and filled with homogenous material, whereas the others less frequent but larger in size (about 400nm) (Fig. 10 A and B).Stimulation with NEI (100 x 10^{-8} and 400 x 10^{-8}) for 2 and 4 hour, promoted several subtle structural changes, particularly in the

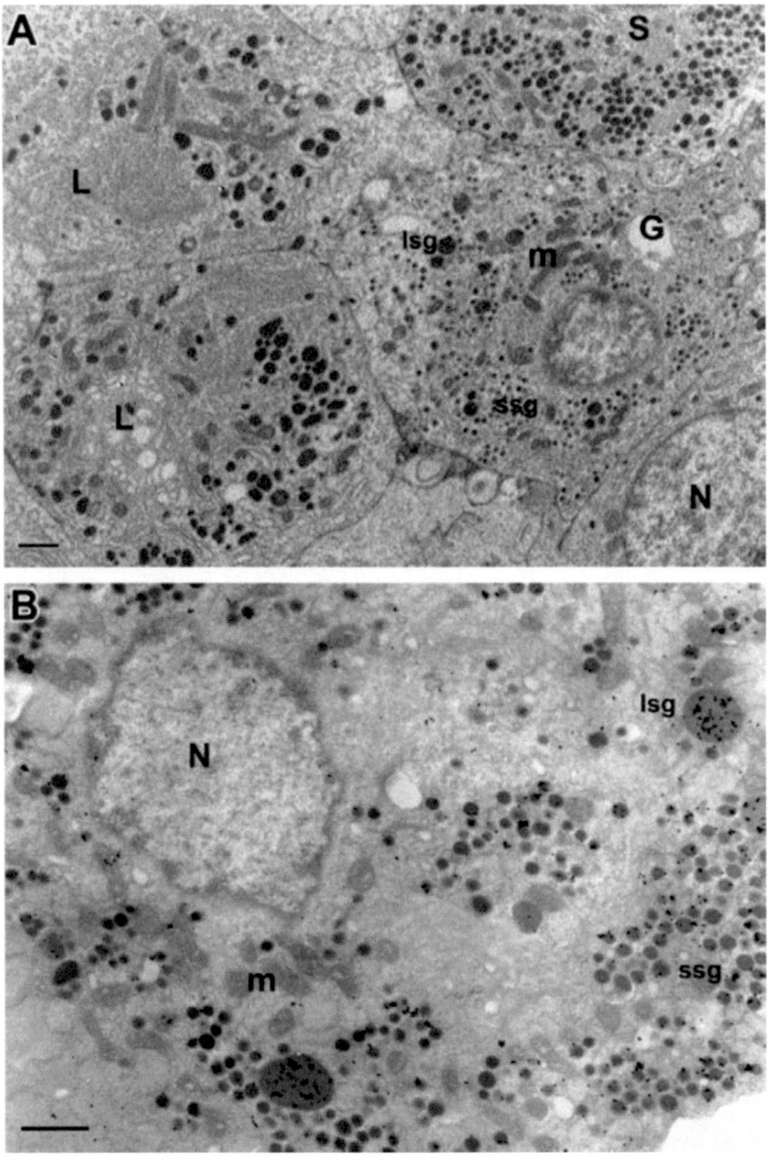

Figure 9. (A) Electron micrograph of a pituitary cell culture from control rats illustrating different pituitary cell populations. Two lactotroph cells (L) exhibit an accumulation of large and polymorphic mature secretory granules (about 500– 900 nm in diameter) in the cytoplasm. The somatotroph cell (S) can be easily recognized by the mature, round GH secretory granules ranging from 200 to 350 nm in diameter and scattered throughout the cytoplasm. In close contact with both secretory cell types, a gonadotroph cell (G) displays small (ssg) and large (lsg) round secretory granules (about 150 or 400 nm in diameter respectively, with different electron densities, homogeneously disseminated in the cytoplasm (m = mitochondria, N = nucleus). Bar: 1 μm. (B) Gonadotroph cell specifically immunostained for LH. The cytoplasm shows a noticeable accumulation of characteristic small (ssg) and large (lsg) round secretory granules (m = mitochondria, N = nucleus). Bar: 0.5 μm. – Reproduced from De Paul et al, 2009, with permission from Peptides.

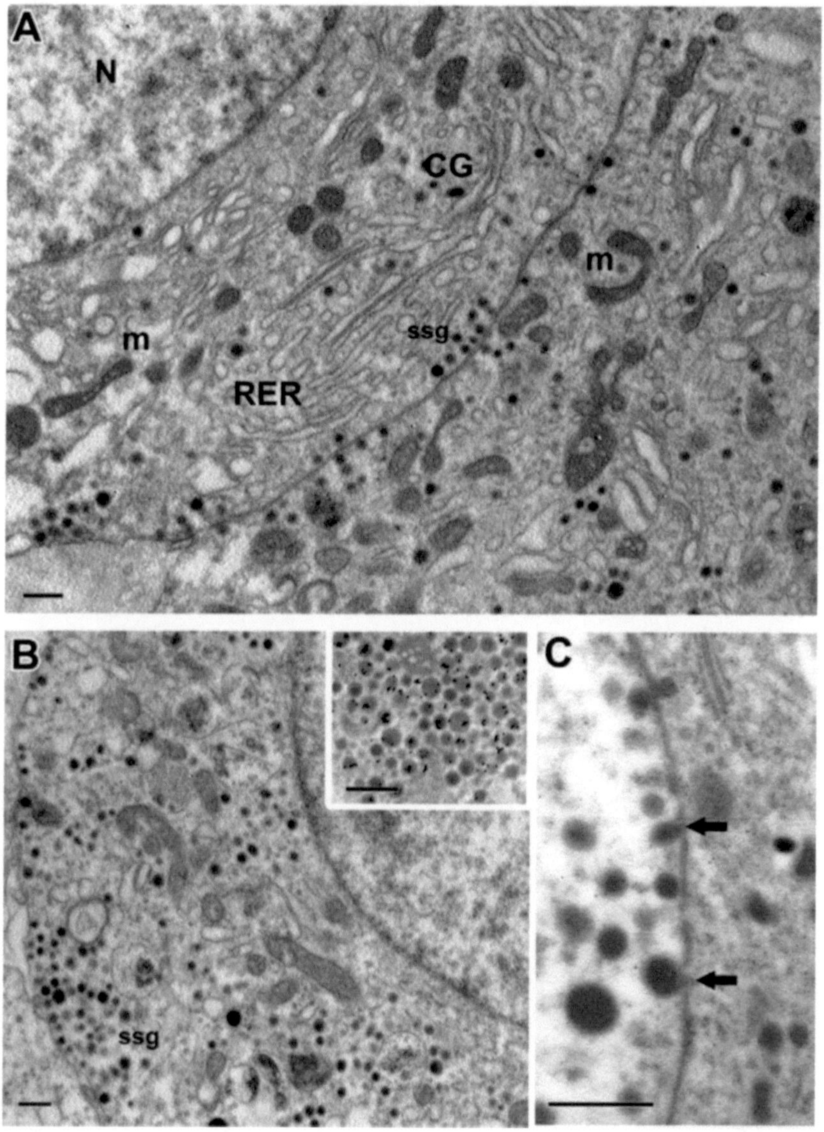

Figure 10. (A) Electron microscopy of two cultured gonadotroph cells treated with 400 x 10^{-8} M NEI for 4 h. The cytoplasm contains a remarkably well developed rough endoplasmic reticulum (RER) and Golgi complex (GC) and also scarce small secretory granules (ssg) that are mostly in contact with the plasma membrane. Bar: 0.5 μm. (B) Electron micrograph of a cultured gonadotroph cell (G) after exposition to 100 x 10^{-8} M NEI for 2 h which is shown exhibiting small secretory granules (ssg) mobilized toward the plasmalemma, where they will then be subsequently discharged by exocytosis. Bar: 0.5 mm. Inset: small round secretory granules from a gonadotroph cell specifically identified by immunocytochemistry for LH. Bar: 0.5 mm. (C) Detail of two adjacent gonadotroph cells after NEI treatment displaying evidence of secretory activity. The secretory granules are aligned alongside the cell membrane and are in the process of exocytosis (arrows). Bar: 0.5 μm. – Reproduced from De Paul et al, 2009, with permission from Peptides.

gonadotroph cell population. For this cell type, the most prominent changes consisted of a striking development of the rough endoplasmic reticulum (RER) and Golgi complex (Fig 10B) when compared to the control group. Many secretory granules were located to the cell membrane and presented images of exocytosis after NEI treatment (Fig. 10 C) Other pituitary cell populations, the lactotrophs, thyrotrophs and somatotrophs, did not exhibit any features indicating a significant activation of hormone release after NEI treatment.

The present results were the first demonstration of a specific and direct action of NEI in cultured pituitary cells without modifying other pituitary hormones. Moreover, the analysis of the electron microscope images taken 2 and 4h after NEI treatment was indicative of the stimulation of LH release occurring at these times.

From the present study, it is possible to conclude that NEI is effective when injected into the brain to release LH in male and female rats. The anatomical substrate underlying this effect was identified using combined methods of immunohistochemistry. A schematic representation of the proposed pathways by which NEI participates in LH secretion is depicted in Figure 11.

NEI is also capable of inducing a marked release of LH without modifying the other pituitary hormones in the pituitary cultured cells. There is an interaction between NEI and GnRH in vivo and in vitro.

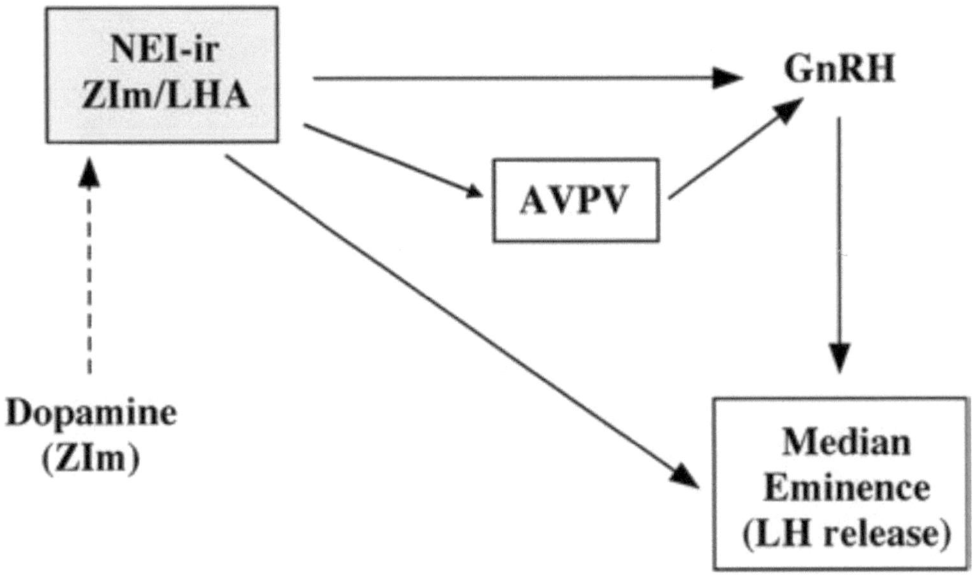

Figure 11. Schematic representation of the proposed pathways by which NEI participates in LH secretion. NEI-ir neurons in the medial zona incerta (ZIm) or LHA receive dopaminergic innervation from TH neurons located in the ZIm and project directly to the median eminence or to GnRH neurons in the preoptic area. In addition, NEI might modulate LH secretion by innervating the AVPV. – Reproduced from Attademo et al, 2006, with permission from Neuroendocrinology.

Author details

María Ester Celis
Laboratorio de Ciencias Fisiológicas, Cátedra de Bacteriología y Virología, Facultad de Ciencias Médicas, Universidad Nacional de Córdoba, Santa Rosa, Córdoba, Argentina

Acknowledgement

First of all I wish to thank to Dr. Paul Hobson for critical reading of this manuscript. I also wish to thank Dr. Jorge Paván, Miss Laura Alazraki and Miss Marina Juarez for editing the manuscript. Thanks for the grants from CONICET; SECyT and FONCyT. MEC is member of CONICET.

8. References

[1] Attademo AM, Sanchez-Borzone M, Lasaga M, Celis ME. Intracerebroventicular injection or neuropeptide El increases serum LH in male and female rats. Peptides 2004; 25:1995-9

[2] Berberian V, Sanchez MS, Celis ME. Participation of the cholinergic system in the exesesive grooming behavior induced by neuropeptide (N) glutamic acid (E) isoleucine (I) amide (NEI). Neurochem Res 2002; 27:1713-1717.

[3] Sanchez M, Baker BI, Celis M: Melanin-concentrating hormone (MCH) antagonizes the effects of alpha-MSH and neuropeptide E-I on grooming and locomotor activities in the rat. Peptides 1997; 18:393-396.

[4] Sanchez MS, Barontini M, Armando I, Celis ME: Correlation of increasing grooming and motor activity with alterations in nigrostriatal and mesolimbic catecholamines after alpha melanocortin and neuropeptide glutamine-isoleucine injection in the tegmental area. Cell Mol Neurobiol 2001; 21(5):523-33.

[5] Sánchez- Borzone M, Attademo AM, Baiardi G, Celis ME: Effect of β- adrenoceptors on the behavior induced by the neuropeptide glutamic acid isoleucine amide. Eur J Pharmacol 2007; 568:186-91.

[6] Gonzales MI, Baker BI, Hole DR, Wilson CA: Behavioral effects of neuropeptide E-I (NEI) in the female rat: Interactions with α- MSH, MCH and dopamine. Peptides 1998;19:1007-1016.

[7] Nahon JL, Presse F, Bittencourt JC, Sawchenko PE, Vale W. The rat melanin-concentrating hormone messenger ribonucleic acid encodes multiple putative neuropeptides coexpressed in the dorsolateral hypothalamus. Endocrinology 1989; 125:2056-65.

[8] Parkes DG, ValeW. Secretion of melanin-concentrating hormone and neorupeptide- EI from cultured rat hypothalamic cells. Endocrinology 1992;131:1826-31.

[9] Presse F, Nahon JL, Fischer WH, Vale W. Structure of the human melanin- concentrating hormone mRNA. Mol Endocrinol 1990;4:632-7.

[10] Nahon JL, Presse F, Bittencourt JC, Sawchenko PE, Vale W.The rat melanin-concentrating hormone messengerribonucleic acid encodes multiple putatives neuropeptides coexpressed in the dorsolateral hypothalamus. Endocrinology 1989;125:2056-65.

[11] ParkesDG.,Constracting actionsVale W. Secretion of melanin-concentrating hormone and neuropeptide-EI from cultured rat hypothamic cells. Endocrinology 1992; 131:1826-31.

[12] Parkes DG., Vale W Constrasting actions of melanin-concentrating hormone and neuropeptide –E-I on posterior pituitary function. Ann NY Acad Sci 1993;680:580-90.

[13] SitaLV, ElíasCF; bittencourt JC. Connectivity pattern suggests that incero-hypothalamic area belongs to the medial hypothalamic system. Neuroscience 2007;148(4):949-69.

[14] Swanson LW.Brainmaps: structure of the rat brain, 3rd edition, Academic Press; 2004

[15] Bittencourt JC, Presse F, Arias C, Peto C, Vaughan J, Nahon JL, Vale W, Sawchenko PE: The melanin-concentrating hormone system of the rat brain: an inmuno-and hybridization histochemical characterization. J Comp. Neurol 1992; 319:218-245.

[16] Presse F, Nahon J. Differential regulation of melanin- concentrating hormone gene expression in distinct hypothalamic areas under osmotic stimulation in rat. Neuroscience 1993,55:709-720.

[17] Bittencourt JC, Elias CF. Melanin- concentrating hormone and neuropeptide EI projections from the lateral hypothalamic area and zona incerta to the medial septal nucleus and spinal cord: a study using multiple neuronal traces. Brain Res 1998; 805(1-2):1-19.

[18] Viale A, Kerdelhue B, Nahon JL: 17beta-estradiol regulation of melanin-concentrating hormone and neuropeptide- E-I contents in cynomolgus monkeys: a preliminary study. Peptides 1999; 20:553-559.

[19] Murray JF, Baker BI, Levy A, Wilson CA: The influence of gonadal steroids on pre-promelanin-concentrating hormone m RNA in female rats. Neuroendocrinol 2000; 12:53-59.

[20] MacKenzie FJ, James MD, Wilson CA: Changes in dopamine activity in the zona incerta (ZI) over the rat oestrous cycle and the effect of lesion of the ZI on cyclicity: further evidence that the incerto- hypothalamic tract has a stimulatory role in the control of LH release. Brain Res 1988; 444:75-83.

[21] Murray JF, Adan RA, Walker R, Baker BI, Thody AJ, Nijenhuis WA, Yukitake J, Wilson CA: Melanin- concentrating hormone, melacortin receptors and regulation of luteinizing hormone release. J Neuroendocrinol 2000; 12:217-223.

[22] Murray JF, Hahn JD, Kennedy AR, Small CJ, Bloom SR, Haskell-Luevano C, Coen CW, Wilson CA: Evidence for stimulatory action of melanin-concentrating hormone on luteinising hormone release involving MCH1 and melanocortin-5 receptors. J Neuroendocrinol 2006; 18:157-167.

[23] Murray JF, Mercer JG, Adan RA, Datta JJ, Aldairy C, Moar KM, Baker BI, Stock MJ, Wilson CA: The effect of leptin on luteinizing hormone release is exerted in the zona incerta and mediated by melanin-concentrating hormone. J Neuroendocrinol 2000; 12:1133-1139.

[24] Chiocchio SR, Gallardo MG, Louzan P, Gutnisky V, Tramezzani JH: Melanin-Concentrating hormone stimulates the release of luteinizing hormone-releasing hormone and gonadotropins in the female rat acting at both median eminence and pituitary levels. Biol Reprod 2001; 64:1466-1472.

[25] Williamson- Hughes PS, Grove KL, Smith MS: Melanin concentrating hormone (MCH): a novel neutral pathway for regulation of GnRH neurons. Brain Res 2005; 1041:117-124.

[26] Gonzales MI, Baker BI, Wilson CA: Stimulatory effect of melanin-concentrating hormone on luteinising hormone release. Neuroendocrinology 1997; 66:254-262.

[27] Schlumberger SE, Talke- Messerer C, Zumsteg U, Eberle AN: Expression of receptors for melanin-concentrating hormone (MCH) in different tissues and cell lives. J Recept Signal Transd Res 2002; 22: 509-531.

[28] Attademo AM, Rondini TA, Rodrigues BC, Bittencourt JC, Celis ME, Elias CF. Neuropeptide glutamic acid-isoleucine may induce luteinizing hormone secretion via multiple pathways. Neuroendrocrinology 2006; 83:313-24.

[29] Hoffman GE, Lee WS, Attardi B, Yann V, Fitzsimmons MD. Luteinizing hormone releasing hormone neurons express c-fos antigen after steroid activation. Endocrinology 1990; 126:1736-1741.

[30] Hoffman GE, Smith MS, Verbalis JG: C-fos and related immediate early gene products as makers of activity in neuroendocrine systems. Front Neuroendocrinol 1993; 14:173-213.

[31] Le WW, Attardi B, Berghorn KA, Blaustein J, Hoffman GE: Progesterone blockade of a luteinizing hormone surge blocks luteinizing hormone-releasing hormone fos activation and activation of its preoptic area afferents. Brain Res 1997; 778:272-280.

[32] Le WW, Berghorn KA, Rassnick S, Hoffman GE: Periventricular preoptic area neurons coactived whit luteinizing hormone (LH) releasing hormone (LHRH) neurons at the time of the LH surge are LHRH afferents. Endocrinology 1999;140:510-519.

[33] Lee WS, Smith MS, Hoffman GE: Luteinizing hormone- releasing hormone neurons express fos protein during the proestrous surge of luteinizing hormone. Proc Natl Acad Sci USA 1990; 87:5163-5167.

[34] Wang HJ, Hoffman GE, Smith MS: Increased GnRH mRNA in the GnRH neurons expressing cFos during the proestrous LH surge. Endocrinology 1995; 136:3673-3676.

[35] Hoffman GE, Lyo D: Anatomical markers of activity in neuroendocrine systems: are we all "fos-ed out"? J. Neuroendocrinol 2002; 14:259-268.

[36] Bittencourt JC, Elias CF: Melanin- Concentrating hormone and neuropeptide EI projections from the lateral hypothalamic area and zona incerta to medial septal nucleus and spinal cord: a study using multiple neuronal tracers. Brain res 1998;805:1-9.

[37] Levine JE, Pau KY, Ramirez VD, Jackson GL: Simultaneous measurement of luteinizing hormone- releasing hormone and luteinizing hormone release in unanesthetized, ovariectomized sheep. Endocrinology 1982; 111: 1449-1455.

[38] Negro-Vilar A, Ojeda SR, McCann SM: Catecholaminergic modulation of luteinizing hormone-releasing hormone release by median eminence terminals in vitro. Endrocrinology 1979; 104: 1749-1757.

[39] Rasmussen DD, Kennedy BP, Ziegler MG, Nett TM: Endogenous opioid inhibition and facilitation of gonadotropin-releasing hormone release from the medial eminence in vitro: potencial role of catecholamines. Endocrinology 1988; 123: 2916-2921.

[40] Bourguignon JP, Gerard A, Franchimont P: Direct activation of gonadotropin-releasing hormone secretion through different receptors to neuroexitatory amino acids. Neuroendocrinology 1989; 49: 402-408.

[41] Lebrethon MC, Vandermissen E, Gerard A, Parent AS, Junien JL, Bourguignon JP: In vitro stimulations of the prepubertal rat gonadotropin-releasing hormone pulse generartor by leptin and neuropeptide Y through distinct mechanism. Endocrinology 2000; 141: 1464-1469.

[42] Parent AS, Lebrethon MC, Gerard A, Vandermissen E, Bourguignon JP: Leptin effects on pulsatile gonadotropin releasing hormone secretion from the adult rat hypothalamus and interaction with cocaine and amphetamine regulated transcript peptide and neuropeptide Y. Regul Pept 2000; 92: 17-24.

[43] Lebrethon MC, Vandermissen E, Gerard A, Parent AS, Bourguignon JP: Cocaine and amphetamine-regulated-transcript peptide mediation of leptin stimulatory effect on the rat gonadotropin-releasing hormone pulse generator in vitro. J Neuroendocrinol 2000; 12: 383-385.

[44] Leslie RA, Sanders SJ, Anderson SI, Schuhler S, Horan TL, Ebling FJ: Appositions between cocaine and amphetamine-related transcript- and gonadotropin releasing hormone-immunoreactive neurons in the hypothalamus of the Siberian hamster. Neurosci Lett 2001; 314: 111-114.

[45] Rondini TA, Baddini SP, Sousa LF, Bittencourt JC, Elias CF: Hypothalamic cocaine and amphetamine-regulated transcript neurons project to areas expressing gonadotropin releasing hormone immunoreactivity and to the anteroventral periventricular nucleus in male and female rats. Neuroscience 2004; 125:735-748.

[46] Elias CF, Lee CE, Kelly JF, Ahima RS, Kuhar M, Saper CB, Elmquist JK: Characterization of CART neurons in the rat and human hypothalamus. J Comp Neurol 2001; 432:1-19.

[47] Broberger C: Hypothalamic cocaine- and amphetamine- regulated transcript (CART) neurons: Histochemical relationship to thyrotropin-releasing hormone, melanin-concentrating hormone, orexin/hypocretin and neuropeptide Y. Brain Res 1999;848:101-113.

[48] Hahn J, Coen C: Comparative study of the sources of neuronal projections to the site of gonadotropin- releasing hormone perikarya and to the anteroventral periventricular nucleus in female rats. J Comp Neurol 2006; 494: 190-214.

[49] De Paul AL, Attademo AM, Torres AI, Jahn GA, Celis ME. Neuropeptide glutamic-isoleucine (NEI) specifically stimulates the secretory activity of gonadotropes in primary cultures of female rat pituitary cells. Peptides 2009; 30: 2081-2087.

[50] De Paul Al, Pons P, Auki A, Torres A: Different behavior of lactotroph cell in response to angiotensin II and thyrotropin-releasing hormone. Cell Mol Neurobiol 1997; 17: 245-258.

Chapter 5

Regulation and Differential Secretion of Gonadotropins During Post Partum Recovery of Reproductive Function in Beef and Dairy Cows

Mark A. Crowe and Michael P. Mullen

Additional information is available at the end of the chapter

http://dx.doi.org/10.5772/48654

1. Introduction

Reproductive efficiency in dairy and beef cows is dependent on achieving high submission rates and high conception rates per service. However, to achieve good submission and conception rates cows must resume ovarian cyclicity, have normal uterine involution, be detected in estrus, and inseminated at an optimum time. In seasonally calving herds the aim is to achieve conception by 85 days following parturition so that calving to calving intervals are maintained at 365 days. Reproductive performance of cows affects the efficiency of milk production in the herd because of its influence on the calving to first service interval, calving pattern, length of lactation and culling rate.

The pattern of resumption of ovarian function in both dairy and beef cows was recently reviewed (Crowe 2008). Resumption of ovarian cyclicity is largely dependent on LH pulse frequency. Both dairy and beef cows have early resumption of follicular growth within 7 to 10 days post partum. The fate of the dominant follicle within the first follicular wave is dependent on LH pulsatility. This chapter will focus on the factors contributing to resumption of ovulation in postpartum dairy and beef cows.

2. Ovarian follicle growth in cattle

Ovarian follicle growth takes a period of 3-4 months and can be categorized into gonadotropin independent and gonadotropin dependent stages (Webb et al. 2004). Gonadotropin dependent follicle growth in cattle occurs in waves (Rajakoski 1960; Matton et al. 1981; Ireland and Roche 1987; Savio et al. 1988; Sirois and Fortune 1988). Each wave of growth involves emergence, selection and dominance followed by either atresia or ovulation. Emergence of a follicle wave is defined as growth of a cohort of follicles ≥ 5mm in diameter and coincides with a transient increase in FSH secretion (Adams et al. 1992; Sunderland et al. 1994). Selection is the process by which the growing cohort of follicles is reduced to the ovulatory quota for the species (in cattle it is generally one), selection occurs in the face of declining FSH concentrations (Sunderland et al. 1994). The selected follicle survives in an environment of reduced FSH due to the development of LH receptors in granulosa cells (Xu et al. 1995, Bao et al. 1997) and increased intrafollicular bioavailable insulin-like growth factor-I (IGF-I; Austin et al. 2001; Canty et al. 2006). The increased bioavailable IGF-I is achieved by reduced IGF-I binding proteins (IGFBP) due to increased IGFBP protease activity. Dominance is the phase during which the single selected follicle actively suppresses FSH concentrations and ensures suppression of all other follicle growth on the ovaries (Sunderland et al. 1994). The fate of the dominant follicle is then dependent on the prevailing LH pulse frequency during the dominance phase. In the presence of elevated progesterone (luteal phase of cyclic animals) LH pulse frequency is maintained at 1 pulse every 4 hours and the dominant follicle undergoes atresia, in the follicular phase (preovulatory period in cyclic animals) the LH pulse frequency increases to one pulse per hour and this stimulates final maturation, increased estradiol concentrations and positive feedback on gonadotropin-releasing hormone (GnRH), LH (and FSH) in a surge that induces ovulation (Sunderland et al. 1994). Normal follicle waves have an inherent lifespan of 7 to 10 days in duration from the time of emergence of a wave until emergence of the next wave (indicating either ovulation or physiological atresia of the dominant follicle). In cyclic heifers during the normal 21 day estrous cycle there are normally 3 waves (sometimes 2 waves and rarely 1 or 4 waves; Savio et al. 1988; Murphy et al. 1991).

2.1. Pattern of gonadotropin secretion and follicle growth during pregnancy

During pregnancy follicular growth continues during the first two trimesters (Ginther et al. 1989; Ginther et al. 1996) at regular 7 to 10 day intervals. In late pregnancy (last 22 days) the strong negative feedback of progestagens (mostly from the CL of pregnancy and partly of placental origin) and estrogens (mostly placental in origin) suppresses the recurrent transient FSH rises that stimulate follicle growth (Ginther et al. 1996; Crowe et al. 1998; Figure 1) so that the ovaries during the last 20 – 25 days are largely quiescent.

2.2. Resumption of gonadotropin secretion and follicle growth post partum

At the time of parturition progesterone and estradiol concentrations cascade to basal concentrations. This allows for the almost immediate resumption of recurrent transient increases in FSH concentrations (within 3 to 5 days of parturition) that occur at 7 to 10 day intervals (Crowe et al. 1998). The first of these increases stimulates the first postpartum wave of follicle growth that generally produces a dominant follicle by 7-10 days post partum (Savio et al. 1990a; Murphy et al. 1990; Crowe et al. 1993). The fate of this first follicular wave dominant follicle is dependent on its ability to secrete sufficient estradiol to induce a gonadotropin surge. The capacity for estradiol secretion is in turn dependent on the prevailing LH pulse frequency during the dominance phase of the follicle wave, the size of the dominant follicle and IGF-I bioavailability (Austin et al. 2001; Canty et al. 2006). So the major driver for ovulation of a dominant follicle during the postpartum period is the LH pulse frequency. This has been tested and validated by the LH pulsatile infusion studies of Duffy et al. (2000) in early postpartum anestrous beef cows. The LH pulse frequency required to stimulate a dominant follicle towards ovulation is one LH pulse per hour. Figure 2 is a schematic indicating the likely fate of the early postpartum dominant follicles in beef and dairy cows. In beef cows the first dominant follicle generally does not ovulate (Murphy et al. 1990, Stagg et al. 1995), but rather it undergoes atresia. With beef cows in good body condition the first postpartum dominant follicle to ovulate is generally from wave 3.2 ± 0.2 (~ 30 days; Murphy et al. 1990); whereas for beef cows in poor body condition there are typically 10.6 ± 1.2 waves of follicular growth before ovulation occurs (~ 70-100 days; Stagg et al. 1995; Figure 3). In the case of dairy cows ovulation of the first postpartum dominant follicle typically occurs in 50 to 80% of cows, it undergoes atresia in 15 to 60% of cows or becomes cystic in 1-5% of cows (Savio et al. 1990b; Beam and Butler 1997; Sartori et al. 2004; Sakaguchi et al. 2004).

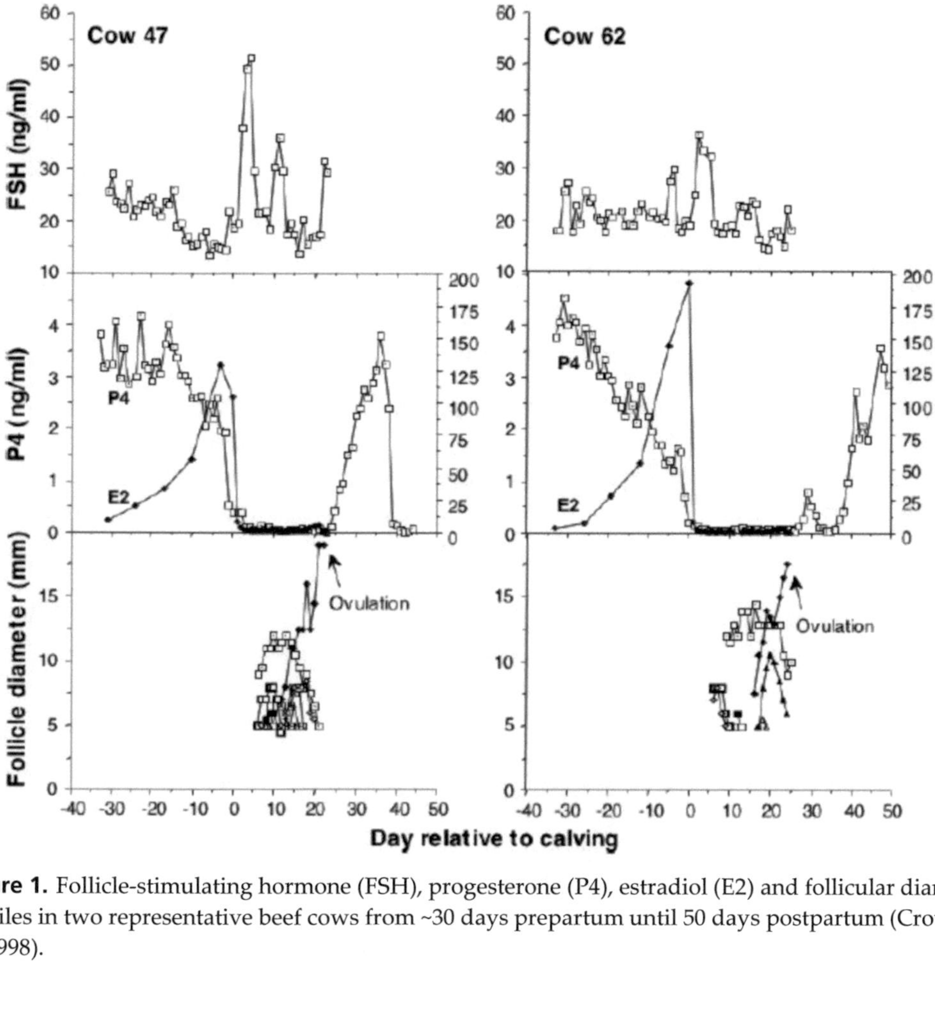

Figure 1. Follicle-stimulating hormone (FSH), progesterone (P4), estradiol (E2) and follicular diameter profiles in two representative beef cows from ~30 days prepartum until 50 days postpartum (Crowe et al. 1998).

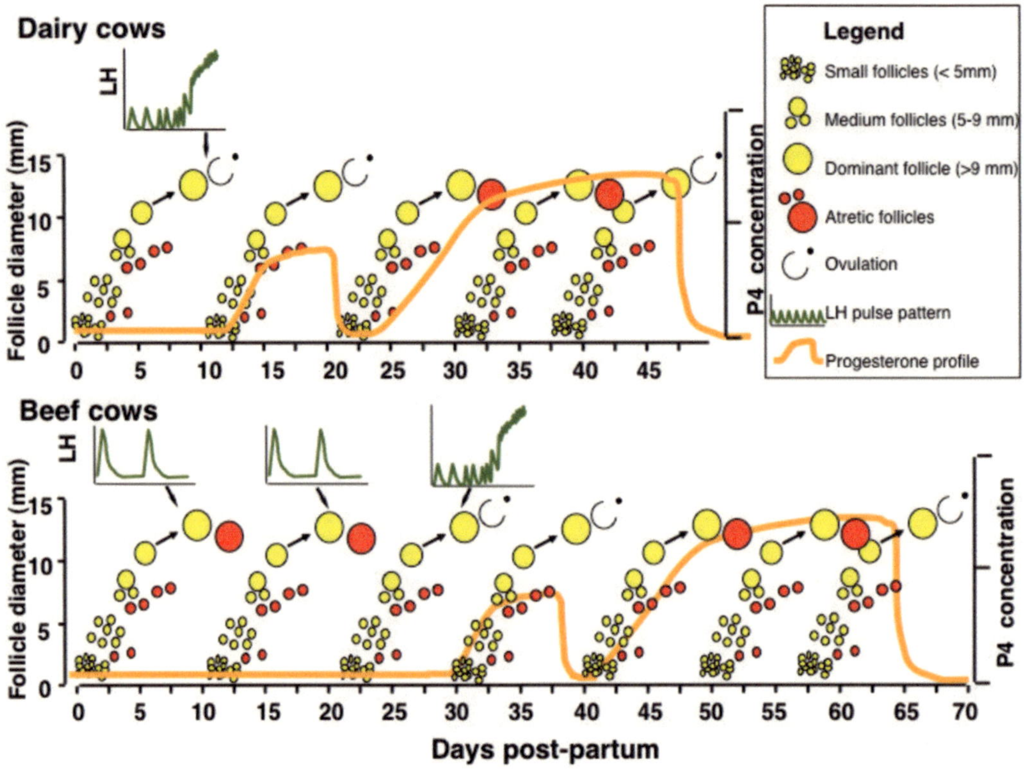

Figure 2. Diagrammatic scheme of resumption of dominant follicles and ovarian cycles during the postpartum period in dairy and beef suckler cows not nutritionally stressed. LH pulse frequency is that occurring during an 8 h window where cows are blood sampled every 15 min. Short cycles occur in most (70%), but not all cows after first ovulation (Reprinted with permission Crowe, 2008).

First ovulation in both dairy and beef cows is generally silent (i.e., no behavioural estrus; Kyle et al. 1992) and is generally (>70%) followed by a short cycle, usually containing just one follicle wave. This first luteal phase is reduced in length due to the premature release of prostaglandin F2α (PGF2α; Peter et al. 1989) presumably arising from the increased estradiol produced from the formation of the post-ovulatory dominant follicle on days 5-8 of the cycle inducing premature estradiol and oxytocin (Zollers et al., 1993) receptors. Thus the corpus luteum regresses prematurely around days 8-10 of the cycle, with the second ovulation (of this post-ovulatory dominant follicle) occurring around days 9-11 after the first ovulation. This second ovulation is generally associated with the expression of estrus and a normal length luteal phase.

Cyclic postpartum cows may have 2, 3 or occasionally 4 follicle waves during the estrous cycles that occur in the postpartum period (Savio et al. 1990a; Sartori et al. 2004). Unlike non-lactating heifers, lactating Holstein postpartum dairy cows tend to have two follicle waves per 18-23 day cycle (Sartori et al. 2004). Progesterone concentration is the major factor that affects LH pulse frequency in cyclic animals. Generally lactating Holstein dairy cows tend to have lower progesterone concentrations during the cycle than cyclic heifers (Sartori et al. 2004; Wolfenson et al. 2004). These lower progesterone concentrations tend to allow a subtle increase in LH pulse frequency and allows for prolonged growth of each dominant follicle rather than the faster atresia that occurs in cyclic heifers. Cows with prolonged luteal phases tend to have a fourth follicle wave (Savio et al. 1990a). The number of follicle waves or rate of turnover of dominant follicles are directly related to the duration of dominance of each dominant follicle, and cattle with shorter durations of dominance for the ovulatory dominant follicles tend to have higher conception rates (Austin et al. 1999). Therefore nutrition, by altering metabolic clearance of progesterone can affect the duration of dominance of a dominant follicle, the number of follicle waves per cycle and have an indirect effect on conception rates.

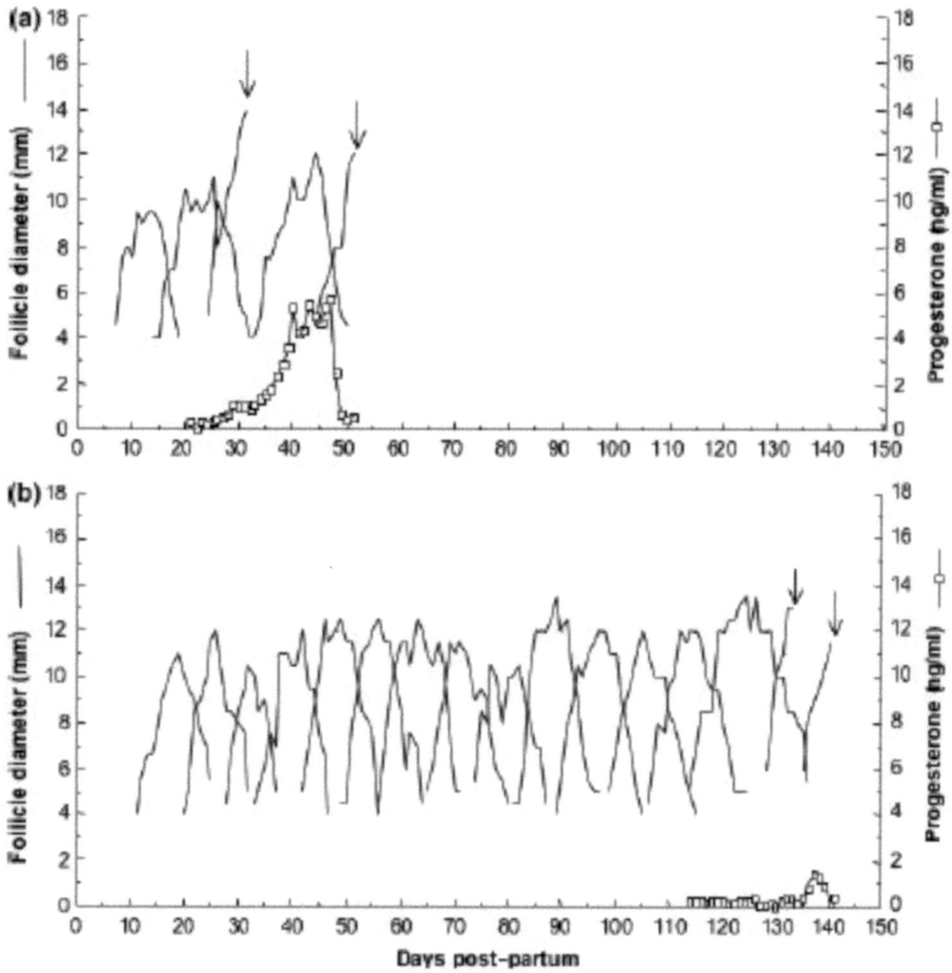

Figure 3. Pattern of growth and regression of dominant follicles from calving to second ovulation in (a) a beef suckler cow with two non-ovulatory follicle waves prior to first ovulation, and (b) a beef suckler cow with 14 non-ovulatory waves prior to first ovulation. Arrows indicate ovulation. Reproduced with permission Stagg et al. (1995); Crowe 2008.

3. Post-partum anestrus

3.1. Factors contributing to LH pulse frequency in early post-partum beef cows

The major factors that control LH pulse frequency (and therefore the fate of early postpartum dominant follicles) in postpartum beef cows include maternal bond / calf presence (presumably due to effects on opioid release), suckling inhibition (Myers et al. 1989), and poor body condition (Canfield and Butler 1990). Calf presence has a very clear negative effect on resumption of ovulation in beef suckler cows nursing calves. Restricted suckling of beef cows (once per day) from day 30, where calves were in an isolated pen away from sight of the cows, significantly advanced the interval from calving to first ovulation (51 days) compared with *ad libitum* suckled control cows (79 days). The effect of calf presence can be further compartmentalized into suckling stimuli (mammary sensory pathways) and maternal behaviour / bonding effects (Silveira et al. 1993; Williams et al. 1993) but requires positive calf identification by either sight or olfaction (Griffith and Williams 1996). Beef cows that calve down in poor BCS (<2.5; scale 1-5 as described by Lowman et al. 1976) are more likely to have a prolonged anestrous period (Stagg et al. 1995) due presumably to lower LH pulse frequency (Stagg et al. 1998). Similarly anestrus can be induced by chronic nutrition restriction in post-partum beef cows, and occurs when cows lose 22-24% of their initial body weight (Richards et al, 1989).

As beef suckler cows (with prolonged anovulatory anestrus) approach their first postpartum ovulation LH pulse frequency increases (observed during each sequential follicle wave from 6 waves before ovulation until the ovulatory wave; Stagg et al. 1998). Concentrations of IGF-I increased linearly from 75 days before first ovulation until ovulation which was associated with a linear decrease in growth hormone concentrations during the same period (Stagg et al. 1998). Thus postpartum beef cows require increased LH pulse frequency that is mediated largely by suckling inhibition and plane of nutrition, in addition to increased IGF-I concentrations to help stimulate dominant follicle maturation and growth so that there is sufficient secretion of estradiol to induce an LH surge and ovulation. Management may be used to encourage earlier ovulation by restricting suckling / access of the cows to the calves from approximately day 30 post partum (Stagg et al. 1988) or by increased plane of nutrition and body condition.

3.2. Factors contributing to LH pulse frequency in early postpartum dairy cows

In dairy cows the major factors affecting resumption of ovulation include BCS and energy balance (yield and dry matter intake), parity, season and disease (Bulman and Lamming 1978; Beam and Butler 1997; Beam and Butler 1999; Opsomer et al. 2000; Wathes et al. 2007). Energy intake, BCS and milk yield interact to affect energy balance in dairy cows. There is evidence to link many of these factors to reduced LH pulse frequency; indeed a negative association between energy balance and prolonged post-partum anestrous interval is well established for dairy cows (Butler et al. 1981; Canfield and Butler 1990; Staples et al. 1990) and is mediated by reduced LH pulse frequency (Canfield and Butler, 1990). A number of studies have been conducted in dairy cows of various yield potential that have categorised the pattern of resumption of ovarian function with the use of milk progesterone. These range from a study by Fagan and Roche (1986) using what would now be classified as traditional moderate yielding Friesian cows (4,000 – 5,000 kg milk per lactation) to that of Opsomer et al. (1998) using modern high yielding Holstein type cows (6,900 – 9,800 kg milk per lactation). The data from these two studies are summarised in Table 1. Furthermore, this pattern of resumption of ovarian function has been validated in a series of equivalent papers and the two key problem categories (prolonged interval to first ovulation and prolonged luteal phase) are summarized in Figure 4. Risk factors for these two ovarian abnormalities have been determined in a large epidemiological study by Opsomer et al. (2000). The major risk factors for a prolonged interval to first ovulation included (odds ratio in parentheses): acute body condition score loss up to 60 days post calving (18.7 within 30 days, 10.9 within 60 days), clinical ketosis (11.3), clinical diseases (5.4), abnormal vaginal discharge (4.5), and difficult calving (3.6).

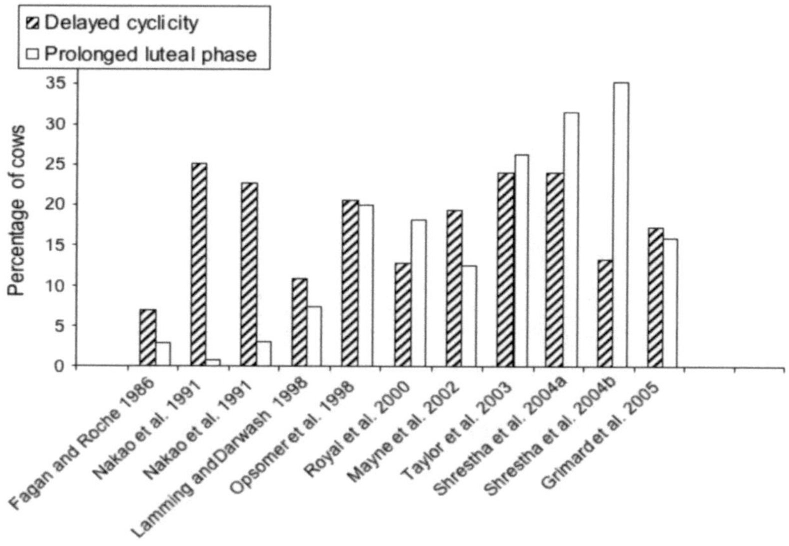

Figure 4. Percentage of cows defined as having either i) delayed resumption of ovulation or ii) prolonged luteal phases based on evaluation of milk progesterone profiles across a number of studies in dairy cows (compiled by Benedicte Grimard, France, personal communication; Reproduced with permission, Crowe 2008).

The greatest of these risk factors is acute body condition score loss. Current evidence suggests that dairy cows should calve down in a BCS of 2.75 – 3.0 (Scale 1-5; as described by Edmonson et al. 1989) and not lose more than 0.5 of a BCS unit between calving and first service (Overton and Waldron 2004; Mulligan et al. 2006) rather than earlier recommendations of 3.0 – 3.5 (Buckley et al. 2003). Cows that lose excessive body condition (≥ 1.0 BCS unit) have a longer postpartum interval to first ovulation. Thus monitoring BCS from before calving to first service is essential to good reproductive management. Body condition score changes are good indicators of energy balance and reflect milk yield and dry matter intake. It is necessary to prevent a steep decline in energy balance and shorten the duration of postpartum negative energy balance. This is best achieved by ensuring that dry matter intake in the early postpartum period is maximized and by having cows in appropriate BCS (2.73 – 3.0) at calving. Cows that are mobilizing tissue at a high rate have increased blood non-esterified fatty acids, and β-hydroxy butyrate, but reduced concentrations of insulin, glucose and IGF-I (Grummer et al. 2004). The metabolic status associated with high rates of tissue mobilization increases the risk of hypocalcaemia, acidosis, fatty liver, ketosis and displaced abomasa (Gröhn and Rajala-Schultz 2001; Overton and Waldron 2004, Maizon et al. 2004). Cows affected by these metabolic disorders are more prone to anestrus, mastitis, lameness and reduced conception rate to AI (Fourichon et al. 1999; Gröhn and Rajala-Schultz 2001; Lucy 2001; Lopez-Gatius et al. 2002; Maizon et al. 2004). It is hypothesized that serum IGF-I concentrations could be useful as a predictor of nutritional status and hence reproductive efficiency in dairy cows (Zulu et al. 2002a). Plasma IGF-I concentrations before calving and in the first few weeks of lactation have been linked to subsequent cyclicity and conception rate (Taylor et al. 2006). This emphasizes the critical role of correct nutritional management to ensure that the deficit in energy balance post calving is mild rather than severe. Current approaches to minimize the energy balance deficit post calving includes: the optimization of body condition score at calving (2.75 - 3.0), shorter dry periods and maintenance of normal rumen function (Mulligan et al. 2006).

Item	Fagan and Roche 1986 Moderate yielding Friesian cows	Opsomer et al. 1998 High yielding Holstein cows
No. of cows / postpartum periods	463	448
Normal cyclic patterns (%)	78	53.5*
Prolonged interval to 1st ovulation (%)	7	20.5*
Prolonged luteal phase (%)	3	20*
Temporary cessation of ovulation (%)	3	3
Short cycles (%)	4	0.5
Other irregular patterns (%)	4	2.5

Table 1. Pattern of resumption of ovarian cyclicity in postpartum dairy cows (traditional moderate yielding Friesians vs modern high yielding Holsteins), using milk progesterone profiling (samples collected twice weekly). *Categories with a major disparity between the two studies.

Disease state may also regulate follicle fate via LH and other mechanisms. Uterine conditions such as retained foetal membranes, endometritis and metritis contribute to reproductive efficiency via various mechanisms. Local infection of the uterus in postpartum cows delays uterine involution, causes inflammation of the endometrium, reduce conception rate to first insemination (Sheldon 2004), but may also affect follicle growth, decrease estradiol secretion from dominant follicles, and delay the interval to first ovulation (LeBlanc et al. 2002; Sheldon et al. 2002; Sheldon and Dobson 2004; Williams et al. 2007;

Sheldon et al. 2008). These effects on follicle growth and ovulation implicate potential roles mediated by either direct effects within follicles and reduced LH secretion / failure of the gonadotropin surge. Indeed the evidence supports both possible mechanisms: uterine disease associated with *E. Coli* or infusion of endotoxins reduces estradiol secretion from dominant follicles (Sheldon et al. 2002; Herath et al. 2007) and delays the LH surge and ovulation (Suzuki et al. 2001). Other diseases such as mastitis (Huzenicza et al. 2005) and lameness (Petersson et al. 2006) delay resumption of luteal activity by 7 to 17 days, respectively. For these there is considerable evidence that this is mediated due to acute stressors reducing GnRH and hence LH pulse frequency, leading to decreased estradiol production by dominant follicles and preventing or reducing the gonadotropin surge, thus delaying ovulation.

4. Abnormal ovarian function during the post-partum period

4.1. Prolonged luteal phases

Irregular estrous cycles in cows once they have resumed ovulation tend to be predominantly prolonged luteal phases. The incidence of prolonged luteal phases has increased from 3% (Fagan and Roche 1986) to 11-22% (Lamming and Darwash 1998; Opsomer et al. 1998; Shrestra et al. 2004; Figure 4). It is generally considered that prolonged luteal phases are associated with an abnormal uterine environment that disrupts prostaglandin production. Interestingly in the study of Opsomer et al. (1998), where the incidence of cows with prolonged luteal phases was 20% (89/448 cows), only 43/89 cows had abnormal uterine content, 2/89 had ovarian cysts and 44/89 had no detectable abnormalities. However in this study abnormalities were identified only by rectal palpation. The major risk factors for a prolonged luteal phase in cows having resumed ovulation included (odds ratio in parentheses; Opsomer et al. 2000): metritis (11.0), abnormal vaginal discharge (4.4), retained placenta (3.5), parity (2.5 for parity 4+ vs primiparous), earlier resumption of ovulation (2.8 for resumption < 19 days post partum, 2.4 for resumption 19-24 days post partum). These data support the concept that prolonged luteal phases are related to uterine problems rather than ovarian problems.

4.2. Follicular cysts

These occur where dominant follicles in the early postpartum period (often the first dominant follicle postpartum) fail to ovulate. Cysts typically continue to grow to diameters >20-25 mm over a 10 to 40 day period in the absence of a CL (Savio et al. 1990a; Gümen et al. 2002, Hatler et al. 2003). This continued growth appears to be due to lack of positive feedback induced by estradiol and thus failure of the LH/FSH pre-ovulatory surge, despite increased LH pulse frequency (to an intermediate level). At this time progesterone concentrations are low, while estradiol concentrations are elevated above normal pro-estrus concentrations (Savio et al. 1990b; Hatler et al. 2003), resulting in many cases in strong exhibition of estrous behaviour by cows in the early phases of a follicular cyst. This is followed by a period of time when there is an absence of estrous behaviour in the second half of the cysts lifespan. The elevated estradiol in conjunction with elevated inhibin suppresses FSH concentrations, so that no new follicle waves emerge during the early active phase of a follicular cyst. The cyst then becomes estrogen inactive (despite being morphologically still present) and a new follicle wave emerges. The dominant follicle of this new wave may either ovulate, undergo atresia or become cystic. Many cows with follicular cysts correct themselves, but some develop sequential follicular cysts. The metabolic risk factors associated with cows that develop cysts in the early postpartum period are over conditioned cows, a reduction in insulin (Vanholder et al. 2005) and IGF-I, and increased non-esterified fatty acids (Zulu et al. 2002b).

5. Induction of estrus and ovulation in anovulatory anestrous cows

From the previous sections it is clear that in many cases (especially with dairy cows) anovulatory anestrus is associated with management risk factors and other diseases (excessive loss of BCS, severe lameness, uterine disease, displaced abomasum, etc). Therefore before embarking on a specific treatment for anestrus, the underlying factors and diseases should be first addressed before commencement of specific treatments for the ovarian problems.

5.1. GnRH

The major cause of delayed ovulation in postpartum cows is an infrequent LH pulse frequency (and by inference GnRH pulse frequency). GnRH treatment was used with variable effectiveness in numerous studies of postpartum cows when the follicle status of the animals was unknown. A single injection, two injections 10 days apart, or frequent low dose injections at 1- to 4-h intervals of GnRH or GnRH analogues failed consistently to induce ovulation in over 90% of treated anestrous cows (Mawhinney et al. 1979; Riley et al. 1981; Walters et al. 1982; Edwards et al. 1983). However, when a GnRH analogue (20 μg Buserelin) was used at known stages of follicle growth (determined by daily ultrasound scanning) of the first postpartum DF, all cows ovulated when administered during the growing phase of the DF (12/12) and the majority (7/10) ovulated when the first postpartum DF was in its plateau / early declining phase of growth (Crowe et al. 1993). In a further study conducted by Ryan et al. (1998), 250 μg GnRH resulted in ovulation in 20 of 20 cows when given at dominance of a follicular wave, this was followed by emergence of a new wave of ovarian follicular growth 1.6 ± 0.3 days later and dominance of the subsequent wave was attained in 5 ± 0.3 days. However, there was no effect of GnRH on follicular dynamics when given at emergence of a follicular wave. The existing cohort of follicles continued to develop unaffected in 17 of 17 cows, and dominance occurred 3.6 ± 0.5 days later. Thus, GnRH may cause ovulation or no effect on follicle development depending on the animal's stage of follicle development at treatment. Thus when GnRH is used as part of an ovsynch protocol (GnRH-PGF2α-GnRH treatment) in postpartum anestrous cows the effectiveness of the treatment is wholly dependent on the presence or absence of a DF at the time the first GnRH injection is administered.

5.2. Progesterone

Treatment of anestrous cows with progesterone (and estradiol) will induce estrus and shorten the postpartum interval to conception (Rhodes et al. 2003). Anestrous cows require progesterone treatment to ensure that the first ovulation is associated with expression of estrus and a normally functioning luteal phase. The use of eCG may accompany progesterone treatment in cows that are in deep anovulatory anestrus to ensure ovulation (Mulvehill and Sreenan 1977), but care must be taken not to induce too high an ovulation rate.

5.3. Restricted suckling (beef cows)

Earlier onset of ovulation in beef cows may be induced by restricting suckling by calves from 30 days post partum (Stagg et al. 1998). Restricted suckling involves once or twice daily access of calves to cows for suckling and at other times of the day the calves are isolated and out of sight of the cows (Stagg et al. 1998).

6. Conclusions

Follicular growth generally resumes within 7-10 days post partum in the majority of cows associated with a transient FSH rise that occurs within 3 to 5 days of parturition. A summary of reproductive parameters for beef and dairy cows is presented in Table 2. Delayed resumption of ovulation is invariably due to a lack of LH pulse frequency whether it is due to suckling inhibition in beef cows or metabolic related stressors in high yielding dairy cows. First ovulation in both dairy and beef cows is generally silent and followed by a short cycle. The key to optimizing resumption of ovulation in both beef and dairy cows is appropriate pre-calving nutrition and management so that cows calve down in optimal body condition (body condition score 2.75-3.0) with postpartum body condition loss restricted to <0.5 body condition score units.

	Dairy cows	Beef cows
Emergence of the 1st follicle wave (days post partum)	5-10	5-10
% cows that ovulate the 1st dominant follicle	50-80	20-35
Postpartum interval to first estrus (days)	25-45	30-130
Nature of 1st ovulation	silent	silent
% short cycles after 1st ovulation	>70	>70
Regulation of LH pulse frequency	• declining energy balance • BCS at calving • dry matter intake	• suckling • maternal bond • declining energy balance • BCS at calving

Table 2. Reproductive parameters in the early postpartum period of dairy and beef suckler cows

Author details

Mark A. Crowe* and Michael P. Mullen
School of Veterinary Medicine, University College Dublin, Ireland

7. References

Adams, G.P., Matteri, R.L., Kastelic, J.P., Ko, J.C.H. & Ginther, O.J. (1992). Association between surges in follicle-stimulating hormone and emergence of follicular waves in heifers. *Journal of Reproduction and Fertility* 94: 177-188.

Austin, E.J., Mihm, M., Evans, A.C.O., Knight, P.G., Ireland, J.L.H., Ireland, J.J. & Roche, J.F. (2001). Alterations in intrafollicular regulatory factors and apoptosis during selection of follicles in the first follicular wave of the bovine oestrous cycle. *Biology of Reproduction* 64: 839-848.

Austin, E.J., Mihm, M., Ryan, M.P., Williams, D.H. & Roche, J.F. (1999). Effect of duration of dominance of the ovulatory follicle on the onset of estrus and fertility in heifers. *Journal of Animal Science* 77: 2219-2226.

Bao, B., Garverick, H.A., Smith, G.W., Smith, M.F., Salfen, B.E. & Youngquist, R.S. (1997). Changes in messenger ribonucleic acid encoding luteinizing hormone receptor, cytochrome P450-side chain cleavage, and aromatase are associated with recruitment and selection of bovine ovarian follicles. *Biology of Reproduction* 56: 1158-1168

Beam, S.W. & Butler, W.R. (1997). Energy balance and ovarian follicle development prior to the first ovulation postpartum in dairy cows receiving three levels of dietary fat. *Biology of Reproduction* 56: 133-142.

Beam, S.W. & Butler, W.R. (1999). Effects of energy balance on follicular development and first ovulation in post-partum dairy cows. *Journal of Reproduction and Fertility* Supplement 54: 411–424.

Buckley, F., O'Sullivan, K., Mee, J.F., Evans, R.D. & Dillon, P. (2003). Relationships among milk yield, body condition, cow weight, and reproduction in spring-calved Holstein-Friesians. *Journal of Dairy Science* 86: 2308-2319.

Bulman, D.C. & Lamming, G.E. (1978). Milk progesterone levels in relation to conception, repeat breeding and factors influencing acyclicity in dairy cows. Journal of Reproduction and Fertilty 54: 447-458.

Butler, W.R., Everett, R.W. & Coppock, C.E. (1981). The relationships between energy balance, milk production and ovulation in post-partum Holstein cows. *Journal of Animal Science* 53: 742–748

Canfield, R.W. & Butler, W.R. (1990). Energy balance and pulsatile LH secretion in early postpartum dairy cattle. *Domestic Animal Endocrinology* 7: 323-330.

Canty, M.J., Boland, M.P., Evans, A.C.O. & Crowe, M.A. (2006). Alterations in follicular IGFBP-2, -3 and –4 mRNA expression and intrafollicular IGFBP concentrations during the first follicle wave in beef heifers. *Animal Reproduction Science* 93: 199-217.

---

* Corresponding Author

Crowe, M.A., Goulding, D., Baguisi, A., Boland, M.P. & Roche, J.F. (1993). Induced ovulation of the first postpartum dominant follicle in beef suckler cows using a GnRH analogue. *Journal of Reproduction and Fertilty* 99: 551-555.

Crowe, M.A., Padmanabhan, V., Mihm, M., Beitins, I.Z. & Roche, J.F. (1998) Resumption of follicular waves in beef cows is not associated with periparturient changes in follicle-stimulating hormone heterogeneity despite major changes in steroid and luteinizing hormone concentrations. *Biology of Reproduction* 58: 1445-1450.

Duffy, P., Crowe, M.A., Boland, M.P. & Roche, J.F. (2000). Effect of exogenous LH pulses on the fate of the first dominant follicle in postpartum beef cows nursing calves. *Journal of Reproduction and Fertilty* 118: 9-17.

Edmonson, A.J., Lean, I.J., Weaver, L.D., Farver, T. & Webster, G., 1989. A body condition scoring chart for Holstein dairy cows. *Journal of Dairy Science* 72, 68–78.

Edwards, S., Roche, J.F. & Niswender, G.D. (1983). Response of suckling beef cows to multiple, low-dose injections of Gn-RH with or without progesterone pretreatment. *Journal of Reproduction and Fertilty* 69: 65-72.

Fagan, J.G. & Roche, J.F. (1986). Reproductive activity in postpartum dairy cows based on progesterone concentrations in milk or rectal examination. *Irish Veterinary Journal* 40: 124-131.

Fourichon, C., Seegers, H. & Malher, X. (1999). Effects of disease on reproduction in the dairy cow. A meta-analysis. *Theriogenology* 53: 1729-1759.

Ginther, O.J., Knopf, L. & Kastelic, J.P. (1989). Ovarian follicular dynamics in heifers during early pregnancy. *Biology of Reproduction* 41: 247-254.

Ginther, O.J., Kot, K., Kulick, L.J., Martin, S. & Wiltbank, M.C. (1996). Relationship between FSH and ovarian follicular waves during the last six months of pregnancy in cattle. *Journal of Reproduction and Fertilty* 108: 271-279.

Griffith, M.K. & Williams, G.L. (1996) Roles of maternal vision and olfaction in suckling-mediated inhibition of luteinizing hormone secretion. Expression of maternal selectivity, and lactational performance of beef cows. *Biology of Reproduction* 54: 761-768.

Grimard, B., Touze, J.L., Laigre, P. & Thomeret, F. (2005) Abnormal patterns of resumption of ovarian postpartum cyclicity in Prim'Holstein dairy cows: risk factors ad consequences on reproductive efficiency. *Reproduction in Domestic Animals* (Abstract) 40: 342.

Gröhn, Y.T. & Rajala-Schult, P.J. (2000). Epidemiology of reproductive performance in dairy cows. *Animal Reproduction Science* 60/61: 605-614.

Grummer, R.R., Mashek, D.G. & Hayirli, A. (2004). Dry matter intake and energy balance in the transition period. *Veterinary Clinics of North America: Food Animal Practice* 20: 447-470.

Herath, S., Williams, E.J., Lilly, S.T., Gilbert, R.O., Dobson, H., Bryant, C.E. & Sheldon, I.M. (2007). Ovarian follicular cells have innate immune capabilities that modulate their endocrine function. *Reproduction* 134: 683-693.

Huszenicza, G., Janosi, S., Kulcsar, M., Korodi, P., Reiczigel, J., Katai, L., Peters, A.R. & de Rensis, F. (2005). Effects of clinical mastitis on ovarian function in post-partum dairy cows. *Reproduction in Domestic Animals* 40: 199-204.

Ireland, J.J. & Roche, J.F. (1987). Hypothesis regarding development of dominant follicles during a bovine estrous cycle. In: Roche, J.F. and O'Callaghan, D. (eds), *Follicular growth and ovulation rate in farm animals*. Martinus Nijhoff The Netherlands, pp. 1-18.

Kyle, S.D., Callahan, C.J. & Allrich, R.D. (1992). Effect of progesterone on the expression of estrus at the first postpartum ovulation in dairy cattle. *Journal of Dairy Science* 75: 1456-1460.

Lamming, G.E. & Darwash, A.O. (1998). The use of milk progesterone profiles to characterize components of subfertility in milked dairy cows. *Animal Reproduction Science* 52: 175-190.

LeBlanc, S.J., Duffield, T.F., Leslie, K.E., Bateman, K.G., Keefe, G.P., Walton, J.S. & Johnson, W.H. (2002). Defining and diagnosing postpartum clinical endometritis and its impact on reproductive performance in dairy cows. *Journal of Dairy Science* 85: 2223-2236.

López-Gatius, F., Santolaria, P., Yániz, J., French, M. & López-Béjar, M. (2002). Risk factors for postpartum ovarian cysts and their spontaneous recovery or persistence in lactating dairy cows. *Theriogenology* 58: 1723-1632.

Lowman, B.G., Scott, N.A. & Somerville S.H. (1976). Condition scoring of cattle. *Review Edition Bulletin, East of Scotland College of Agriculture*, no. 6, Scotland.

Lucy, M.C. (2001). Reproductive loss in high-producing dairy cattle: where will it end? *Journal of Dairy Science* 84: 1277-1293.

Maizon, D.O., Oltenacu, P.A., Gröhn, Y.T., Strawderman, R.L. & Emanuelson, U. (2004). Effects of diseases on reproductive performance in Swedish red and white dairy cattle. *Preventive Veterinary Medicine* 66: 113-126.

Matton, P., Adelakoun, V., Couture, Y. & Dufour, J. (1981). Growth and replacement of the bovine ovarian follicles during the estrous cycle. *Journal of Animal Science* 52: 813-818.

Mawhinney, S., Roche, J.F., Gosling, J.P. (1979). The effects of oestradiol benzoate (OB) and gonadotrophin releasing hormone (GnRH) on reproductive activity in beef cows at different intervals post partum. *Annales de Biologie Animale, Biochimie, Biophysique* 19: 1575-1587.

Mayne, C.S., McCoy, M.A., Lennox, S.D., Mackey, D.R., Verner, M., Catney, D.C., McCaughey, W.J., Wylie, A.R., Kennedy, B.W. & Gordon, F.J. (2002). Fertility of dairy cows in Northern Ireland. *Veterinary Record* 150: 707-713.

Mulligan, F.J., O'Grady, L., Rice, D.A. & Doherty, M.A. (2006) A herd health approach to dairy cow nutrition and production diseases of the transition cow. *Animal Reproduction Science* 96: 331-353.

Mulvehill, P. & Sreenan, J.M. (1977) Improvement of fertility in postpartum beef cows by treatment with PMSG and progestagen. *Journal of Reproduction and Fertilty* 50: 323-325.

Murphy, M.G., Boland, M.P. & Roche, J.F. (1990) Pattern of follicular growth and resumption of ovarian activity in post-partum beef suckler cows. *Journal of Reproduction and Fertility* 90: 523-533.

Murphy, M.G., Enright, W.J., Crowe, M.A., McConnell, K., Spicer, L.J., Boland, M.P. & Roche, J.F. (1991). Effect of dietary intake on pattern of growth of dominant follicles during the oestrous cycle in beef heifers. *Journal of Reproduction and Fertilty* 92 333-338.

Myers, T.R., Myers, D.A., Gregg, D.W. & Moss, G.E. (1989). Endogenous opioid suppression of release of luteinizing hormone during suckling in postpartum anestrous beef cows. *Domestic Animal Endocrinology* 6: 183-190.

Nakao, T., Tomita, M., Kanbayashi, H., Takagi, H., Abe, T., Takeuchi, Y., Ochiai, H., Moriyoshi, M. & Kawata, K. (1991). Comparisons of several dosages of a GnRH analog with the standard dose of hCG in the treatment of follicular cysts in dairy cows. *Theriogenology* 38: 137-145.

Opsomer, G., Coryn, M., Deluyker, H., de Kruif, A. (1998). An analysis if ovarian dysfunction in high yielding dairy cows after calving based on progesterone profiles. *Reproduction in Domestic Animals* 33: 193-204.

Opsomer, G., Grohn, Y.T., Hertl, J., Coryn, M., Deluyker, H. & de Kruif, A. (2000). Risk factors for post partum ovarian dysfunction in high producing dairy cows in Belgium: a field study. *Theriogenology* 53: 841-857.

Overton, T.R. & Waldron, M.R. (2004). Nutritional management of transitions dairy cows: strategies to optimize metabolic health. *Journal of Dairy Science* 87: E105-E119.

Peter, A.T., Bosu, W.T., Liptrap, R.M. & Cummings, E. (1989). Temporal changes in serum prostaglandin F(2alpha) and oxytocin in dairy cows with short luteal phases after the first postpartum ovulation. *Theriogenology* 32: 277-284.

Petersson, K.J., Strandberg, E., Gustafsson, H. and Berglund, B. (2006). Environmental effects on progesterone profile measures of dairy cow fertility. *Animal Reproduction Science* 91: 201-214.

Rajakoski, E. (1960). The ovarian follicular system in sexually mature heifers with special reference to seasonal, cyclical. and left-right variations. *Acta Endocrinology* 51: 1-68.

Rhodes, F.M., McDougall, S., Burke, C.R., Verkerk, G.A. and Macmillan, K.L. (2003). Invited review: treatment of cows with an extended postpartum anestrous interval. *Journal of Dairy Science* 86: 1876-1918.

Richards, M.W., Wettemann, R.P. & Schoenemann, H.M. (1989). Nutritional anestrus in beef cows: body weight change, body condition, luteinizing hormone in serum and ovarian activity. *Journal of Animal Science* 67: 1520–1526

Riley, G.M., Peters, A.R. and Lamming, G.E. (1981). Induction of pulsatile LH release and ovulation in post partum cyclic beef cows by repeated small doses of GnRH. *Journal of Reproduction and Fertility* 63: 559-565.

Royal, M.D., Darwash, A.O., Flint, A.P.F., Webb, R., Woolliams, J.A. & Lamming, G.E. (2000) Declining fertility in dairy cattle: changes in traditional and endocrine parameters of fertility. *Animal Science* 70: 487-501.

Ryan, M., Mihm, M., and Roche, J.F. (1998). Effect of GnRH given before or after dominance on gonadotrophin response and the fate of that follicle wave in postpartum dairy cows. *Journal of Reproduction and Fertilty* Abstract Series 21: 28.

Sakaguchi, M., Sasamoto, Y., Suzuki, T., Takahashi, Y. and Yamada, Y. (2004). Postpartum ovarian follicular dynamics and estrous activity in lactating dairy cows. *Journal of Dairy Science* 87: 2114-2121.

Sartori, R., Haughian, J.M., Shaver, R.D., Rosa, G.J.M. and Wiltbank, M.C. (2004). Comparison of ovarian function and circulating steroids in estrous cycles of Holstein heifers and lactating cows. *Journal of Dairy Science* 87: 905-920.

Savio, J.D., Boland, M.P. and Roche, J.F. (1990a). Development of dominant follicles and length of ovarian cycles in post-partum dairy cows. *Journal of Reproduction and Fertilty* 88: 581-591.

Savio, J.D., Boland, M.P., Hynes, N. and Roche, J.F. (1990b). Resumption of follicular activity in the early post-partum period of dairy cows. *Journal of Reproduction and Fertilty* 88: 569-579.

Savio, J.D., Keenan, L., Boland, M.P. and Roche, J.F. (1988). Pattern of dominant follicles during the oestrous cycle of heifers. *Journal of Reproduction and Fertilty* 83: 663-671.

Schallenberger, E. (1985). Gonadotrophins and ovarian steroids in cattle. III. Pulsatile changes of gonadotrophin concentrations in the jugular vein post partum. *Acta Endocrinology* (Copenh) 109: 37-43.

Sheldon, I.M. & Dobson, H. 2004. Postpartum uterine health in cattle. *Animal Reproduction Science* 82/83: 295-306.

Sheldon, I.M. (2004). The postpartum uterus. *Veterinary Clinics of North America Food Animal Practice* 569-591.

Sheldon, I.M., Noakes, D.E., Rycroft, A.N., Pfeiffer, D.U. & Dobson, H. (2002). Influence of uterine bacterial contamination after parturition on ovarian dominant follicle selection and follicle growth and function in cattle. *Reproduction* 123: 837-845.

Sheldon, I.M., Williams, E.J., Miller, A.N.A., Nash, D.M. & Herath, S. (2008). Uterine diseases in cattle after parturition. The Veterinary Journal 176: 115-121.

Shrestha, H.K., Nakao, T., Higaki, T., Suzuki, T. & Akita, M. (2004). Effects of abnormal ovarian cycles during pre-service period postpartum on subsequent reproductive performance of high-producing Holstein cows. Theriogenology 61: 1559-1571.

Shrestha, H.K., Nakao, T., Higaki, T., Suzuki, T. & Akita, M. (2004). Resumption of postpartum ovarian cyclicity in high-producing Holstein cows. *Theriogenology* 61: 637-649.

Silveira, P.A., Spoon, R.A., Ryan, D.P. & Williams, G.L. (1993). Evidence for maternal behavior as a requisite link in suckling-mediated anovulation in cows. *Biology of Reproduction* 49: 1338-1346.

Sirois, J. & Fortune, J.E. (1988). Ovarian follicular dynamics during the estrous cycle in heifers monitored by real-time ultrasonography. *Biology of Reproduction* 39: 308-317.

Stagg, K., Diskin, M.G., Sreenan, J.M. & Roche, J.F. (1995). Follicular development in long-term anestorus suckler beef cows fed two levels of energy postpartum. *Animal Reproduction Science* 38: 49-61.

Stagg, K., Spicer, L.J., Sreenan, J.M., Roche, J.F. & Diskin, M.G. (1998). Effect of calf isolation on follicular wave dynamics, gonadotropin, and metabolic hormone changes, and interval to first ovulation in beef cows fed either of two energy levels postpartum. *Biology of Reproduction* 59: 777-783.

Staples, C.R., Thatcher, W.W. & Clark, J.R. (1990). Influence of supplemental fats on reproductive tissues and performance of lactating cows. Journal of Dairy Science 81: 856–871

Sunderland, S.J., Crowe, M.A., Boland, M.P., Roche, J.F. & Ireland, J.J. (1994). Selection, dominance and atresia of follicles during the oestrous cycle of heifers. *Journal of Reproduction and Fertilty* 101: 547-555.

Suzuki, C., Yoshioka, K., Iwamura, S. & Hirose, H. (2001). Endotoxin induces delayed ovulation following endocrine aberration during the proestrous phase in Holstein heifers. *Domestic Animal Endocrinology* 20: 267-278.

Taylor, V.J., Beever, D.E., Bryant, M.J. & Wathes, D.C. (2003). Metabolic profiles and progesterone cycles in first lactation dairy cows. *Theriogenology* 59: 1661-1677.

Taylor, V.J., Beever, D.E., Bryant, M.J. & Wathes, D.C. (2006). Pre-pubertal measurements of the somatotrophic axis as predictors of milk production in Holstein-Friesian dairy cows. *Domestic Animal Endocrinology* 31: 1-18.

Vanholder, T., Leroy, J.L.M.R., Dewulf, J., Duchateau, L., Coryn, M., deKruif, A. and Opsomer, G. (2005). Hormonal and metabolic profiles of high-yielding dairy cows prior to ovarian cyst formation or first ovulation post-partum. *Reproduction in Domestic Animals* 40: 460-467.

Walters, D.L., Short, R.E., Convey, E.M., Staigmiller, R.B., Dunn, T.G. & Kaltenbach, C.C. (1982). Pituitary and ovarian function in postpartum beef cows. II. Endocrine changes prior to ovulation in suckled and nonsuckled postpartum cows compared to cycling cows. *Biology of Reproduction* 26: 647-654.

Wathes, D.C., Bourne, N., Cheng, Z., Mann, G.E., Taylor, V.J. & Coffey, M.P. (2007). Multiple correlation analyses of metabolic and endocrine profiles with fertility in primiparous and multiparous cows. *Journal of Dairy Science* 90: 1310-1325.

Webb, R, Garnsworthy, P.C., Gong, J-C., Armstrong, D.G. (2004). Control of follicular growth: local interactions and nutritional influences. *Journal of Animal Science* 82: E63-E74.

Williams, E.J., Fischer, D.P., Noakes, D.E., England, G.C.W., Rycroft, A., Dobson, H. & Sheldon, I.M. (2007). The relationship between uterine pathogen growth density and ovarian function in the postpartum dairy cow. *Theriogenology* 68: 549-559.

Williams, G.L., Mcvey, W.R. & Hunter JF, 1993: Mammary somatosensory pathways are not required for suckling-mediated inhibition of luteinizing hormone secretion and delay of ovulation of cows. *Biology of Reproduction* 49 1328-1337.

Wolfenson, D., Inbar, G., Roth, Z., Kaim, M., Bloch, A. & Braw-Tal, R. (2004). Follicular dynamics and concentrations of steroids and gonadotropins in lactating cows and nulliparous heifers. *Theriogenology* 62: 1042-1055.

Xu, Z.Z., Garverick, H.A., Smith, G.W., Smith, M.E., Hamilton, S.A. & Youngquist, R.S. (1995) Expression of follicle-stimulating hormone and luteinizing hormone receptor messenger ribonucleic acids in bovine follicles during the first follicular wave. *Biology of Reproduction* 52: 464-469

Zollers, W.G. Jr., Garverick, H.A., Smith, M.F., Moffatt, R.J., Salfen, B.E., Youngquist, R.S. (1993) Concentrations of progesterone and oxytocin receptors in endometrium of postpartum cows expected to have a short or normal oestrous cycle. Journal of Reproduction and Fertilty 97: 329-337.

Zulu, V.C., Nakao, T. & Sawamukai, Y. (2002a). Insulin-like growth factor-I as a possible hormonal mediator of nutritional regulation of reproduction in cattle. *Journal of Veterinary Medical Science* 64: 657-665.

Zulu, V.C., Sawamukai, Y., Nakada, D., Kida, K. & Moriyoshi, M. (2002b). Relationship among insulin-like growth factor-I blood metabolites and postpartum ovarian function in dairy cows. *Journal of Veterinary Medical Science* 64: 879-885.

Chapter 6

Relative Roles of FSH and LH in Stimulation of Effective Follicular Responses in Cattle

Mark A. Crowe and Michael P. Mullen

Additional information is available at the end of the chapter

http://dx.doi.org/10.5772/50272

1. Introduction

The growth development and maturation of ovarian follicles is a fundamental process for effective reproduction in farm animals. Initial stages of follicle growth occur independent of gonadotropic hormones, antral follicles then become responsive to and subsequently dependent on FSH. In heifers, there are usually 2-3 waves of gonadotropin dependent follicle growth during the estrous cycle (Ireland and Roche, 1987; Savio et al., 1988; Sirois and Fortune, 1988; Knopf et al., 1989) each involving emergence of the wave, selection of the dominant follicle (DF) and a period of dominance, followed by either atresia or ovulation of the DF. The objective is to review some of the data on the mechanisms of gonadotropic control of antral follicle growth in cattle.

2. Pattern of follicle growth in cattle

The pattern of follicle growth in cattle has been clearly characterized with the use of ultrasound. Several reports (Savio et al., 1988; Sirois and Fortune, 1988; Knopf et al., 1989; Ginther et al., 1989) have shown that there are either two, three or occasionally four waves of follicle growth during the estrous cycle of cattle. During each wave of follicle growth, a cohort of 2 to 5 follicles emerges to grow beyond 4 mm in diameter to medium (5-9 mm) size classes (emergence). From the pool of medium follicles that emerge a single follicle is selected to become the dominant follicle (selection). Selection is a fundamental process that determines the species-specific ovulation rate in females (Goodman and Hodgen, 1983) thereby playing a major role in determining the number of offspring born per pregnancy. The selected DF continues to grow in size, while other follicles in the cohort undergo atresia. Finally the DF will either undergo atresia (during the luteal phase) or ovulate (during the follicular phase).

3. Association between gonadotropin concentrations and follicle growth

The initial stages of folliculogenesis occur independently of gonadotropic hormones. Antral follicles initially become responsive to and then dependent on FSH for their continued growth. In cattle, follicle growth above 4 mm in diameter is considered to be gonadotropin dependent (Campbell et al., 1995).

Associated with each new wave of follicular development, FSH concentrations increase as emergence occurs (Adams et al., 1992; Sunderland et al., 1994; Hamilton et al., 1995). This transient rise in FSH concentrations occurs over a period of 1 to 2 days during emergence of each new wave of follicle growth (Sunderland et al., 1994; Cooke et al., 1997). Thus, in a typical 3-wave estrous cycle, recurrent FSH rises occur on days 0.5 to 1.5, 8 to 10, and 13.5 to 15; each follicular wave lasts for approximately 7 days. Whereas in a 2-wave estrous cycle only the first two recurrent FSH rises occur; with each wave of follicular growth lasting approximately 10 days. The process of selection of the DF occurs during a period when FSH returns to nadir concentrations. It has now been clearly demonstrated that during all physiological states where follicle waves occur, associated transient increases in FSH concentrations coincide with follicle wave emergence (cyclic cattle: Adams et al., 1992; Sunderland et al., 1994; Cooke et al., 1997; pregnancy: Ginther et al., 1996; post-partum cows during anestrus: Crowe et al., 1998; and pre-pubertal heifers: Adams et al., 1994a).

The precise pattern of pulsatile LH during each wave of follicle growth has been less clearly characterized. The earlier studies of Rahe et al. (1980) characterized the pattern of LH secretion on days 3 (early luteal), 10 or 11 (mid luteal) and 18 or 19 of the estrous cycle of cows. During the early luteal phase pulses were low amplitude and high frequency (20-30 pulses / 24 h), in the mid-luteal period pulses were high amplitude and low frequency (6-8 pulses / 24 h) and pre-ovulatory surges occurred on day 18 / 19 with high frequency and high amplitude pulses occurring during the surge. However, this study was performed before characterization of the pattern of follicular growth, so no recognition regarding stage of follicular development was possible. A more recent study demonstrated that LH pulse frequency is at a minimum during the mid-luteal phase (days 7 through 13 of the estrous cycle; 2.7 to 3.4 pulses per 12 h window); LH pulse amplitude increases from early (0.5 ng / ml) to mid luteal phase (1.04 to 1.3 ng / ml on days 8-11); subsequently decreases to 0.7 to 0.8 ng / ml on days 12-14; and recovers to about 1.0 ng/ml from days 15 - 19 (Cupp et al., 1995). However, this study also failed to align animals by stage of the follicle wave before analyzing the LH pulse characteristics. In a study reported by Mihm et al. (1995), the pattern of pulsatile secretion of LH was characterized at three stages of the first DF: first day of dominance (day 5 of estrous cycle), end of growth phase of the first DF (day 8 of estrous cycle) and at emergence of the second follicle wave (loss of dominance of the first wave DF; day 11 of estrous cycle). LH pulse frequency decreased ($p = 0.08$) between day 5 and 8 (7.5 ± 0.4 vs 5.7 ± 0.8 pulses per 12 hours) and LH pulse amplitude increased ($p < 0.05$) between days 5 and 11 (0.45 ± 0.04 vs 1.1 ± 0.2 ng /ml). These data are largely confirmed by a similar study (Evans et al., 1997), where LH pulse amplitude and frequency were characterized on days 3 or 4 (early dominance), 7 or 8 (end of growth phase) and 11, 12 or 13 (loss of dominance) of the estrous cycle. LH pulse frequency was lower at the end of the growth phase than at early dominance, with an intermediate LH pulse frequency at loss of dominance; LH pulse amplitude was greater at the end of the growth phase of the first DF than at either early dominance or at loss of dominance. Thus, while there are good characterizations of the pattern of LH secretion during the estrous cycle, the relationship of LH pulse pattern to the stage of the follicle wave has only been characterized for the first wave, so the precise role of LH in controlling follicular dynamics throughout the entire estrous cycle remains unclear. These data, however, support the hypothesis that LH pulse frequency decreases once a follicle is selected to become dominant, with an associated increase in LH pulse amplitude; an increase in LH pulse frequency and a decrease in amplitude occurs when a non-ovulatory DF undergoes atresia (Roche, 1996) or both frequency and amplitude increase as a DF proceeds to ovulate during the follicular phase (Rahe et al., 1980). Further evidence for the role of increased LH pulse frequency at later stages of follicular development is provided by studies where dominant follicles were maintained for prolonged periods of time during artificial induction of luteal phases using low levels of progesterone, in the absence of endogenous CL, and associated increased LH pulse frequencies (Sirois and Fortune, 1990; Savio et al., 1993; Mihm et al., 1994). Thus the pattern of secretion of LH at the time when a DF is selected is responsible for determination of the fate of that DF. Luteal phase LH pulse frequencies allow dominant follicles to turnover and undergo atresia; whereas, follicular phase LH pulse frequencies are associated with DF that ovulate. Experimental induction of intermediary LH pulse frequencies induces persistent DF that maintains their physiological health for an extended time period, but when ovulated is associated with reduced pregnancy rates (Mihm et al., 1994). This reduction in pregnancy rate, associated with oocytes from persistent DF, appears to be due to loss of developmental competence due to premature resumption of meiosis relative to time of ovulation (Mihm et al., 1999).

4. Models to study the role of gonadotropins in folliculogenesis in cattle

While the characterization studies mentioned in the previous section relate stage of the estrous cycle (and / or follicle wave) to gonadotropin concentrations, little work has been done to demonstrate cause and effect in terms of how gonadotropins control the process of follicle growth. There are some appropriate *in vivo* models to address these fundamental issues.

4.1. GnRH immunization

GnRH immunization involves immunization of animals against GnRH conjugated to a carrier protein (to render it immunogenic) and then administration of this immunogen mixed with an adjuvant to a subcutaneous injection site. For example, Prendiville et al. (1995) used human serum albumin (HSA)-Cys-Gly-GnRH as immunogen in DEAE-dextran adjuvant injected subcutaneously as a primary and booster (28 days post primary immunization) immunization. Vizcarra et al. (2012) has used subcutaneous and intra dermal immunizations into the mammary gland using various conjugates (GnRH-Ovalbumin, GnRH human serum albumin, or GnRH- keyhole limpet hemocyanin) along with various adjuvants (Freunds complete, Freunds incomplete, DEAE-dextran and mineral oil) in various combinations. Optimal immunization responses (decent antibody titers, estrous cycle suppression and minimal granulomas at the injection sites) were achieved using GnRH-Ovalbumin as adjuvant and Freunds incomplete adjuvant in conjunction with DEAE-dextran. Recombinant DNA techniques to fuse GnRH to carrier proteins has also been used with success as part of the approach to achieving an efficacious vaccination protocol against GnRH (Stevens et al., 2005). Following GnRH immunization pulsatile secretion of LH is reduced (Adams and Adams, 1986; Prendiville et al., 1996), pituitary content of LH and LHRH-receptors are reduced by approximately 50% (Adams and Adams, 1990); resulting in anestrus with follicular growth arrested at ≤ 4 mm in diameter for at least 80 days (Prendiville et al., 1995). It has also been demonstrated that GnRH immunization prevents recurrent transient increases in FSH concentrations (Crowe et al., 2001a).

Administration of 12 mg recombinant bovine FSH (rbFSH) as 24 equal doses over 6 days to GnRH-immunized anestrous heifers caused a significant increase in serum FSH concentrations (Figure 1) and emergence of 4.3 ± 1.1 medium (5-9 mm diameter) and 2.0 ± 1.1 large (≥ 10 mm) follicles. Using a higher dose of rbFSH (24 mg administered as 16 equal doses over 4 days) stimulated emergence of 9.2 ± 0.9 medium and 8.4 ± 1.2 large follicles (Crowe et al., 2001a). However, regardless of dose of FSH used, selection of a single DF failed to occur. The failure of selection of a single DF in this study can be explained by either the lack of pulsatile LH secretion or excessive dose or duration of rbFSH treatment. Furthermore, growth of medium and large follicles following FSH treatment was not associated with any change in estradiol concentrations (Crowe et al., 2001a). The lack of estradiol secretion in animals where large follicles are present on the ovary is likely associated with the absence of LH to stimulate the synthesis of androgen precursor required for estradiol secretion from the granulosa cells of large healthy follicles.

A further study was performed to determine the specific roles of FSH and LH in the process of follicle selection (Crowe et al., 2001b). Seventeen GnRH-immunized anestrous heifers, were assigned to receive either i) FSH alone (1.5 mg pFSH i.m.; Folltropin, Vetrepharm Inc., Ontario, Canada; every 6 hours for 48 hours), ii) pulses of LH alone (150 μg pLH; Lutropin, Vetrepharm Inc., Ontario, Canada; every 4 hours for 132 hours) or iii) a combination of FSH and LH (at the same doses and schedules as in treatments (i) and (ii), respectively). Ovaries were collected following slaughter 134 - 137 hours after initiation of gonadotropin treatments. Heifers treated with FSH and LH grew substantial numbers of medium and estrogen active large follicles (some of which had associated aromatase activity), those treated with FSH alone grew large numbers of medium sized follicles, but much fewer large follicles (Table 1) and those treated with LH alone grew no follicles greater than 4 mm in diameter. Serum estradiol concentrations were 10- to 14-fold higher in heifers treated with both pFSH and pLH than in heifers treated with either pFSH alone or pLH alone (Figure 2). Follicular fluid taken from heifers treated with a combination of pFSH and pLH had E_2

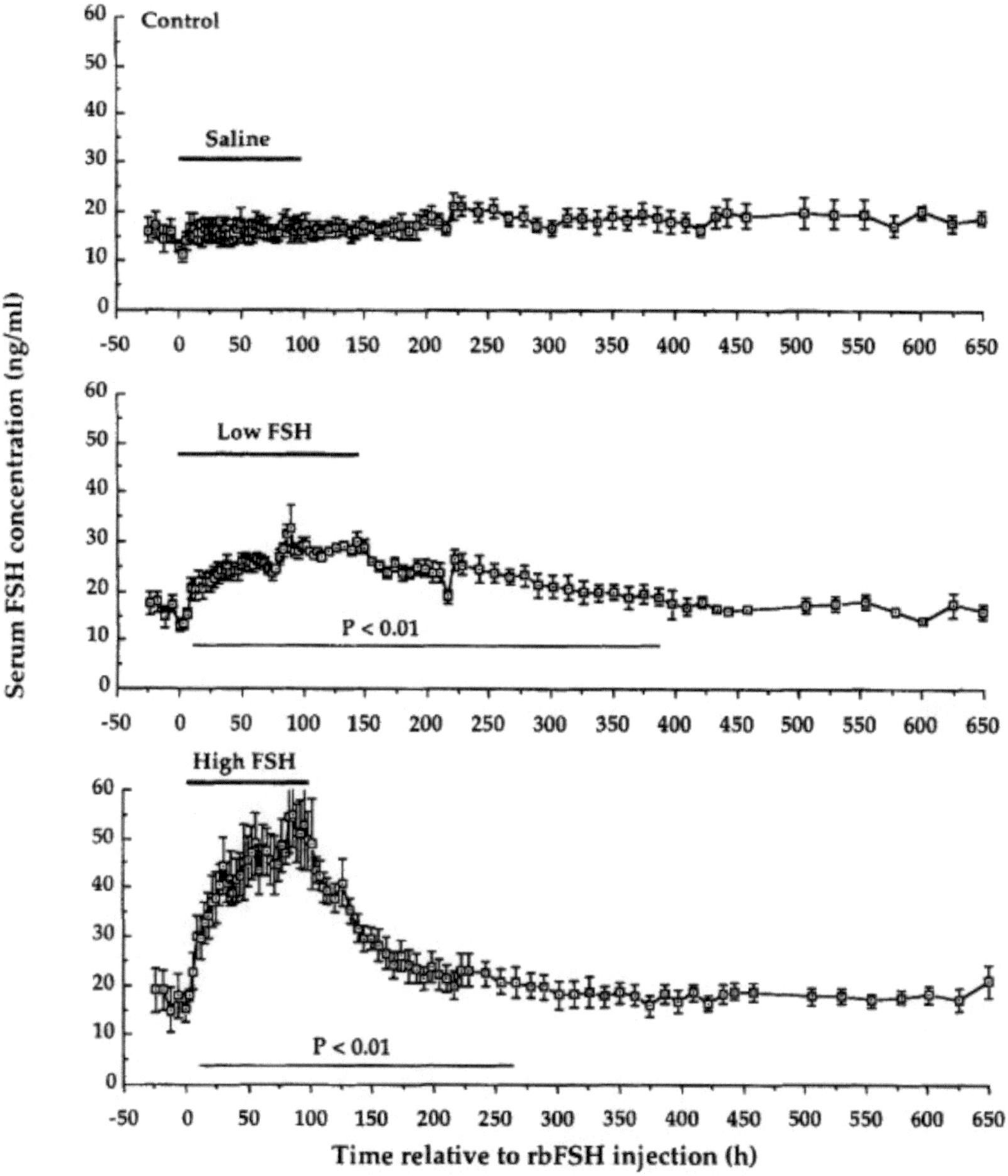

Figure 1. Mean ± SEM FSH concentrations in GnRH-immunized anestrous heifers treated with either saline 4 x/d for 4 d (n = 5), 0.5 mg equivalent (USDA bFSH BP 1) of recombinant bovine FSH (rbFSH) 4 x/d for 6 d (n = 6; 12 mg in total; LOW FSH) or 1.5 mg rbFSH 4 x/d for 4 d (n = 5; 24 mg in total; HIGH FSH). Line with P value indicates period during which a significant elevation above pre-treatment baseline occurred (Modified and reprinted with permission, Animal Science, Crowe et al., 2001a).

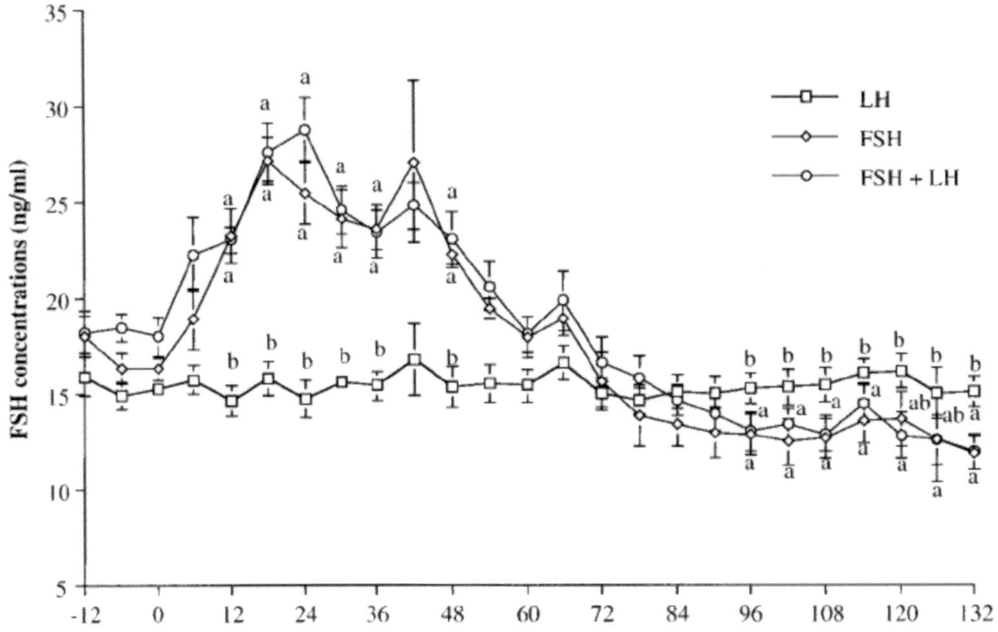

(a)

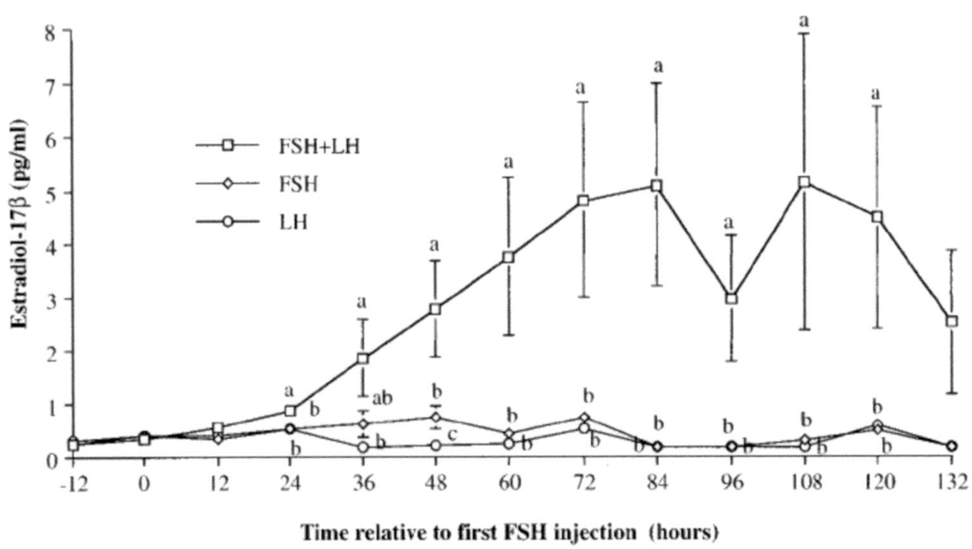

(b)

Figure 2. Changes in mean ± SEM serum concentrations of a) FSH and b) estradiol in GnRH-immunized anestrous heifers treated with pFSH alone (1.5 mg porcine FSH; pFSH; injected i.m. 4 x/d for 2d), pLH alone (150 μg pLH infused i.v. 6 x/d for 6d) or pFSH and pLH (combination of FSH alone and LH alone treatments; reprinted with permission from Biology of Reproduction, Crowe et al., 2001b).

	Medium Follicles		Large Follicles	
Day	pFSH	pFSH+pLH	pFSH	pFSH+pLH
-1	0	0	0	0
0	0	0	0	0
1	0	1.0 ± 0.6	0	0
2	5.0 ± 1.4a	11.7 ± 2.6b	0	0.2 ± 0.2
3	7.2 ± 2.7	12.2 ± 2.6	0.6 ± 0.4a	7.5 ± 2.4b
4	4.0 ± 2.0	5.4 ± 2.2	2.4 ± 1.0a	13.0 ± 4.4b
5	3.4 ± 1.5	5.8 ± 2.0	3.4 ± 1.1a	12.7 ± 3.2b
6	2.8 ± 1.0	3.5 ± 1.2	4.4 ± 1.6a	14.8 ± 3.0b

Table 1. Mean ± SEM number of medium (5-9 mm) and large (≥ 10 mm) sized follicles, detected by daily ultrasonography, in GnRH-immunized anestrous heifers treated with pFSH alone (1.5 mg porcine FSH; pFSH; injected i.m. 4 x/d for 2d) or both pFSH and pLH (FSH as for FSH alone and 150 μg pLH infused i.v. 6 x/d for 6d). Heifers treated with pLH alone (150 μg pLH infused i.v. 6 x/d for 6d) failed to grow follicles > 4 mm in diameter (Crowe et al., 2001b). [a,b]Means, within follicle class and rows, with different superscripts are different ($P < 0.05$ for medium follicles; $P < 0.01$ for large follicles).

concentrations and E_2:P_4 ratios that were highly correlated with aromatase activity. This was not the case with follicular fluid taken from heifers treated with pFSH alone. In the study of Crowe et al. (2001b) the dose of FSH used and/or the pattern of administration of LH was still inappropriate to induce physiological selection of a single DF, despite stimulating follicles that were estrogen active using a combination of both FSH and LH. The lack of ability to achieve normal DF selection may reflect an excessive dose of FSH used or an inappropriate pattern of LH infusion. In a further study using GnRH-immunized anestrous heifers administered a lower dose of FSH (1 mg oFSH i.m.; Ovagen, ICP, Auckland, New Zealand; every 6 hours for 30 hours) which gave rise to a transient increase in serum FSH concentration which was similar in both amplitude (although marginally higher peak concentrations were attained) and duration to that seen in cyclic animals (Figure 3a; DJ Cooke and MA Crowe, unpublished observations). A second treatment group received the same dose of FSH coupled with pulses of LH (50 mg pLH; Lutropin; every hour for 48 or 96 hours) generating a high frequency, low amplitude LH pulse pattern similar to that seen during the follicular phase of the normal estrous cycle. A greater ($p < 0.05$) number of animals treated with FSH and LH produced large follicles (8-12 mm size class) compared with those treated with FSH alone (10/14 vs. 4/14 respectively). As with the previous study (Crowe et al., 2001b) an increase in serum estradiol concentrations was observed in response to FSH and LH treatment compared with controls or with the FSH only group (Figure 3b). Interestingly, the dynamics of this increase in serum estradiol were very similar to that seen during the early luteal phase of the cyclic heifer (Cooke et al., 1997), following emergence of the first follicle wave and selection of the first dominant follicle. Intriguingly, despite an almost "ideal" physiological gonadotropin treatment, and indeed a near perfect follicular response in terms of cohort emergence and presumably activation of steroid biosynthesis, as evidenced by the increase in serum estradiol, a morphologically dominant follicle (as previously defined, Cooke et al., 1997) was not formed. This may indicate that either i) further manipulation of the replacement pattern of FSH may be required to more precisely mimic a normal recurrent FSH increase in terms of the peak amplitude, the declining phase and / or the nadir pattern of FSH attained, or ii) perhaps a vital "selection factor" has not been provided through mere replacement of gonadotropin support.

4.2. GnRH analogue administration

Similar to GnRH immunization, chronic GnRH agonist administration (Gong et al., 1995) prevents pulsatile release of LH. However, the effect of GnRH agonist on FSH concentrations is variable depending on the treatment regime used. Chronic treatment with 5 or 10 μg buserelin (a GnRH analog) twice a day for 21 days blocks pulsatile LH, but maintains elevated FSH concentrations with follicles progressing to 7-9 mm in diameter (Gong et al., 1995). Furthermore, extended treatment with buserelin infused for a 48-day period using a 28-day minipump followed by replacement with a second minipump for a further 20 days resulted in a reduction of FSH concentrations following insertion of the second minipump and prevention of follicle growth above 4 mm in diameter (Gong et al., 1996). This approach to suppressing gonadotropin secretion from the anterior pituitary gland is more acute than GnRH immunization, but for long-term studies it has the limitation of requiring continuous administration of the GnRH agonist. To date, no studies in the literature are reported where various combinations of gonadotropin hormones have been replaced to cattle treated with this method of achieving a gonadotropin deficient model.

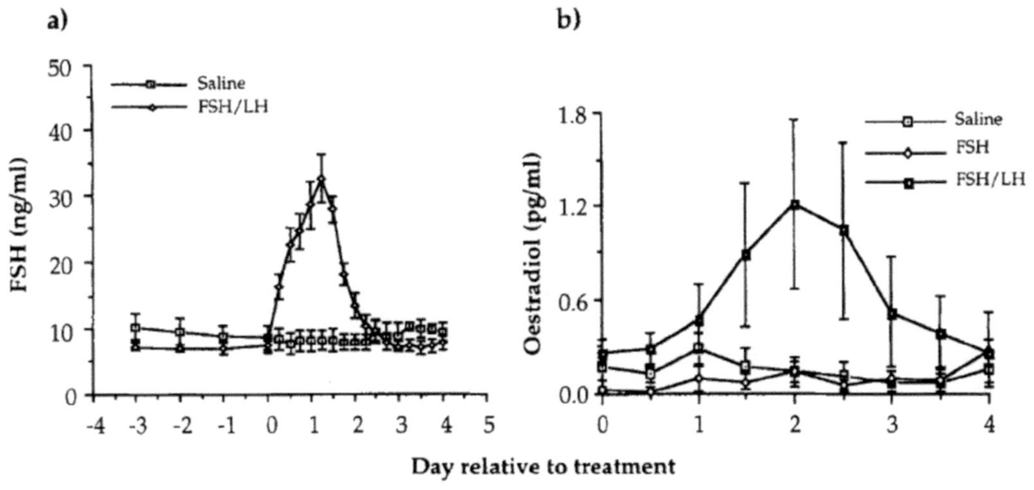

Figure 3. Mean ± SEM serum FSH (a) and estradiol (b) concentrations in GnRH-immunized anestrous heifers treated with either saline, FSH (1 mg ovine FSH i.m. every 6 hours for 30 hours; panel b only) or FSH and pulsatile LH (50 mg porcine LH every hour for 96 hours; DJ Cooke and MA Crowe, unpublished observations).

4.3. Requirement for LH to stimulate androgens and ovulation in post-partum anestrus cows

Post-partum beef cows are an interesting model for study of the mechanisms by which FSH and LH interact to control folliculogenesis. It is now clear that, during post-partum anestrus, recurrent, non-ovulatory follicle waves occur. In cows in good body condition score (BCS) there are typically two non-ovulatory waves of follicle growth before ovulation occurs (Murphy et al., 1990; Crowe et al., 1993), whereas cows in poor BCS have a mean of 9.6 ± 1.2 non-ovulatory follicle waves post-partum before ovulation occurs (Stagg et al., 1995). This lack of ovulation of dominant follicles in post-partum beef cows is associated with a lack of LH pulses, assumed to be required to induce sufficient androgen precursor for FSH stimulated estradiol secretion and subsequently a pre-ovulatory gonadotropin surge and ovulation (Crowe, 2008).

The first post-partum DF is capable of ovulating provided a sufficient gonadotropin signal is available. Crowe et al. (1993) demonstrated that administration of 20 µg Buserelin during the growing/plateau phase of the first postpartum DF in beef cows will induce it to ovulate. Thus, to test the hypothesis that failure of ovulation of dominant follicles during post-partum anestrus in beef cows is due to inadequate LH pulse frequency to stimulate androgen precursor for estradiol synthesis, Duffy et al. (1998) assigned post-partum beef cows to receive either saline, 50 or 100 µg pLH hourly (administration via pulse infusion pumps) for 3 days commencing on the second day of dominance of the first post-partum DF. In 3 of 7 cows receiving 100 µg pLH / hour, ovulation of the first post-partum DF occurred. This result suggests that if sufficient LH is present to stimulate androgen precursor for FSH-induced estradiol production, a positive feedback effect of estradiol on GnRH release can occur, causing an LH surge and hence ovulation of the first DF post-partum. The inconsistent response may be due to a number of possible factors: i) the time of initiation of LH pulses (second day of dominance) may be borderline; ii) the dose of LH may have been inadequate to stimulate sufficient estradiol secretion in some animals or iii) the fact that porcine LH was used in this study rather than bovine LH may have resulted in a lower biopotency of the LH administered than predicted from the dose used. In any event, this study helps confirm the hypothesis that failure of ovulation of early dominant follicles during the post-partum period of beef cows is due to inadequate secretion of LH.

Alternatively studies using nutritional restriction to induce a state of anestrus in cows and then subsequent administration of GnRH has be used to determine the appropriate GnRH pulse frequency to stimulate LH, FSH and ovarian follicular responses. Pulsatile infusion of GnRH once every hour induced ovulation in 6 of 8 nutritionally anestrous cows, whereas continuous infusion of the equivalent amout of GnRH or infusion of a GnRH pulse every 4 hours was much less effective at stimulating resumption of ovulation (Vizcarra et al., 1997). In a further study using nutritionally restricted ovariectomized cows, pulsatile infusion of 2 µg GnRH at a low frequency (once per 4 h) predominantly stimulated LH release only, where as pulsatile infusion of 2 μg GnRH every hour stimulated LH and FSH. At higher doses of GnRH (4 μg) a downregulation of the LH and FSH responses occurred with LH and FSH release only occurring on the 1st and 3rd days of treatment (Vizcarra et al., 1999). These studies suggest that concentrations of LH and FSH in blood of cows, and the ratio of LH to FSH, can be altered by the frequency and amount of GnRH stimulation. Changes in the ratio of LH to FSH that occur in cows in different physiological states may be due to the frequency that GnRH pulses are released from the hypothalamus. Furthermore the ability to induce follicle growth and ovulation is dependent on the pattern and frequency of GnRH pulses and the concomitant effect on differential secretion of LH and FSH.

4.4. Delayed follicle selection

Adams et al. (1993) and Mihm et al. (1997) demonstrated that administration of FSH, before the end of selection, delays the end of selection and attainment of dominance by 1.5 days. Indeed Mihm et al. (1997) concluded that exogenous FSH administered in physiological amounts on days 2 and 3 of the estrous cycle of cattle delayed selection of the first DF and atresia of subordinate follicles and blocked most of the alterations in intrafollicular hormones and growth factors that normally occur during the selection process. These data support the hypothesis that the decline in FSH concentrations to basal levels, following an FSH increase, causes the diverse alterations in FSH-dependent growth factors and hormones within the cohort of pre-selection follicles that lead to the end of the selection process and thus is responsible for differentially inducing both continued growth and enhanced estradiol-producing capacity of the DF and atresia of the subordinate follicles in the cohort.

5. Superovulation in cattle

Superovulation is used as part of commercial multiple ovulation and embryo transfer (MOET) programs as the major method to produce embryos as part of cattle breeding improvement. Superovulatory responses are highly variable ranging from 2 to 80 ovulations and producing 0 to 60 blastocysts following non-surgical flushing. Various factors contribute to the variability in response to superovulatory treatments. These include choice of gonadotropin, animal condition and health, follicle population associated with each wave emergence, presence or absence of a dominant follicle at the time of initiation of gonadotropin treatment, and presence or absence of a CL while treating with FSH.

The options for gonadotropins for use with superovulation in cattle is really between FSH products or equine chorionic gonadotropin (eCG). FSH has a relatively short half-life and must be administered as twice daily injections over 4 days. eCG is predominantly FSH like in action, but has a longer half life and therefore a single injection is sufficient. One problem with eCG is that the prolonged half life can mean that residual FSH activity continues to stimulate follicle growth after ovulation occurs. This has a negative effect on fertilization rate and/or zygote development (likely due to the high estradiol concentrations from these additional growing follicles). For this reason eCG gives high variability when used for superovulation. Therefore repeated FSH injections are generally the preferred treatment to use in cattle.

Traditionally superovulation treatments commenced between days 8 and 12 post estrus. This required synchronization of estrus and then commencing gonadotropin treatment 8 to 12 days after the onset of estrus. Generally the protocols required observation for the synchronized estrus so that day of commencement of treatment was accurately determined. The initiation of superovulation treatment on days 8 to 12 was considered to be optimal. But the mechanisms as to why were not understood. None of the early studies actually monitored follicular status as this work was generally completed before the advent of ultrasound scanning of ovaries for follicle structures. With the advent of transrectal ultrasonography in the late 1980s studies have characterized the pattern of follicular growth throughout the estrous cycle in cattle (Savio et al., 1988; Knopf et al., 1989; Sirois and Fortune 1988). Days 8 to 12 coincides with emergence of the second follicular wave, and the FSH used for ovarian stimulation augments the spontaneous FSH rise that stimulates emergence of the second follicular wave of the cycle (reviewed by Bo et al., 1995). However the precise day of emergence of the second follicular wave is actually dependent on whether the animal has 2 or 3 waves of follicles per cycle. With animals having a 3 wave cycle the day of emergence of the second wave is typically 1-2 days earlier (ie day 7 / 8 of the cycle) than those having a 2-wave cycle (ie days 9/10 of the cycle). It has been clearly shown that initiation of the gonadotropin treatment for superovulation at follicle wave emergence gives a better response than at a later stage of follicle wave development (Adams et al., 1994; Nasser et al., 1993). Starting the FSH treatment as little as one day after emergence of the wave reduced the superovulatory response compared with commencement on the day of follicle wave emergence (Adams et al., 1994b; Nasser et al., 1993).

One approach to manipulating the time of follicle wave emergence is to ablate all follicles (≥5mm diameter) across both ovaries by transvaginal ultrasound guided follicle aspiration. Then superovulation treatment with gonadotropin can commence 1-2 days later at the time of emergence of the next follicle wave (Baracaldo et al., 2000; Bergfelt et al., 1997). This treatment is quite difficult to implement routinely on farm. Therefore manipulation of follicle waves by hormonal treatments is preferered. Estradiol treatment at the commencement of a progesterone based treatment (CIDR or PRID) will suppress FSH and allow FSH to rebound to stimulate follicle wave emergence 48-72 h after administration of estradiol (Lane et al., 2000). However use of estradiol as part of an estrous synchronization program in cattle is now not permitted in many countries (Lane et al., 2008). While GnRH may be used to control follicle waves at the start of a progesterone based treatment, it will only have an effect if there is a healthy dominant follicle (≥10 mm) at the time of GnRH administration, so this is not an ideal option (Lane et al., 2008) to regulate follicle waves before commencement of a superovulatory treatment.

An alternative strategy is to initiate the superovulatory treatment at the start of a synchronized cycle (day 1 after estrus) when the first follicle wave is emerging, but requires use of a CIDR device to be inserted during the gonadotropin treatments, and PGF treatments on day 4 (pm) and day 5 (am). This treatment strategy was reviewed by Bo et al. (2008), and provides an acceptable alternative where estrus observation is not going to be done to aid with superovulation by the conventional approach of initiating FSH treatment on days 10 – 12 of a previously synchronized cycle.

It has been shown that following the administration of an experimental GnRH agonist in cattle, follicles grew to ~8 mm in diameter, when pulsatile LH release was inhibited, and to ~4 mm in diameter, when both FSH release and LH pulses were inhibited (Gong et al., 1996; section 4.2 this chapter). Similarly, when an anti-GnRH vaccine was administered (Prendiville et al., 1995; Crowe et al., 2001a; Crowe et al., 2001b; section 4.1 this chapter), follicles grew to 3 mm, but not larger. The growth of follicles to a larger size resumed upon treatment with exogenous FSH and their growth rate in response to exogenous FSH was similar to controls (Crowe et al., 2001a), but with FSH treatment alone the follicles were not estrogen active (Crowe et al., 2001b). Stimulation with a combination of FSH and pulsatile LH stimulated estrogen active follicles to grow (Crowe et al., 2001b), and this would be an appropriate strategy for superovulation. Both approaches provides for the possibility of preparing donor cows that are in a constant state of readiness with follicles that never achieve dominance unless exogenous gonadotropins are administered.

D'Occhio et al. (1997) developed a model in which two implants impregnated with the GnRH agonist, deslorelin, were inserted to desensitize the pituitary gland to GnRH and block the endogenous LH surge. Each implant released 20 mg of deslorelin per 24 h. Seven days after treatment at random stages of the estrous cycle, superstimulatory FSH treatments were initiated and 2 days later PGF2α was administered; 60 h after the PGF2α treatment, ovulation was induced with an injection of pLH (D'Occhio et al., 1997). This treatment protocol was compared with the EB-CIDR superstimulation protocol in Nelore cows and the number of transferable embryos did not differ (Barros and Nogueira, 2001). Unfortunately, deslorelin implants are not commercially available for use in cattle.

6. Conclusions

In conclusion, the mechanisms by which FSH and LH control follicle growth in cattle are complex. Recent models have started to tease apart some of the mechanisms involved. Certainly emergence of follicles > 4 mm in size is FSH dependent and the subsequent fate of selected dominant follicles is dependent on the LH environment present during the dominance phase. Growth of normal estrogen-active follicles beyond 8-9 mm in size is dependent on the presence of adequate LH. Normal luteal phase LH pulse frequencies / amplitudes are required to cause DF turnover (atresia of DF); increased LH pulse frequencies maintained by the presence of continuous progestogens (in the absence of a corpus luteum) will maintain estrogen-active DF for an extended period of time; and follicular phase LH pulse frequencies stimulate final maturation and ovulation of DF.

The precise mechanisms by which follicles achieve the capacity to be selected to become dominant, while subordinates undergo atresia in the face of declining FSH concentrations is still somewhat unclear. However, it can be hypothesized that the follicle destined to become dominant maintains an ability to grow in the presence of declining FSH concentrations due to a number of possible mechanisms: i) increased bioavailability of insulin-like growth factor-I (IGF-I) in that follicle due to reduced total IGF-I binding protein activity (Mihm et al., 1997; Stewart et al., 1996; Canty et al., 2006); ii) expression of LH-receptor messenger RNA (Bao et al., 1997) and LH-receptors (Ireland and Roche, 1983) in granulosa cells of that follicle rendering it more responsive to LH than other follicles in the cohort. Further use of the models discussed in this paper along with identification of expression of key genes involved with these processes should provide further insights in the near future.

Gonadotropin treatments to achieve superovulation are best achieved when administered at the time of emergence of a follicle wave. While strategies have been developed to facilitate this, precise protocols that minimize the need for observation of estrous behavior and achieving optimal superovulatory responses are still being developed.

Author details

Mark A. Crowe* and Michael P. Mullen
School of Veterinary Medicine, University College Dublin, Ireland

7. References

Adams, G.P., Matteri, R.L., Kastelic, J.P., Ko, J.C.H, & Ginther, O.J. (1992). Association between surges of follicle-stimulating hormone and the emergence of follicular waves in heifers. *Journal of Reproduction and Fertility* 94: 177-188.

Adams, T.E. & Adams, B.M. (1986). Gonadotrope function in ovariectomized ewes actively immunized against gonadotropin-releasing hormone (GnRH). *Biology of Reproduction* 35: 360-367.

Adams, T.E. & Adams, B.M. (1990). Reproductive function and feedlot performance of beef heifers actively immunized against GnRH. *Journal of Animal Science* 68: 2793-2802.

Adams, G.P., Kot, K., Smith, C.A. & Ginther, O.J. (1993). Selection of a dominant follicle and suppression of follicular growth in heifers. *Animal Reproduction Science* 30: 259-271.

Adams, G.P., Evans, A.C.O. & Rawlings, N.C. (1994a). Follicular waves and circulating gonadotrophins in 8-month-old prepubertal heifers. *Journal of Reproduction and Fertility* 100: 27-33.

* Corresponding Author

Adams, G.P., Nasser L.F., Bo, G.A., Mapletoft, R.J., Garcia, A, Del Campo, M.R. (1994b). Superstimulatory response of ovarian follicles of wave 1 versus wave 2 in heifers. *Theriogenology* 42: 1103-1113.

Baracaldo, M.I., Martinez, M., Adams, G.P. & Mapletoft R.J. 2000. Superovulatory response following transvaginal follicle ablation in cattle. Theriogenology 53: 1239-1250.

Bao, B., Garverick, H.A., Smith, G.W., Smith, M.F., Salfen, B.E. & Youngquist, R.S. (1997). Changes in messenger ribonucleic acid encoding luteinizing hormone receptor, cytochrome P450-side chain cleavage, and aromatase are associated with recruitment and selection of bovine ovarian follicles. *Biology of Reproduction* 56: 1158-1168.

Barros, C.M. and Nogueira, M.F.G. (2001). Embryo transfer in Bos indicus cattle. *Theriogenology* 56: 1483-1496.

Bergfelt, D.R., Bo, G.A., Mapletoft R.J. & Adams, G.P. (1997). Superovulatory response following ablation-induced follicular wave emergence at random stages of the oestrous cycle in cattle. *Animal Reproduction Science* 49: 1-12.

Bo, G.A., Adams, G.P., Pierson, R.A. & Mapletoft, R.J. (1995). Exogenous control of follicular wave emergence in cattle. *Theriogenology* 43: 31-40.

Bo, G.A., Guerrero, D.C. & Adams, G.P. (2008). Alternative approaches to setting up donar cows for superstimulation. *Theriogenology* 69: 81-87.

Campbell, B.K., Scaramuzzi, R.J. & Webb, R. (1995). Control of antral follicle development and selection in sheep and cattle. *Journal of Reproduction and Fertility* Supplement 49: 335-350.

Canty, M.J., Boland, M.P., Evans, A.C.O. & Crowe, M.A. (2006). Alterations in follicular IGFBP-2, -3 and –4 mRNA expression and intrafollicular IGFBP concentrations during the first follicle wave in beef heifers. *Animal Reproduction Science* 93: 199-217.

Cooke, D.J., Crowe, M.A. and Roche, J.F. (1997). Circulating FSH isoform patterns during recurrent increases in FSH throughout the oestrous cycle of heifers. *Journal of Reproduction and Fertility* 110: 339-345.

Crowe, M.A. (2008). Resumption of ovarian cyclicity in postpartum beef and dairy cows. *Reproduction in Domestic Animals* 43 (Suppl. 5): 20-28.

Crowe, M.A., Goulding, D., Baguisi, A., Boland, M.P. & Roche, J.F. (1993). Induced ovulation of the first postpartum dominant follicle in beef suckler cows using a GnRH analogue. *Journal of Reproduction and Fertility* 99: 551-555.

Crowe, M.A., Padmanabhan, V., Mihm, M., Beitins, I.Z. & Roche, J.F. (1998). Resumption of follicular waves in beef cows is not associated with periparturient changes in follicle-stimulating hormone heterogeneity despite major changes in steroid and luteinizing hormone concentrations. *Biology of Reproduction* 58, 1445-1450.

Crowe, M.A., Enright, W.J., Boland, M.P. & Roche, J.F. (2001a). Follicular growth and serum follicle-stimulating hormone (FSH) responses to recombinant bovine FSH in GnRH-immunized heifers. *Animal Science* 73: 115-122.

Crowe, M.A., Kelly, P., Driancourt, M.A., Boland, M.P. & Roche, J.F. (2001b). Effects of FSH with and without LH on serum hormone concentrations, follicle growth and intra-follicular estradiol and aromatase activity in GnRH-immunized heifers. *Biology of Reproduction* 64: 368-374.

Cupp, A.S., Stumpf, T.T., Kojima, F.N., Werth, L.A., Wolfe, M.W., Roberson, M.S., Kittok, R.J. & Kinder, J.E. (1995). Secretion of gonadotrophins change during the luteal phase of the bovine oestrous cycle in the absence of corresponding changes in progesterone or 17 β-oestradiol. *Animal Reproduction Science* 37: 109-119.

D'Occhio, M.J., Sudha, G., Jillella, D., White, T., MacLellan, L.J., Walsh, J., Trigg, T .E. & Miller, D. (1997). Use of GnRH agonist to prevent the endogenous LH surge and injection of exogenous LH to induce ovulation in heifers superstimulated with FSH: a new model for superovulation. *Theriogenology* 47:601–613.

Duffy, P., Crowe, M.A., Boland, M.P. & Roche, J.F. (2000). The effect of exogenous LH pulses on the fate of the first dominant follicle in post-partum beef cows nursing calves. *Journal of Reproduction and Fertility* 118: 9-17.

Evans, A.C.O., Komar, C.M., Wandji, S-A., Fortune, J.E. (1997). Changes in androgen secretion and luteinizing hormone pulse amplitude are associated with the recruitment and growth of ovarian follicles during the luteal phase of the bovine estrous cycle. *Biology of Reproduction* 57: 394-401.

Ginther, O.J., Kastelic, J.P. & Knopf, L. (1989). Composition and characteristics of follicular waves during the bovine estrous cycle. *Animal Reproduction Science* 20: 187-200.

Ginther, O.J., Kot, K., Kulick, L.J., Martin, S. & Wiltbank, M.C. (1996). Relationships between FSH and ovarian follicular waves during the last six months of pregnancy in cattle. *Journal of Reproduction and Fertility* 108: 271-279.

Gong, J.G., Bramley, T.A., Gutierrez, C.G., Peters, A.R. & Webb, R. (1995). Effects of chronic treatment with a gonadotrophin-releasing hormone agonist on peripheral concentrations of FSH and LH, and ovarian function in heifers. *Journal of Reproduction and Fertility* 105: 263-270.

Gong, J.G., Campbell, B.K., Bramley, T.A., Gutierrez, C.G., Peters, A.R. & Webb, R. (1996). Suppression in the secretion of follicle-stimulating hormone and luteinizing hormone, and ovarian follicle development in heifers continuously infused with a gonadotrophin-releasing hormone agonist. *Biology of Reproduction* 55: 68-74.

Goodman, A.L. and Hodgen, G.D. (1983). The ovarian triad of the primate menstrual cycle. *Recent Progress in Hormone Research* 39: 1-73.

Hamilton, S.A., Garverick, H.A., Keisler, D.H., Xu, Z.Z., Loos, K., Youngquist, R.S. & Salfen, B.E. (1995). Characterization of ovarian follicular cysts and associated endocrine profiles in dairy cows. *Biology of Reproduction* 53: 890-898.

Ireland, J.J. & Roche, J.F. (1983). Development of nonovulatory antral follicles in heifers: changes in steroids in follicular fluid and receptors for gonadotropins. *Endocrinology* 112: 150-156.

Ireland, J.J. and Roche, J.F. (1987). Hypothesis regarding development of dominant follicles during a bovine estrous cycle. In *Follicular Growth and Ovulation Rate in Farm Animals*, pp 1-18 Eds J.F. Roche & D. O'Callaghan. Martinus Nijhoff, The Hague.

Knopf, L., Kastelic, J.P., Schallenberger, E. & Ginther, O.J. (1989). Ovarian follicular dynamics in heifers: test of two-wave hypothesis by ultrasonically monitoring individual follicles. *Domestic Animal Endocrinology* 6: 111-119.

Lane, E.A., Austin, E.J., Roche, J.F. & Crowe, M.A. (2001). The effect of estradiol benzoate or a synthetic gonadotropin-releasing hormone used at the start of a progesterone treatment on estrous response in cattle. *Theriogenology* 56: 79-90.

Lane, E.A., Austin, E.J. & Crowe, M.A. (2008). Oestrous synchronisation in cattle - current options following the EU regulations restricting use of oestrogenic compounds in food producing animals: a review. *Animal Reproduction Science* 109: 1-16.

Mihm, M., Baguisi, A., Boland, M.P. & Roche, J.F. (1994). Association between the duration of dominance of the ovulatory follicle and pregnancy rate in beef heifers. *Journal of Reproduction and Fertility* 102: 123-130.

Mihm, M., Curran, N., Hyttel, P., Knight, P.G., Boland, M.P. & Roche, J.F. (1999). Effect of dominant follicle persistence on follicular fluid oestradiol and inhibin and on oocyte maturation in heifers.. *Journal of Reproduction and Fertility* 116: 293-304.

Mihm, M., Boland, M.P., Knight, P.G. & Roche, J.F. (1995). Relationship between gonadotrophins and follicular fluid oestradiol and inhibin during the loss of dominance of the first dominant follicle in beef heifers *Proceedings of the A.E.T.E. 11th Scientific Meeting*, Hannover p. 208.

Mihm, M., Good, T.E.M., Ireland, J.L.H., Ireland, J.J., Knight, P.G. & Roche, J.F. (1997). Decline in serum follicle-stimulating hormone concentrations alters key intrafollicular growth factors involved in selection of the dominant follicle in heifers. *Biology of Reproduction* 57: 1328-1337.

Murphy, M.G., Boland, M.P. & Roche, J.F. (1990). Pattern of follicular growth and resumption of ovarian activity in post-partum beef suckler cows. *Journal of Reproduction and Fertility* 90: 523-533.

Nasser, L., Adams, G.P., Bo, G.A. & Mapletoft R.J. (1993). Ovarian superstimulatory response relative top follicular wave emergence in heifers. *Theriogenology* 40: 713-724.

Prendiville, D.J., Enright, W.J., Crowe, M.A., Finnerty, M., Hynes, N. & Roche, J.F. (1995). Immunization of heifers against gonadotropin-releasing hormone: antibody titers, ovarian function, body growth, and carcass characteristics. *Journal of Animal Science* 73: 2382-2389.

Prendiville, D.J., Enright, W.J., Crowe, M.A., Finnerty, M. & Roche, J.F. (1996). Normal or induced secretory patterns of luteinising hormone and follicle-stimulating hormone in anoestrous gonadotrophin-releasing hormone-immunized and cyclic control heifers. *Animal Reproduction Science* 45: 177-190.

Rahe, C.H., Owens, R.E., Fleeger, J.L., Newton, H.J. & Harms, P.G. (1980). Pattern of plasma luteinizing hormone in the cyclic cow: dependence upon the period of the cycle. *Endocrinology* 107: 498-503.

Roche, J.F. (1996). Control and regulation of folliculogenesis - a symposium in perspective. *Reviews of Reproduction* 1: 19-27.

Savio, J.D., Keenan, L., Boland, M.P. & Roche, J.F. (1988). Pattern of growth of dominant follicles during the oestrous cycle of heifers. *Journal of Reproduction and Fertility* 83: 663-671.

Savio, J.D., Thatcher, W.W., Morris, G.R., Entwistle, K., Drost, M. & Mattiacci, M.R. (1993). Effects of induction of low plasma progesterone concentrations with a progesterone-releasing intravaginal device on follicular turnover and fertility in cattle. *Journal of Reproduction and Fertility* 98: 77-84.

Sirois, J. & Fortune, J.E. (1988). Ovarian follicular dynamics during the estrous cycle in heifers monitored by real-time ultrasonography. *Biology of Reproduction* 39: 308-317.

Sirois, J. & Fortune, J.E. (1990). Lengthening of the bovine estrous cycle with two levels of exogenous progesterone: a model for studying ovarian follicular dominance. *Endocrinology* 127: 916-925.

Stagg, K., Diskin, M.G., Sreenan, J.M. & Roche, J.F. (1995). Follicular development in long-term anoestrous suckler beef cows fed two levels of energy postpartum. *Animal Reproduction Science* 38: 49-61.

Stevens, J. D., Sosa, J. M., deAvila, D. M., Oatley, J. M., Bertrand, K. P., Gaskins, C. T. & Reeves, J. J. (2005). Luteinizing hormone-releasing hormone fusion protein vaccines block estrous cycle activity in beef heifers. *Journal of Animal Science* 83: 152-159.

Stewart, R.E., Spicer, L.J., Hamilton, T.D., Keefer, B.E., Dawson, L.J., Morgan, G.L. & Echternkamp, S.E. (1996). Levels of insulin-like growth factor (IGF) binding proteins, luteinizing hormone and IGF-I receptors, and steroids in dominant follicles during the first follicular wave in cattle exhibiting regular estrous cycles. *Endocrinology* 137: 2842-2850.

Sunderland, S.J., Crowe, M.A., Boland, M.P., Roche, J.F. & Ireland, J.J. (1994). Selection, dominance and atresia of follicles during the oestrous cycle of heifers. *Journal of Reproduction and Fertility* 101: 547-555.

Vizcarra, J.A., Wettemann, R.P., Braden, T., Turzillo, A.M. & Nett, T. (1997). Effect of gonadotropin-releasing hormone (GnRH) pulse frequency on serum and pituitary concentrations of luteinizing hormone and follicle-stimulating hormone, GnRH receptors, and messenger ribonucleic acid for gonadotropin subunits in cows. *Endocrinology* 138: 594-601.

Vizcarra, J.A., Wettemann, R.P. & Morgan, G.L. (1999). Influence of dose, frequency and duration of infused gonadotropin releasing hormone on secretion of luteinizing hormone and follicle-stimulating hormone in nutritionally anestrous beef cows. *Domestic Animal Endocrinology* 16: 171-181.

Vizcarra, J.A., Wettemann, R.P. & Karges S.L. (2012). Immunization of beef heifers against gonadotropin-releasing hormone prevents luteal activity and pregnancy: Effect of conjugation to different proteins and effectiveness of adjuvants. *Journal of Animal Science* 90: 1479-1488.

Chapter 7

Regulation and Function of Gonadotropins Throughout the Bovine Oestrous Cycle

Mark A. Crowe and Michael P. Mullen

Additional information is available at the end of the chapter

http://dx.doi.org/10.5772/53870

1. Introduction

Gonadotropins are protein hormones secreted by the pituitary gland and include luteinizing hormone (LH) and follicle stimulating hormone (FSH). Both LH and FSH govern the estrous cycle i.e. the cyclical pattern of ovarian activity that facilitates the transition of female animals between periods of reproductive non-receptivity to receptivity enabling mating and subsequent pregnancy. The onset of estrous cycles occurs at the time of puberty. In heifers puberty occurs at 6–12 months of age, generally at a weight of 200–250 kg. The normal duration of an estrous cycle in cattle is 18–24 days. The cycle consists of two discrete phases: the luteal phase (14–18 days) and the follicular phase (4–6 days). The luteal phase is the period following ovulation when the corpus luteum (CL) is formed (often further designated as met-estrus and diestrus), while the follicular phase is the period following the demise of the corpus luteum (luteolysis) until ovulation (often further designated as pro-oestrus and oestrus). During the follicular phase, final maturation and ovulation of the ovulatory follicle occurs, the oocyte is released into the oviduct allowing the potential for fertilization.

2. Gonadotropin regulation of follicle growth during the estrous cycle

Cattle are polyestrous animals and display estrous behavior approximately every 21 days. The estrous cycle is regulated by the hormones of the hypothalamus (gonadotropin-releasing hormone; GnRH), the anterior pituitary (follicle-stimulating hormone; FSH and luteinizing hormone; LH), the ovaries (progesterone; P4, estradiol; E2 and inhibins) and the uterus (prostaglandin F2α; PGF). These hormones function through a system of positive and negative feedback to govern the estrous cycle of cattle [1]. GnRH was first isolated from the hypothalamus of pigs and is a decapeptide [2, 3]. Its control of the estrous cycle is mediated via its actions on the anterior pituitary which regulates the secretion of the gonadotrophs, LH and FSH [4].

The pulsatile secretion of basal levels of GnRH from the tonic center of the hypothalamus and the pre-ovulatory surge of GnRH from the surge center of the hypothalamus prevents the desensitisation of the GnRH receptor on the gonadotroph cells of the anterior pituitary. After transportation of GnRH from the hypothalamus to the pituitary gland via the hypophyseal portal blood system [5], GnRH binds to its G-protein coupled receptor on the cell surface of the gonadotroph cells [6]. This binding releases intracellular calcium which activates intermediaries in the mitogen activated protein kinases (MAPK) signaling pathway culminating in the release of FSH and LH from storage compartments in the cytoplasm [7]. FSH is only stored in secretory granules in the cytoplasm for short periods of time, whereas LH is stored for longer periods during the estrous cycle [8]. During the follicular phase of the estrous cycle there is a hormonal environment of basal progesterone due to the regression of the corpus luteum (CL). The increased E2 concentrations, derived from the rapid proliferation of the pre-ovulatory dominant follicle (DF), concomitant with the decrease in circulating concentrations of progesterone, induces a surge in GnRH and allows the display of behavioral estrus during which heifers/cows are sexually receptive and will stand to be mounted [9]. This pre-ovulatory GnRH surge induces a coincidental LH and FSH surge [10]. Only when serum progesterone concentrations are basal and LH pulse frequency increases to one per hour for 2–3 days does the DF ovulate [1]. Ovulation occurs 10–14 h after estrus and is followed by the luteal phase of the estrous cycle. The beginning of the luteal phase is also known as met-estrus and typically lasts 3–4 days. It is characterised by the formation of the CL from the collapsed ovulated follicle (corpus haemorragicum). Following ovulation, progesterone concentrations begin to increase due to the formation of the CL in which the granulosa and theca cells of the ovulated DF lutenize and produce progesterone in readiness for the establishment and maintenance of pregnancy and/or resumption of the estrous cycle [11]. During the di-estrous phase, progesterone concentrations remain elevated and recurrent waves of follicle development continue to be initiated by release of FSH from the anterior pituitary. However, these DFs that grow during the luteal phase of the estrous cycle do not ovulate, due to inadequate LH pulse frequency.

The progesterone dominant luteal phase of the estrous cycle, through negative feedback, only allows the secretion of greater amplitude but less frequent LH pulses (one pulse per 3 to 4 hours) that are inadequate for ovulation of the DF [12]. Finally, during the pro-estrous period, progesterone concentrations decrease when the CL regresses in response to PGF secretion from the uterus [13].

3. Gonadotropin regulation of final maturation of the pre-ovulatory follicle and ovulation

The growth, development and maturation of ovarian follicles are fundamental processes for high reproductive efficiency in farm animals. A fixed number of primordial follicles are established during fetal development with ovarian follicle growth taking a period of 3–4 months and categorized into gonadotropin independent and gonadotropin dependent stages [14]. Gonadotropin dependent follicle growth in cattle occurs in waves with 2–3 waves per estrous cycle [15, 16 Fig.1].

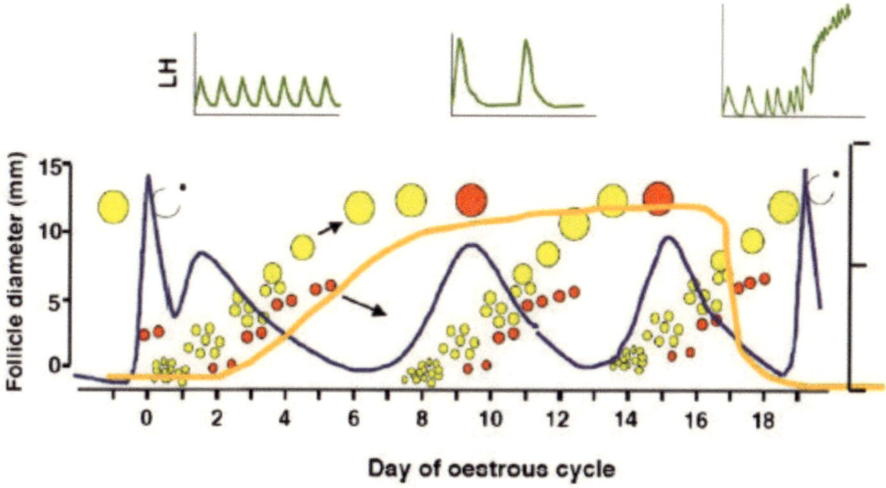

Figure 1. Schematic depiction of the pattern of secretion of follicle-stimulating hormone (FSH; blue line), luteinizing hormone (LH; green lines), and progesterone (P4; orange line); and the pattern of growth of ovarian follicles during the estrous cycle in cattle. Each wave of follicular growth is preceded by a transient rise in FSH concentrations. Healthy growing follicles are shaded in yellow, atretic follicles are shaded red. A surge in LH and FSH concentrations occurs at the onset of estrus and induces ovulation. The pattern of secretion of LH pulses during an 8-h window early in the luteal phase (greater frequency, lesser amplitude), the mid-luteal phase (lesser frequency, lesser amplitude) and the follicular phase (high frequency, building to the surge) is indicated in the inserts in the top panel. Taken from [17].

Each wave of growth involves emergence, selection and dominance followed by either atresia or ovulation of the DF. As mentioned above both FSH and LH have a prominent role in ovarian follicle development. Given that follicles are involved in the positive and negative feedback mechanisms of the hypothalamic–pituitary–gonadal (HPG) axis (estradiol and inhibins), these hormones have a governing role in the regulation of the estrous cycle of cattle. The beginning of gonadotropin dependent follicle development is typified by the emergence of a follicle cohort typically consisting of 5–20 follicles ≥5mm and is correlated with a transient increase in FSH concentrations [10, 18]. This marks the beginning of dependency of follicle growth on FSH [19] with FSH receptors (FSH-R) localized within the granulosa cells of the follicles by Day 3 of the follicle wave [20, 21]. This enables FSH to perform its required down stream signalling effects including promoting cellular growth and proliferation [22, 23]. These transient increases in FSH concentrations also leads to an increase in aromatase enzyme activity (P450arom; CYP19), in the granulosa cells of ovarian follicles, which converts androgen to estrogen [24]. As the DF is selected from the cohort of follicles, the diameter increases and it is recognized as the largest healthy follicle in the cohort [25]. This increase in size leads to an increase in follicular fluid estradiol and inhibin concentrations [24]. Dominance occurs when the the DF reaches 9 mm in diameter, and it actively suppresses FSH, thus preventing further follicle wave emergence until the DF either undergoes atresia or ovulated. The increase in estradiol concentrations in concert with inhibin are the key endocrine signals that suppress FSH concentrations from the anterior pituitary gland via negative feedback reducing FSH to basal concentrations [10, 26, 27]. The selected DF becomes increasingly responsive to LH [27] and continues growth in the face of decreasing FSH concentrations. Irrespective of the stage of the estrous cycle during which follicles develop, the switch from FSH [18] to LH dependency [28] is propagated through the presence of LH receptors (LH-R) on the granulosa cells [29]. LH-R are localised to the theca and granulosa cells of healthy follicles, at different stages of follicle development [20]. As the follicle grows, the theca cell LH-R increases and LH-R is acquired by the granulosa cells of the follicle undergoing selection to become the DF [29-31]. Moreover, evidence suggests transient increases in circulating LH concentrations that occur at or around the time of follicle selection [32], allows the DF to continue E2 production and grow in the face of declining FSH concentrations [33]. During the early luteal phase lesser amplitude and greater frequency (20–30 pulses/24 h) LH pulses occur, in the mid-luteal period LH pulses are of greater amplitude and lesser frequency (6–8 pulses/24 h) both of which are of insufficient amplitude and frequency for final maturation and subsequent ovulation of the DF [12]. Thus, the DFs produced during the luteal phase of the estrous cycle undergo atresia, E2 and inhibin production decreases, and removes this negative feedback block to the hypothalamus/pituitary, FSH secretion can increase and a new follicle wave emerges. The production of high concentrations of estradiol is a defining characteristic of the DF [33, 34] and prior to visible differences in follicle diameter; the putative DF has greater follicular fluid concentrations of estradiol compared with other follicles in its cohort [10, 35, 36]. The synthesis of estradiol is dependent on the production of androgens in the theca cells and subsequent aromatisation of these androgens to estrogens in the granulosa cells known as the two cell/two gondatropin model [37]. Production of estradiol from growing follicles is dependent on sufficient LH pulse frequency [38, 39]. The binding of LH to its receptors in the theca cells drives the conversion of cholesterol to testosterone through a series of catalytic reactions [40]. Testosterone, once produced in the theca cells, diffuses out into the granulosa cells where it is converted to estrogens by the aromatase enzyme [40]. Estradiol not only has a local effect on follicle development, but it also has a systemic role via a positive feedback mechanism to the hypothalamus and pituitary gland. During the follicular phase of the estrous cycle, when progesterone concentrations are basal, this large concentration of estradiol produced by the pre-ovulatory DF induces a GnRH surge from the hypothalamus. The resulting LH surge is of sufficient amplitude and frequency to stimulate final maturation and ovulation of the DF [10]. The increased estradiol concentrations also induces expression of estrous behavour, required for successful mating [41]. Other intra-ovarian produced factors play a role in regulating the estrous cycle either indirectly by altering the synthesis of estradiol or via direct negative feedback mechanisms to the hypothalamus and the anterior pituitary gland. The insulin like growth factor (IGF) super-family consisting of its two ligands IGF-I and IGF-II [42-44], two receptors IGFR-I and IGFR-II [45], and it numerous binding proteins and proteases (IGFBP 1-6, pregnancy-associated plasma protein-A: PAPP-A) are responsible for the bioavailability of IGF-1 in the ovarian follicle. The bioavailability of IGF-I contributes to the growth, proliferation and steroidogenic capacity of the future DF [36, 46, 47], indirectly affecting the estradiol induced negative feedback mechanism to the hypothalamus and pituitary. This in addition to early acquisition of LH receptors by the granulosa cell layer of the follicle undergoing selection are considered to be the main mechanisms facilitating the process of follicle selection [48]. The transforming growth factor beta (TGF) super-family contains over 30 structurally related proteins including ligands (TGF, anti-mullerian hormone, inhibins, activins, and bone morphogenetic proteins (BMP's), receptors (TGFRI and II, activin receptor-like kinases; ALK's, accessory receptors (TGF-RIII) and downstream signaling molecules (similar to mothers against decapentaplegic; SMADS). The ligand members of this super-family were first identified in follicular fluid through their modulation of secreted FSH [49]. Activin can increase the production of estradiol in follicular fluid [50] whereas follistatin impedes activins' positive steroidogenic effects, both of which can alter the estradiol feedback mechanism to the hypothalamus and pituitary [51]. Inhibins which have been detected in granulosa cells in cattle play a role in the suppression of FSH secreted in the anterior pituitary also regulating the oestrous cycle [52].

4. Estrous behavior

A recent review of the literature [53] reported mean inter-ovulatory intervals of 22.9 and 22.0 days for lactating dairy cows and heifers, respectively. Standing to be mounted by a bull or herd mate is the primary and most definitive sign of oestrus in cattle. Estrogen, specifically, estradiol, is the primary signal to the brain that induces expression of estrus, but only in the absence of progesterone [54]. It appears that stressors which elevate blood concentrations of cortisol are capable of delaying or blocking the pre-ovulatory LH surge and affecting the expression of estrus without altering pro-oestrous concentrations of blood oestradiol (see review by [55]). In a recent review, Diskin [56] calculated that for dairy cows the average duration of standing estrus was 8.1 h with 9.1 standing events or mounts recorded during standing estrus. There is evidence [57] that the duration of standing estrus decreases as milk production increases (14.7 and 2.8 h in cows yielding 25 or 55 kg milk, respectively). For heifers it would appear that the duration of standing estrus is somewhat longer, 12–14 h [56]. For beef cows, kept indoors, the average duration of standing estrus has been reported to be less than 8.5 h [56]. Both the duration of standing estrus and intensity of estrous expression are affected by a range of environmental factors including under foot surface type, size of the sexually active group and the presence of a bull [56]. Breaks or quiescent interludes in standing activity have also been observed in 30% of dairy cows at [58] while breaks with an average duration of 2.6 h in 67% of beef heifers have been recorded [59]. There is no evidence from dairy cows [60], beef cows or heifers [56] that either the onset of standing estrus or end of estrus follows any distinct diurnal pattern.

5. Gonadotropin regulation of Corpus luteum function

The CL originates from the cells of the ovulatory follicle. LH, the major luteotropic hormone in cattle [61], is responsible for stimulating luteinization of the theca and granulosa cells of the pre-ovulatory follicle into luteal cells [62]. The function of the CL is to produce sufficient concentrations of progesterone throughout the luteal phase of the estrous cycle to maintain pregnancy (if a conceptus is present) and during pregnancy, to decrease gonadotropin secretion and prevent behavioral oestrus occurring. Progesterone is required for the maintenance of pregnancy with many studies reporting a positive association between progesterone concentrations and the probability of embryo survival [63-66]. The proposed mechanisms by which progesterone affects embryo survival are indirect, not acting on the embryo itself but via effects on the uterine endometrium [67, 68]. Available evidence in both cattle and sheep, has identified that sustained increased concentrations of progesterone during the luteal phase of the estrous cycle alters the expression pattern of genes in the uterus [69-73] which in turn alters the composition of the uterine histotroph i.e. availability of enzymes, carrier proteins, hormones and nutrients to the developing embryo prior to implantation [68]. Moreover, alterations in systemic progesterone during the early luteal phase have been shown to have significant effects on conceptus elongation [67, 71, 74]. During the mid-luteal phase, these sustained high concentrations of circulating progesterone down regulate the nuclear progesterone receptor in the luminal epithelium of the endometrium [75]. This is a critical switch in allowing the synchronous increase or decrease in genes of the endometrium that are required to initiate uterine receptivity – regardless of the pregnancy status of the animal [76]. If, by Day 16 of the estrous cycle, the maternal recognition of pregnancy signal (interferon tau) has not been detected in sufficient quantities, luteolysis of the CL occurs. PGF is secreted by the uterus in the bovine [77] and is the major luteolytic hormone in ruminants [78-80]. Oxytocin receptors in the uterus binds oxytocin which propagates the episodic secretion of PGF from the uterus. PGF then mediates the luteolytic mechanism via countercurrent exchange between the uterine vein and the ovarian artery (Fig. 2), inducing regression of the CL. This reduces circulating progesterone concentrations, estradiol concentrations increase and GnRH in the hypothalamus is stimulated as the animal enters the follicular phase of the estrous cycle.

6. Conclusions

The estrous cycle in cattle is typically 18–24 days in duration, with estrous behavior expressed for a 2–24-h period during the late follicular phase. During normal estrous cycles there are typically two to three and occasionally four waves of follicular growth each involving a period of emergence, selection and dominance followed by either atresia or ovulation of the DF. The gonadotropin hormones FSH and LH are the main regulators of folliculogenesis and steroidogenesis with LH being the major luteotrophic hormone. LH pulse frequency is the major determinant affecting the ultimate fate of a selected DF. Pulsatile PGF of uterine origin is the main hormonal signal that induces luteolysis of the CL and the switch from the luteal to the follicular phase of the estrous cycle.

Author details

Mark A. Crowe* and Michael P. Mullen
School of Veterinary Medicine, University College Dublin, Ireland

---

* Corresponding Author

7. References

[1] Roche JF. Control and regulation of folliculogenesis--a symposium in perspective. Rev Reprod. 1996 January 1, 1996;1(1):19-27.

[2] Baba Y, Matsuo H, Schally AV. Structure of the porcine LH- and FSH-releasing hormone. II. Confirmation of the proposed structure by conventional sequential analyses. Biochem Biophys Res Commun. 1971;44(2):459-63.

[3] Schally AV, Arimura A, Baba Y, Nair RMG, Matsuo H, Redding TW, et al. Isolation and properties of the FSH and LH-releasing hormone. Biochem Biophys Res Commun. 1971;43(2):393-9.

[4] Schally AV, Arimura A, Kastin AJ, Matsuo H, Baba Y, Redding TW, et al. Gonadotropin-Releasing Hormone: One Polypeptide Regulates Secretion of Luteinizing and Follicle-Stimulating Hormones. Science. 1971 September 10, 1971;173(4001):1036-8.

[5] Moenter SM, Brand RC, Karsch FJ. Dynamics of gonadotropin-releasing hormone (GnRH) secretion during the GnRH surge: insights into the mechanism of GnRH surge induction. Endocrinology. 1992 May 1, 1992;130(5):2978-84.

[6] Kakar SS, Rahe CH, Neill JD. Molecular cloning, sequencing, and characterizing the bovine receptor for gonadotropin releasing hormone (GNRH). Domest Anim Endocrinol. 1993;10(4):335-42.

[7] Weck J, Fallest PC, Pitt LK, Shupnik MA. Differential Gonadotropin-Releasing Hormone Stimulation of Rat Luteinizing Hormone Subunit Gene Transcription by Calcium Influx and Mitogen-Activated Protein Kinase-Signaling Pathways. Mol Endocrinol. 1998 March 1, 1998;12(3):451-7.

[8] Farnworth PG. Gonadotrophin secretion revisited. How many ways can FSH leave a gonadotroph? J Endocrinol. 1995 June 1, 1995;145(3):387-95.

[9] Frandson R, Wilke WL, Fails AD. Anatomy and physiology of farm animals. Lippincott Williams and Wilkins, Baltimore. 2003.

[10] Sunderland SJ, Crowe MA, Boland MP, Roche JF, Ireland JJ. Selection, dominance and atresia of follicles during the oestrous cycle of heifers. J Reprod Fertil. 1994 August 1, 1994;101(3):547-55.

[11] Niswender G. Mechanisms controlling luteolysis. Raven Press, New York 1981.

[12] Rahe CH, Owens RE, Fleeger JL, Newton HJ, Harms PG. Pattern of Plasma Luteinizing Hormone in the Cyclic Cow: Dependence upon the Period of the Cycle. Endocrinology. 1980 August 1, 1980;107(2):498-503.

[13] Hansel W, Convey EM. Physiology of the Estrous Cycle. J Anim Sci. 1983 July 1, 1983;57(Supplement 2):404-24.

[14] Webb R, Garnsworthy PC, Gong JG, Armstrong DG. Control of follicular growth: Local interactions and nutritional influences. J Anim Sci. 2004 January 1, 2004;82(13 suppl):E63-E74.

[15] Rajakoski E. The ovarian follicular system in sexually mature heifers with special reference to seasonal, cyclical, end left-right variations. Acta Endocrinol Suppl (Copenh). 1960;34(Suppl 52):1-68.

[16] Savio JD, Keenan L, Boland MP, Roche JF. Pattern of growth of dominant follicles during the oestrous cycle of heifers. J Reprod Fertil. 1988 July 1, 1988;83(2):663-71.
[17] Forde N, Beltman ME, Lonergan P, Diskin M, Roche JF, Crowe MA. Oestrous cycles in Bos taurus cattle. Anim Reprod Sci. 2011;124(3–4):163-9.
[18] Adams GP, Matteri RL, Kastelic JP, Ko JCH, Ginther OJ. Association between surges of follicle-stimulating hormone and the emergence of follicular waves in heifers. J Reprod Fertil. 1992 January 1, 1992;94(1):177-88.
[19] Ginther OJ, Bergfelt DR, Beg MA, Kot K. Role of low circulating FSH concentrations in controlling the interval to emergence of the subsequent follicular wave in cattle. Reproduction. 2002 October 1, 2002;124(4):475-82.
[20] Camp TA, Rahal JO, Mayo KE. Cellular Localization and Hormonal Regulation of Follicle-Stimulating Hormone and Luteinizing Hormone Receptor Messenger RNAs in the Rat Ovary. Mol Endocrinol. 1991 October 1, 1991;5(10):1405-17.
[21] Evans ACO, Fortune JE. Selection of the Dominant Follicle in Cattle Occurs in the Absence of Differences in the Expression of Messenger Ribonucleic Acid for Gonadotropin Receptors. Endocrinology. 1997 July 1, 1997;138(7):2963-71.
[22] Richards JS. Hormonal Control of Gene Expression in the Ovary. Endocr Rev. 1994 December 1994;15(6):725-51.
[23] Richards JS, Russell DL, Robker RL, Dajee M, Alliston TN. Molecular mechanisms of ovulation and luteinization. Mol Cell Endocrinol. 1998;145(1–2):47-54.
[24] Hillier SG. Current concepts of the roles of follicle stimulating hormone and luteinizing hormone in folliculogenesis. Hum Reprod. 1994 February 1, 1994;9(2):188-91.
[25] Gougeon A, Lefèvre B. Evolution of the diameters of the largest healthy and atretic follicles during the human menstrual cycle. J Reprod Fertil. 1983 November 1, 1983;69(2):497-502.
[26] Ginther OJ, Bergfelt DR, Kulick LJ, Kot K. Selection of the Dominant Follicle in Cattle: Role of Two-Way Functional Coupling Between Follicle-Stimulating Hormone and the Follicles. Biol Reprod. 2000 April 1, 2000;62(4):920-7.
[27] Ginther OJ, Bergfelt DR, Kulick LJ, Kot K. Selection of the Dominant Follicle in Cattle: Role of Estradiol. Biol Reprod. 2000 August 1, 2000;63(2):383-9.
[28] Kulick LJ, Kot K, Wiltbank MC, Ginther OJ. Follicular and hormonal dynamics during the first follicular wave in heifers. Theriogenology. 1999;52(5):913-21.
[29] Xu Z, Garverick HA, Smith GW, Smith MF, Hamilton SA, Youngquist RS. Expression of follicle-stimulating hormone and luteinizing hormone receptor messenger ribonucleic acids in bovine follicles during the first follicular wave. Biol Reprod. 1995 October 1, 1995;53(4):951-7.
[30] Bao B, Garverick HA, Smith GW, Smith MF, Salfen BE, Youngquist RS. Changes in messenger ribonucleic acid encoding luteinizing hormone receptor, cytochrome P450-side chain cleavage, and aromatase are associated with recruitment and selection of bovine ovarian follicles. Biol Reprod. 1997 May 1, 1997;56(5):1158-68.
[31] Braw-Tal R, Roth Z. Gene expression for LH receptor, 17α-hydroxylase and StAR in the theca interna of preantral and early antral follicles in the bovine ovary. Reproduction. 2005 April 1, 2005;129(4):453-61.

[32] Ginther OJ, Beg MA, Donadeu FX, Bergfelt DR. Mechanism of follicle deviation in monovular farm species. Anim Reprod Sci. 2003;78(3–4):239-57.
[33] Ireland JJ, Roche JF. Development of Nonovulatory Antral Follicles in Heifers: Changes in Steroids in Follicular Fluid and Receptors for Gonadotr opins. Endocrinology. 1983 January 1, 1983;112(1):150-6.
[34] Ireland JJ, Roche JF. Development of Antral Follicles in Cattle after Prostaglandin-Induced Luteolysis: Changes in Serum Hormones, Steroids in Follicular Fluid, and Gonadotropin Receptors. Endocrinology. 1982 December 1, 1982;111(6):2077-86.
[35] Fortune JE. Ovarian follicular growth and development in mammals. Biol Reprod. 1994 February 1, 1994;50(2):225-32.
[36] Mihm M, Austin EJ, Good TEM, Ireland JLH, Knight PG, Roche JF, et al. Identification of Potential Intrafollicular Factors Involved in Selection of Dominant Follicles in Heifers. Biol Reprod. 2000 September 1, 2000;63(3):811-9.
[37] Fortune JE, Quirk SM. REGULATION OF STEROIDOGENESIS IN BOVINE PREOVULATORY FOLLICLES. J Anim Sci. 1988 January 1, 1988;66(Supplement 2):1-8.
[38] Crowe MA, Enright WJ, Boland MP, Roche JF. Follicular growth and serum follicle-stimulating hormone (FSH) responses to recombinant bovine FSH in GnRH-immunized anoestrous heifers. Anim Sci. 2001;73:115-22.
[39] Crowe MA, Kelly P, Driancourt MA, Boland MP, Roche JF. Effects of Follicle-Stimulating Hormone With and Without Luteinizing Hormone on Serum Hormone Concentrations, Follicle Growth, and Intrafollicular Estradiol and Aromatase Activity in Gonadotropin-Releasing Hormone-Immunized Heifers. Biol Reprod. 2001 January 1, 2001;64(1):368-74.
[40] Dorrington JH, Moon YS, Armstrong DT. Estradiol-17beta biosynthesis in cultured granulosa cells from hypophysectomised immature rats; stimulation by follicle-stimulating hormone. Endocrinology. 1975;97:1328–31.
[41] Ireland JJ. Control of follicular growth and development. J Reprod Fertil Suppl. 1987;34:39-54.
[42] Rinderknecht E, Humbel RE. The amino acid sequence of human insulin-like growth factor I and its structural homology with proinsulin. J Biol Chem. 1978 April 25, 1978;253(8):2769-76.
[43] Rinderknecht E, Humbel RE. Primary structure of human insulin-like growth factor II. FEBS Lett. 1978;89(2):283-6.
[44] Spicer LJ, Echternkamp SE. The ovarian insulin and insulin-like growth factor system with an emphasis on domestic animals. Domest Anim Endocrinol. 1995;12(3):223-45.
[45] Hammond JM, Mondschein JS, Samaras SE, Smith SA, Hagen DR. The ovarian insulin-like growth factor system. J Reprod Fertil Suppl. 1991;43:199-208.
[46] Rivera GM, Fortune JE. Proteolysis of Insulin-Like Growth Factor Binding Proteins -4 and -5 in Bovine Follicular Fluid: Implications for Ovarian Follicular Selection and Dominance. Endocrinology. 2003 July 1, 2003;144(7):2977-87.
[47] Canty MJ, Boland MP, Evans ACO, Crowe MA. Alterations in follicular IGFBP mRNA expression and follicular fluid IGFBP concentrations during the first follicle wave in beef heifers. Anim Reprod Sci. 2006;93(3–4):199-217.

[48] Lucy MC. The bovine dominant ovarian follicle. J Anim Sci. 2007 March 1, 2007;85(13 suppl):E89-E99.
[49] Knight PG, Glister C. TGF-beta superfamily members and ovarian follicle development. Reproduction. 2006 Aug;132(2):191-206.
[50] Knight PG, Glister C. Local roles of TGF-beta superfamily members in the control of ovarian follicle development. Anim Reprod Sci. 2003 Oct 15;78(3-4):165-83.
[51] Phillips DJ, de Kretser DM. Follistatin: A Multifunctional Regulatory Protein. Front Neuroendocrinol. 1998;19(4):287-322.
[52] Findlay JK, Drummond AE, Dyson ML, Baillie AJ, Robertson DM, Ethier JF. Recruitment and development of the follicle; the roles of the transforming growth factor-β superfamily. Mol Cell Endocrinol. 2002;191(1):35-43.
[53] Wiltbank M, Lopez H, Sartori R, Sangsritavong S, Gümen A. Changes in reproductive physiology of lactating dairy cows due to elevated steroid metabolism. Theriogenology. 2006;65(1):17-29.
[54] Vailes LD, Washburn SP, Britt JH. Effects of various steroid milieus or physiological states on sexual behavior of Holstein cows. J Anim Sci. 1992 July 1, 1992;70(7):2094-103.
[55] Stevenson JS. A review of oestrous behaviour and detection in dairy cows. In: Diskin, MG (Ed) Proc BSAS Occasional Publication No 26, Fertility in the High-Producing Dairy Cow, vol 1, pp 43–62; 2001; 2001. p. 43-62.
[56] Diskin MG. HeatWatch: a telemetric system for heat detection in cattle. Vet Q. 2008;30: 37-48.
[57] Lopez H, Satter LD, Wiltbank MC. Relationship between level of milk production and estrous behavior of lactating dairy cows. Anim Reprod Sci. 2004;81(3–4):209-23.
[58] O'Farrell KJ. Fertility management in the dairy herd. Irish veterinary journal. 1980;34:160-9.
[59] Stevenson JS, Lamb GC, Kobayashi Y, Hoffman DP. Luteolysis During Two Stages of the Estrous Cycle: Subsequent Endocrine Profiles Associated with Radiotelemetrically Detected Estrus in Heifers. J Dairy Sci. 1998;81(11):2897-903.
[60] Dransfield MBG, Nebel RL, Pearson RE, Warnick LD. Timing of Insemination for Dairy Cows Identified in Estrus by a Radiotelemetric Estrus Detection System. J Dairy Sci. 1998;81(7):1874-82.
[61] Hansel W. Luteotrophic and luteolytic mechanisms in bovine corpora lutea. J Reprod Fertil. 1966:33–48.
[62] Alila HW, Hansel W. Origin of different cell types in the bovine corpus luteum as characterized by specific monoclonal antibodies. Biol Reprod. 1984 December 1, 1984;31(5):1015-25.
[63] Stronge AJH, Sreenan JM, Diskin MG, Mee JF, Kenny DA, Morris DG. Post-insemination milk progesterone concentration and embryo survival in dairy cows. Theriogenology. 2005;64(5):1212-24.
[64] Starbuck GR, Darwash AO, Mann GE, Lamming GE. The detection and treatment of post insemination progesteroneinsufficieny in dairy cows. In: Diskin MG, editor. Fertility in the High Producing Dairy Cow BSAS Occasional Pulication No2; 2001; 2001. p. 447-50.

[65] McNeill RE, Sreenan JM, Diskin MG, Cairns MT, Fitzpatrick R, Smith TJ, et al. Effect of systemic progesterone concentration on the expression of progesterone-responsive genes in the bovine endometrium during the early luteal phase. Reprod Fertil Dev. 2006;18(5):573-83.

[66] Parr MH, Mullen MP, Crowe MA, Roche JF, Lonergan P, Evans ACO, et al. The repeatability of embryo survival, and the relationship between plasma progesterone in the early luteal phase and embryo survival in dairy heifers. J Dairy Sci. 2012;In press.

[67] Clemente M, de La Fuente J, Fair T, Al Naib A, Gutierrez-Adan A, Roche JF, et al. Progesterone and conceptus elongation in cattle: a direct effect on the embryo or an indirect effect via the endometrium? Reproduction. 2009 September 1, 2009;138(3):507-17.

[68] Spencer TE, Johnson GA, Bazer FW, Burghardt RC, Palmarini M. Pregnancy recognition and conceptus implantation in domestic ruminants: roles of progesterone, interferons and endogenous retroviruses. Reprod Fertil Dev. 2006;19(1):65-78.

[69] Simmons RM, Erikson DW, Kim J, Burghardt RC, Bazer FW, Johnson GA, et al. Insulin-Like Growth Factor Binding Protein-1 in the Ruminant Uterus: Potential Endometrial Marker and Regulator of Conceptus Elongation. Endocrinology. 2009 September 1, 2009;150(9):4295-305.

[70] Forde N, Carter F, Fair T, Crowe MA, Evans ACO, Spencer TE, et al. Progesterone-regulated changes in endometrial gene expression contribute to advanced conceptus development in cattle. Biol Reprod. 2009 October 2009;81(4):784-94.

[71] Forde N, Beltman ME, Duffy GB, Duffy P, Mehta JP, O'Gaora P, et al. Changes in the endometrial transcriptome during the bovine estrous cycle: effect of low circulating progesterone and consequences for conceptus elongation. Biol Reprod. 2011 Sep 29(Feb;84(2)):266-78.

[72] Forde N, Spencer TE, Bazer FW, Song G, Roche JF, Lonergan P. Effect of pregnancy and progesterone concentration on expression of genes encoding for transporters or secreted proteins in the bovine endometrium. Physiol Genomics. 2010 March 1, 2010;41(1):53-62.

[73] Satterfield MC, Gao H, Li X, Wu G, Johnson GA, Spencer TE, et al. Select Nutrients and Their Associated Transporters Are Increased in the Ovine Uterus Following Early Progesterone Administration. Biol Reprod. 2010 January 1, 2010;82(1):224-31.

[74] Carter F, Forde N, Duffy P, Wade M, Fair T, Crowe MA, et al. Effect of increasing progesterone concentration from Day 3 of pregnancy on subsequent embryo survival and development in beef heifers. Reprod Fertil Dev. 2008;20(3):368-75.

[75] Kimmins S, Maclaren LA. Oestrous Cycle and Pregnancy Effects on the Distribution of Oestrogen and Progesterone Receptors in Bovine Endometrium. Placenta. 2001;22(8–9):742-8.

[76] Spencer TE, Sandra O, Wolf E. Genes involved in conceptus–endometrial interactions in ruminants: insights from reductionism and thoughts on holistic approaches. Reproduction. 2008 February 1, 2008;135(2):165-79.

[77] Lamothe P, Bousquet D, Guay P. Cyclic variation of F prostaglandins in the uterine fluids of the cow. J Reprod Fertil. 1977 July 1, 1977;50(2):381-2.

[78] Baird DT, Land RB, Scaramuzzi RJ, Wheeler AG. Endocrine changes associated with luteal regression in the ewe; the secretion of ovarian oestradiol, progesterone and androstenedione and uterine prostaglandin F2 alpha throughout the oestrous cycle. J Endocrinol. 1976 May 1, 1976;69(2):275-86.
[79] Kindahl H, Edqvist LE, Granstrom E, Bane A. The release of prostaglandin F2alpha as reflected by 15-keto-13,14-dihydroprostaglandin F2alpha in the peripheral circulation during normal luteolysis in heifers. Prostaglandins. 1976 May;11(5):871-8.
[80] Nett TM, Staigmiller RB, Akbar AM, Diekman MA, Ellinwood WE, Niswender GD. Secretion of Prostaglandin F2α in Cycling and Pregnant Ewes. J Anim Sci. 1976 April 1, 1976;42(4):876-80.

Chapter 8

Structural and Functional Roles of FSH and LH as Glycoproteins Regulating Reproduction in Mammalian Species

Michael P. Mullen, Dara J. Cooke and Mark A. Crow

Additional information is available at the end of the chapter

http://dx.doi.org/10.5772/48681

1. Introduction

The gonadotropins, a family of closely related glycoprotein hormones, include follicle stimulating-hormone (FSH) and luteinizing hormone (LH) which are produced by the same pituitary cells, the gonadotrophs and chorionic gonadotropin (CG) which is of placental origin. Thyroid-stimulating hormone (TSH) is a structurally related glycoprotein hormone produced by pituitary thyrotroph cells. Gonadotropin-releasing hormone (GnRH) is a decapeptide secreted from the pre-optic and arcuate nuclei of the hypothalamus into the hypophyseal-portal blood vessels which transports it to the anterior pituitary. At the anterior pituitary GnRH stimulates the secretion of LH and FSH, both of which play a central role in ovarian function. The classical studies in sheep (conducted by the Karsch lab in University of Michigan, Ann Arbor), that involved collection of hypophyseal portal blood [1], have shown that pulsatile secretion of GnRH from the hypothalamus is virtually 100% coincident with pulsatile secretion of LH from the anterior pituitary. However, increases in serum FSH levels do not always coincide with increases in levels of LH [2], implying that there may be other mechanisms modifying FSH secretory patterns. The growth, development and maturation of ovarian follicles are fundamental to effective reproduction in animals. In heifers, there are two to three periods or cycles of dominant follicle development during the estrous cycle [3-5]. The key hormone regulating follicular growth is FSH, while pulsatile LH appears to be involved in regulating normal follicular turnover. Our knowledge of the chemistry of the gonadotropic hormones has greatly increased our understanding of the mechanisms of mammalian reproduction. The structural features and the biological properties of the gonadotropins have been under intense investigation for many years as illustrated in several reviews [6-8]. For example, the nucleotide and the amino acid sequences of the gonadotropins from many species are now known and there is extensive information regarding the composition and structure of associated carbohydrate moieties [9-12]. Studies using deglycosylated hormones have played a critical role in the elucidation of the functional properties of both carbohydrate and protein components of the hormones. From these studies it has become evident that isoforms of each hormone arise from variations in the carbohydrate moiety present in the hormone, as opposed to varying amino acid sequences. The ability to detect and quantify levels of gonadotropins has been central to their study. The measurement of biological responses in test animals in vivo were the earliest assays used for these hormones. Today, a variety of in vitro bioassays [13-15] and immunoassays [16] are in use. However, a discrepancy exists between bioassays and immunoassays for gonadotropins: i.e. immunologically active hormone may not always be biologically active [16]. Immunogenicity of glycoprotein hormones is, for the most part, dependent on a peptide epitope while the carbohydrate moieties contribute to the overall bioactivity of the hormone [9, 17, 18]. It should follow then, that isoforms of a particular gonadotropin have different bioactivities, due to the variation in carbohydrates found in them.

This book chapter describes the structural features of the gonadotropins, their proposed biosynthetic pathways and the molecular basis for their heterogeneity. It is now widely accepted that the observed heterogeneity is, to a large extent, due to the variation in the carbohydrate component of these molecules. The nature of this carbohydrate has been shown to influence their biopotency. For example, circulatory half-life, receptor binding and ability to stimulate signal transduction have all been shown to be influenced by the oligosaccharides present in the gonadotropins. The influence of various factors, such as age, puberty, pregnancy, estradiol, GnRH and nutrition on heterogeneity patterns in various species is also discussed.

2. Structural features of the gonadotropins

The gonadotropins are glycoprotein hormones consisting of non-covalently associated α- and β-subunits [19, 20]. These heterodimers contain two types of oligosaccharides, N-linked and O-linked. O-linked oligosaccharides are covalently bonded to the hydroxyl oxygen of serine (Ser) or threonine (Thr), while N-linked are covalently bonded to the amide nitrogen of asparagine (Asn) [21]. Both types of oligosaccharide are found in the gonadotropins; however, the N-linked type predominate.

Within a particular species, the α-subunits of all the gonadotropins are identical in amino acid sequence, as a single gene encodes the α-subunit [22, 23]. Target cell specificity arises from the β-subunit [24, 25], which is encoded by a distinct gene. Although the amino acid sequences of the β-subunits of LH, FSH, TSH and CG show some homology, they are not identical. For example, LHβ and CGβ of human origin are approximately 70% homologous, while ovine LHβ and ovine FSHβ are approximately 34% homologous and bovine LHβ and bovine FSHβ are approximately 30% homologous. One exception to this is equine LHβ and equine CGβ, which have identical amino acid sequences [26].

The Asn-linked oligosaccharides of the α and β-subunits of the glycoprotein hormones, of both pituitary and placental origin, consist of a heterogenous array of neutral, sialylated, sulphated and mixed sialylated/sulphated oligosaccharides giving rise to extensive heterogeneity in their molecular forms. Thus, while any one gonadotropin consists of two polypeptide chains, the α and β-subunits, the heterogeneity of the attached carbohydrate gives rise to multiple molecular forms of that particular gonadotropin [11].

3. The α-subunit

Within a given species, the amino acid sequence of the α-subunits of the various glycoprotein hormones is identical, arising from a single mRNA. The molecular heterogeneity generated by variations in carbohydrate content gives rise to gonadotropin isoforms of variable bioactivity [27-29]. The amino acid sequences of the α-subunits of human, bovine, ovine, porcine and equine gonadotropins have been published from data obtained either by direct amino acid sequencing or from the nucleotide sequences of their respective cDNAs [23, 24, 30]. The amino acid sequence is highly conserved across species (Fig. 1), for example, bovine and ovine α-subunits are identical, bovine and equine are approximately 82% homologous and bovine and human α-subunits show approximately 75% amino acid sequence homology. The human α-subunit gene has a 12 base pair deletion that is reflected in the mature protein as having four fewer amino acids close to the N-terminus. The positions of the ten cysteine residues in the α-subunits of various species are highly conserved.

```
            5    10   15   20   25   30   35   40   45   50
            ^    ^    ^    ^    ^    ^    ^    ^    ^    ^
Ovine    FPDGEFTMDGCPECKLKENKYFSKPDAPIYQCMGCCFSRAYPTPARSKKT
Bovine   FPDGEFTMDGCPECKLKENKYFSKPDAPIYQCMGCCFSRAYPTPARSKKT
Porcine  FPDGEFTMQGCPECKLKENKYFSKLGAPIYQCMGCCFSRAYPTPARSKKT
Equine   FPDGEFTTQDCPECKLRENKYFFKLGVPIYQCKGCCFSRAYPTPARSRKT
Human    APD----VQDCPECTLQENPFFSQPGAPILQCMGCCFSRAYPTPLRSKKT

            55   60   65   70   75   80   85   90   95
            ^    ^    ^    ^    ^    ^    ^    ^    ^
Ovine    MLVPKNITSEATCCVAKAFTKATVMGNYRVENHTECHCSTCYYHKS
Bovine   MLVPKNITSEATCCVAKAFTKATVMGNYRVENHTECHCSTCYYHKS
Porcine  MLVPKNITSEATCCVAKAFTKATVMGNARVENHTECHCSTCYYHKS
Equine   MLVPKNITSESTCCVAKAFIRVTVMGNIKLENHTQCYCSTCYHHKI
Human    MLVQKNVTSESTCCVAKSYNRVTVMGGFKVENHTACHCSTCYYHKS
```

Figure 1. The amino acid sequences of the mature alpha subunits of gonadotropic hormones from five species [24, 31, 32] using single letter code (A, alanine; B, either asparagine or aspartic acid; C, cysteine; D, aspartic acid; E, glutamic acid; F, phenylalanine; G, glycine; H, histidine; I, isoleucine; K, lysine; L, leucine; M, methionine; N, asparagine; P, proline; Q, glutamine; R, arginine; S, serine; T, threonine; V, valine; W, tryptophan; Y, tyrosine; Z, either glutamine or glutamic acid). Sequences are aligned with their cysteine residues in register. There is evidence for disulphide bonds linking residue 11 with 35 and 14 with 36 but there is still uncertainty concerning the postulated bonds linking residue 30 with 64, 63 with 91 and 86 with 88 [33, 34].

Data from Cornell and Pierce [33] and from Mise and Bahl [34] provide information for the tentative pairings of cysteine residues in disulphide bridges indicated by the solid lines in Fig. 1. As the positions of cysteine residues are so highly conserved across species, this implies that the disulphide bridges found within the α-subunit are identical among α-subunits of different species. This indicates that the folding of the α-subunits of the different species is likely to be identical. This concept is supported by the fact that it is possible to produce a 'hybrid hormone' containing the α-subunit from one species combined with the β-subunit of another, which displays in vitro biological activity. For example, in studies involving hybrids made from the subunits of human CG gonadotropin (hCG) and ovine and porcine LH, Strickland and Puett [35] have shown that the activity of a given hybrid hormone, as measured by its ability to stimulate steroidogenesis in vitro, has the highest correlation with that of the hormone from which the β-subunit is derived. Indeed, some hybrids show increased activity in in vitro bioassays, as shown by Bousfield et al [36]. In this case, the equine LHα-porcine LHβ hybrid hormone was shown to be 49 times as active as porcine LH in stimulating steroidogenesis by Leydig cells.

While the positions of the various cysteine residues are known, there is little agreement between laboratories on the exact cysteine pairings [33, 34, 37-39]. The alignment of disulphide bridges proposed by Cornell and Pierce [33] for bovine LHα and by Mise and Bahl [34] for human CGα are in exact agreement. Owing to the clustering of cysteine residues in the α-subunit (two groups of two, and two groups of three), definitive identification of disulphide bridges has proven difficult. The positions of the carbohydrate residues on the α-subunits from various species are indicated in Fig. 2. The subunits have been aligned by their cysteine residues as these are so highly conserved. This allows for easy comparison of the homologous regions of the hormones. Hence, the glycosylation sites in the human α-subunit match those in all other α-subunits, even though it contains four fewer amino acids near the N-terminus. Asn-linked glycosylation occurs co-translationally [40, 41] when Asn is encountered in the sequence Asn-X-Ser/Thr, where X is any amino acid, except proline, and the amino acid at the third position is either Ser or Thr. In sharp contrast to their amino acid sequences, the Asn-linked oligosaccharides on the various α-subunits within a species can and do differ significantly. Thus, it is the nature of the carbohydrate residues that distinguish the α-subunits of the various gonadotropins within a species. The α-subunits are found in two forms within the pituitary gland and placenta. These are (i) αβ-dimer-associated α-subunits, and (ii) free α-subunits not combined with a β-subunit (free α). Free α-subunit has been shown to contain one O-linked oligosaccharide at position Thr^{43} [42, 43] which is not present in the α-subunit of αβ-dimers. Hence, the uncombined α-subunit has a higher molecular weight than the α-subunit found in association with β-subunit [44, 45]. Parsons and Pierce [46] have shown that α-subunits with an O-linked oligosaccharide will not combine with β-subunits to form αβ-dimers.

This is in contrast to the α-subunits lacking O-linked oligosaccharides which readily combine with β-subunits forming dimeric structures. Post translational modification of the gonadotropins occurs in the endoplasmic reticulum (ER) and subsequently, further modification occurs in the Golgi apparatus (GA) [21, 40, 41]. As αβ-dimerisation occurs in the ER [47, 48] and O-linked glycosylation is thought to occur in the GA, dimerisation may block a potential O-glycosylation site.

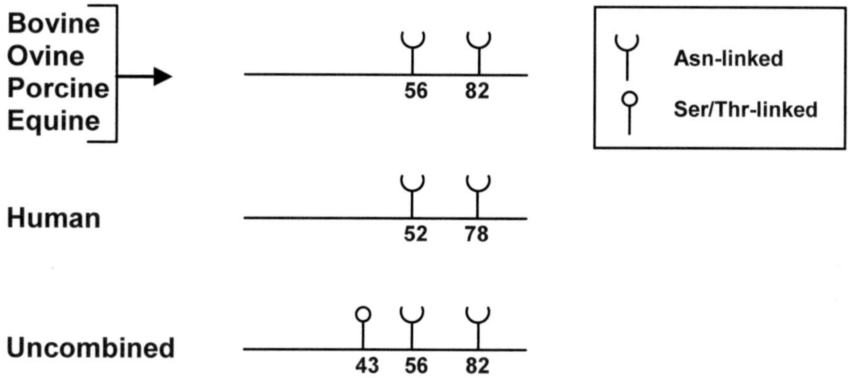

Figure 2. Glycosylation sites on the alpha and uncombined alpha subunits of the gonadotropic hormones [17, 24, 49]. Amino acid sequences are represented by solid horizontal lines. Proteins are aligned with their cysteine residues in register. Numbers indicate the positions of the glycosylated amino acids. For convenience, numbering is based on ovine LH.

4. The β-subunit

As the β-subunit determines the biological specificity of the gonadotropins [24], it is often referred to as the hormone specific subunit. The amino acid sequences of the β-subunits of various gonadotropins from several species are compared in Fig. 3. The β-subunits of LH, FSH, TSH and CG are proteins of varying lengths, ranging from 111 amino acids in bovine FSHβ (one of the shortest), to 149 amino acids in equine CGβ and equine LHβ (the longest). Human and equine CG have additional amino acids at the C-terminal [50, 51], compared with the other hormones (Fig. 3). This C-terminal extension peptide was originally thought to be a characteristic of CG and not of pituitary-derived glycoprotein hormones. However, it was subsequently discovered that equine LH also has a C-terminal extension peptide [52]. No other pituitary derived gonadotropin from any other species has this extension peptide.

The C-terminal extension peptide is heavily glycosylated containing four O-linked oligosaccharides in the case of human CG and five or six in the case of equine CG and equine LH (Fig. 4). Unfortunately, there is no recognised consensus sequence to signal O-linked glycosylation, in contrast to the Asn-X-Ser/Thr sequence which is required for N-linked glycosylation.

It is possible that a single gene may code for both the equine CGβ and equine LHβ subunits, as these have identical amino acid sequences (Fig. 3). Separate genes encode the separate β-subunits of the various gonadotropins in all other animal species and these genes are located on different chromosomes with one exception, the human LH/CG β-subunit gene cluster which is found on chromosome 19 [53]. This cluster consists of a single copy of the human LHβ gene and six copies of the human CGβ gene; however, some of these are not transcribed. In contrast to equine LHβ and equine CGβ, analysis of the amino acid sequences of human LHβ and human CGβ shows these to have different amino acid sequences.

```
         5    10   15   20   25   30   35   40   45   50     55   60   65   70   75
         ^    ^    ^    ^    ^    ^    ^    ^    ^    ^      ^    ^    ^    ^    ^
hCG   SKEPLRPRCRPINATLAVEKEGCPVCITVNTTICAGYCPTMTRVLQGVLPALP--QVVCNYRDVRFESIRLPGCPRG
eCG   SRGPLRPLCRPINATLAAEKEACPICITFTTSICAGYCPSMVRVMPAALPAIP--QPVCTYRELRFASIRLPGCPPG
eLH   SRGPLRPLCRPINATLAAEKEACPICITFTTSICAGYCPSMVRVMPAALPAIP--QPVCTYRELRFASIRLPGCPPG
hLH   SREPLRPWCHPINAILAVEKEGCPVCITVNTTICAGYCPTMMRVLQAVLPPLP--QVVCTYRDVRFESIRLPGCPRG
oLH   SRGPLRPLCQPINATLAAEKEACPVCITFTTSICAGYCPSMKRVLPVILPPMP--QRVCTYHELRFASVRLPGCPPG
bLH   SRGPLRPLCQPINATLAAEKEACPVCITFTTSICAGYCPSMKRVLPVILPPMP--QRVCTYHELRFASVRLPGCPPG
pLH   SRGPLRPLCRPINATLAAENEACPVCITFTTSICAGYCPSMRRVLPAALPPVP--QPVCTYRELSFASIRLPGCPPG
eFSH  ------NSCELTNITIAVEKEGCGFCITINTTWCAGYCYTRDLVYK--DPARPNIQKTCTFKELVYETVKVPGCAHH
hFSH  ------NSCELTNITIAIEKEECRFCISINTTWCAGYCYTRDLVYK--DPARPKIQKTCTFKELVYETVRVPGCAHH
oFSH  ------RSCELTNITITVEKEECSFCISINTTWCAGYCYTRDLVYK--DPARPNIQKACTFKELVYETVKVPGCAHH
bFSH  ------RSCELTNITITVEKEECGFCISINTTWCAGYCYTRDLVYR--DPARPNIQKTCTFKELVYETVKVPGCAHH
pFSH  ------NSCELTNITITVEKEECNFCISINTTWCAGYCYTRDLVYK--DPARPNIQKTCTFKELVYETVKVPGCAHH
hTSH  -------FCIPTEYTMHIERRECAYCLTINTTICAGYCMTRDINGKLFLPKYALSQDVCTYRDFIYRTVEIPGCPLH
bTSH  -------FCIPTEYMMHVERKECAYCLTINTTVCAGYCMTRDVNGKLFLPKYALSQDVCTYRDFMYKTAEIPGCPRH
pTSH  -------FCIPTEYMMHVERKECAYCLTINTTICAGYCMTRDFNGKLFLPKYALSQDVCTYRDFMYKTVEIPGCPHH

          80   85   90   95  100  105  110  115  120  125  130  135  140  145
          ^    ^    ^    ^    ^    ^    ^    ^    ^    ^    ^    ^    ^    ^
eCG   VDPMVSFPVALSCHCGPCQIKTTDCGVFRDQPLACAPQASSSSKDPPSQPLTSTSTPTPGASRRSSHPLPIKTS
hCG   VNPVVSYAVALSCQCALCRRSTTDCGGPKDHPLTCDDPRFQDSSSSKAPPPSLPSPSRLPGPSDTPILPQ
eLH   VDPMVSFPVALSCHCGPCQIKTTDCGVFRDQPLACAPQASSSSKDPPSQPLTSTSTPTPGASRRSSHPLPIKTS
hLH   VDPVVSFPVALSCRCGPCRRSTSDCGGPKDHPLTCDHPQLSGLLFL
oLH   VDPMVSFPVALSCHCGPCRLSSTDCGPGRTQPLACDHPPLPDIL
bLH   VDPMVSFPVALSCHCGPCRLSSTDCGGPRTQPLACDHPPLPDILFL
pLH   VDPTVSFPVALSCHCGPCRLSSSDCGGPRAQPLACDRPLLPGLLFL
eFSH  ADSLYTYPVATACHCGKCNSDSTDCTVRGLGPSYCSFGDMKE
hFSH  ADSLYTYPVATQCHCGKCDSDSTDCTVRGLGPSYCSFGEMKE
oFSH  ADSLYTYPVATECHCGKCDRDSTDCTVRGLGPSYCSFSDIRE
bFSH  ADSLYTYPVATECHCSKCDSDSTDCTVRGLGPSYCSFREIKE
pFSH  ADSLYTYPVATECHCGKCDSDSTDCTVRGLGPSYCSFSENKE
hTSH  VAPYFSYPVALSCKCGKCNTDYSDCIHEAIKTNYCTKPQKSYLVGFSV
bTSH  VTPYFSYPVAISCKCGKCNTDYSDCIHEAIKTNYCTKPQKSYMVGFSI
pTSH  VTPYFSYPVAISCKCGKCNTDYSDCIHEAIKTNYCTKPQKSYVLEFSI
```

Figure 3. Compilation of the reported amino acid sequences of the glycoprotein hormone beta subunits [49]. Original references are cited in several reviews [24, 31, 32]. For single letter code, see legend to Fig. 1.

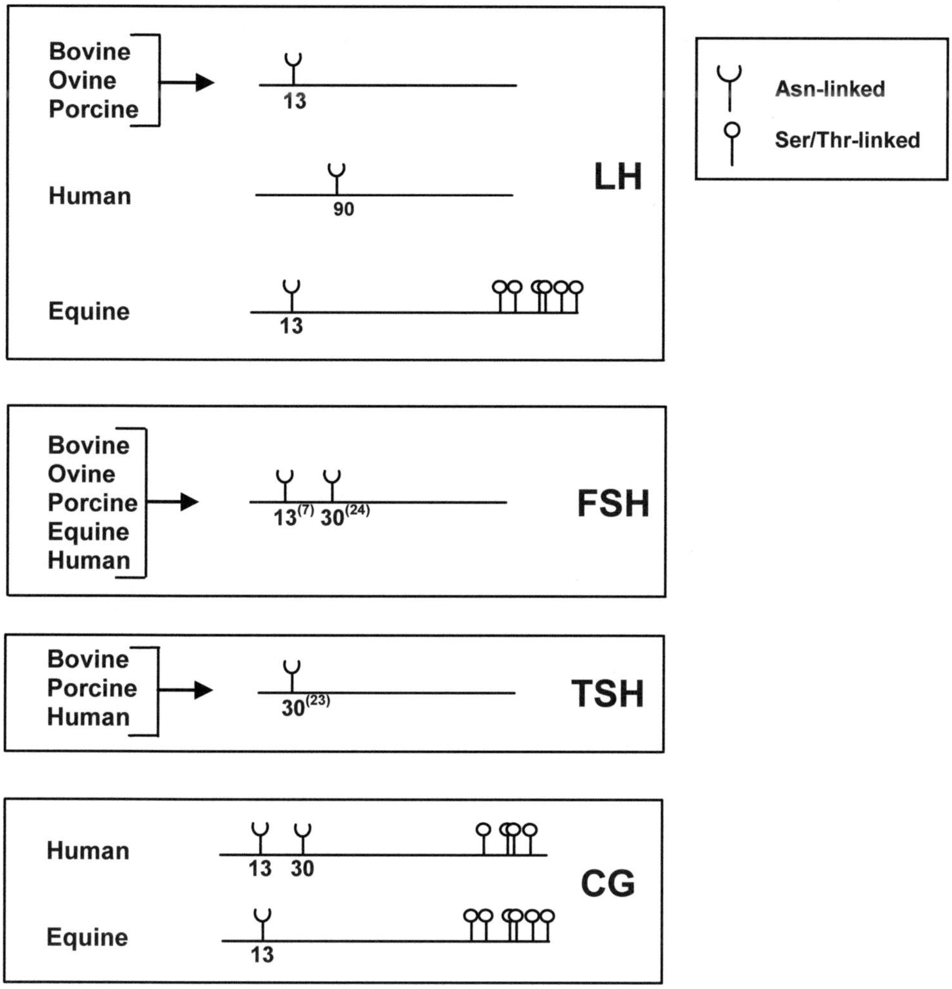

Figure 4. Glycosylation patterns on the beta subunits of the gonadotropic hormones. Proteins are aligned with their cysteine residues in register [49]. Numbers indicate the positions of the glycosylated amino acids and numbering is based on ovine LH. Where actual numbers differ, the positions of the glycosylated amino acids are indicated by the numbers in parentheses.

As in the α-subunit, cysteine residues are located in highly conserved positions in all the β-subunits of all species with one exception, i.e. one cysteine residue from a salmon gonadotropic hormone, (sGTHbl), is not present [26]. Again, as with the α-subunit, alignment of the β-subunit sequences by placing their half cystines in register, allows comparisons of highly conserved regions, although some subunits are shorter at the N-terminus than others. For example, the β-subunits of FSH and TSH from all species are shorter by six and seven amino acid residues, respectively, than the β-subunits of LH. The degree of amino acid sequence homology between β -subunits from different species varies. For example, ovine and bovine LHβ are approximately 96% homologous while equine and human CGβ display an homology of approximately 50%.

Each β-subunit contains 12 cysteine residues making up six intra-disulphide bonds. These 12 cysteine residues are more evenly scattered through the molecule than those found in the α-subunit. Two groups of researchers, using different methodologies, have indicated identical disulphide bridge placements for ovine LHβ and human CGβ [34, 54]. However, agreement exists on only three of six disulphide bridges among all authors. As such, some uncertainty remains as to the exact cysteine pairings in the β-subunit, but this situation is less controversial than that in the case of the α-subunits. As with the α-subunits, the positioning of the cysteine residues among all β-subunits is likely to lead to similar disulphide bridge formation and therefore very similar, or identical, overall three-dimensional structures.

5. Structural features of the Asn-linked carbohydrates

The α- and β-subunits of the gonadotropins contain either one or two Asn-linked oligosaccharides. The positions of the oligosaccharides on the β-subunits of the gonadotropins are indicated in Fig. 4. The position and structure of the Asn-linked carbohydrates found on gonadotropin subunits are varied [17, 24, 55] and consist of four types: (i) neutral, (ii) sialylated, (iii) sulphated and (iv) mixed sialylated/sulphated types. Oligosaccharides differ not only in their degree of sialylation or sulphation, but also in their core structures; these differences are the basis for the microheterogeneous molecular populations of individual hormones with varying biological activities [27, 29, 56-60]. Green and Baenziger [9, 11] have elucidated the structures and distributions of the sulphated (S) and sialylated (N) oligosaccharides on bovine, ovine and human pituitary glycoprotein hormones. The sulphated, sialylated and sulphated/sialylated structures were found to be highly heterogeneous and comprised 67-90% of the N-linked carbohydrate moieties present in pituitary-derived gonadotropins. As the hormone samples used in these studies were pituitary-derived, it should be borne in mind that some of the structures may represent partially synthesised/degraded oligosaccharides and may not correspond to secreted forms of the hormones. Nonetheless, these studies have provided a molecular basis for the observed heterogeneity of the gonadotropins. The oligosaccharides found in the placental gonadotropin, human CG, consist of typical neutral and sialylated di-branched structures [61-63] found in many serum glycoproteins. However, those found in pituitary-derived gonadotropins are more heterogeneous and complex in nature, perhaps reflecting partially processed forms of the molecules.

6. Sulphated oligosaccharides in the pituitary glycoprotein hormones

The oligosaccharide chains of glycoprotein hormones are of the complex type, as opposed to the mannose-rich type. The sulphated carbohydrates on bovine LH were among the first of the pituitary-derived gonadotropins to be fully characterized [55, 64]. The structures of the sulphated oligosaccharides found in the pituitary gonadotropins are illustrated in Fig. 5. These oligosaccharides vary in both the number of sulphate moieties and in the composition of the oligosaccharide structures (Fig. 5).

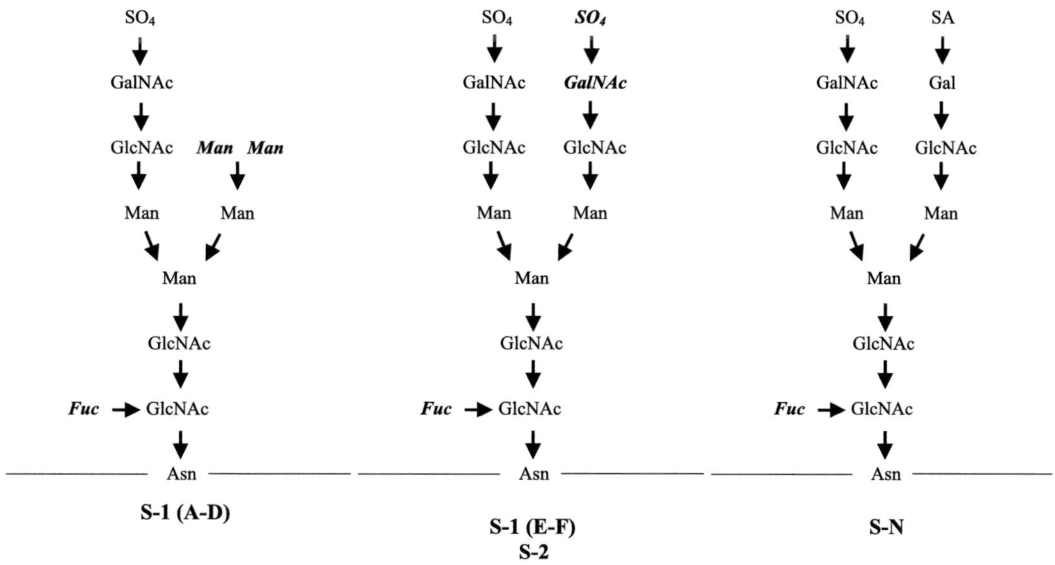

Figure 5. Structures of the sulphated N-linked oligosaccharides found in the pituitary-derived gonadotropins [11, 49]. Residues in bold italics are variably present. Both fucosylated and non-fucosylated forms of oligosaccharide are found in the pituitary hormones.

Each of the sulphated oligosaccharides has a core region consisting of three mannose and two N-acetylglucosamine (GlcNAc) residues [9, 55]. Additionally, each of the sulphated structures has one similar peripheral branch consisting of the sequence SO_4-N-acetylgalactosamine-N-acetylglucosamine-manose (SO_4-GalNAc-GlcNAc-Man). The second peripheral branch always commences with a mannose residue bonded to the core mannose. Sulphated oligosaccharides are either mono-(S-1) or di-(S-2) sulphated. The sulphated/ sialylated (S-N) structure contains both sulphate and sialic acid residues. Sulphate is always found associated with GalNAc while sialic acid is always linked to a galactose residue. The relative amounts of sulphated oligosaccharides varies considerably among the different hormones [64]. For example, the bovine hormones were found to contain very little S-N (0-2% of total oligosaccharides), while human and ovine hormones have relatively large amounts of S-N (10% of ovine FSH and 23% of human LH oligosaccharides are of the S-N type). However, bovine, ovine and human pituitary glycoprotein hormones display a very similar spectrum of sulphated oligosaccharides, i.e. most of the sulphated structures shown in Fig. 5 were isolated from each of the species' pituitary gonadotropins. In terms of the relative biosynthetic and secretory pathways, the presence of significant amounts of S-N on some of the hormones is important. It demonstrates that hormones which receive SO_4 and GalNAc do not traverse a physically distinct pathway to those hormones which receive sialic acid and galactose.

7. Sialylated oligosaccharides in the pituitary glycoprotein hormones

In general, the terminal carbohydrate residue of gonadotropin oligosaccharides is either sulphated or sialylated [17]. Some hormones, for example bFSH and hFSH, contain a much greater proportion of sialic acid and galactose than sulphate and GalNAc [10, 65, 66]. The sialylated oligosaccharides found on the gonadotropins, like the sulphated ones, consist of a heterogeneous array of structures. Three major types of sialylated oligosaccharide exist. These are mono-, di- and tri-sialylated oligosaccharides, containing one (N-1), two (N-2) and three (N-3) sialic acid residues, respectively. These oligosaccharides include both di- and tri-branched structures. The structures of the sialylated di- and tri-branched Asn-linked oligosaccharides found in pituitary gonadotropins are shown in Fig. 6. Additional details of all proposed structures for both sulphated and sialylated oligosaccharides are provided by Green and Baenziger [11].

The spectrum of sialylated structures found among the different hormones varies widely, in sharp contrast to the spectrum of sulphated oligosaccharides associated with each hormone. The relative amounts of particular sialylated structures also varies significantly among the various hormones. Some oligosaccharides are found exclusively associated with one particular hormone from one species. For example, N-3(D) (Fig. 6) and an N-2 form of this oligosaccharide are found exclusively on bovine FSH [12]. Hence, these oligosaccharides are both hormone and species specific. Human TSH was shown to have oligosaccharides bearing exclusively sialic acid residues while bovine TSH does not. Bovine TSH does have small amounts of S-N. Of all the bovine, ovine and human pituitary gonadotropins, only human LH and human FSH contained sialylated oligosaccharides bearing a β1,4 linked 'bisecting' GlcNAc residue attached to the core mannose (Fig. 6, N-2(C)). This implies that the enzyme responsible for the addition of GlcNAc in this position is active only in human and not in bovine or ovine gonadotroph cells.

Follicle-stimulating hormone contains sialylated oligosaccharides which are different to those found on LH or TSH. The most striking difference is the presence of tri-sialylated, N-3 type, oligosaccharides on FSH but not on LH or TSH [12]. This is true for ovine, bovine and human. Hence the study of sialylated oligosaccharide structures has highlighted several examples of both hormone and animal species-specific differences.

The distributions of the various oligosaccharide types in the pituitary glycoprotein hormones are illustrated in Table 1.

It is interesting to note the distribution of sulphated and sialylated structures. Bovine LH bears exclusively sulphated oligosaccharides while, in bovine FSH, the sialylated type predominates. Similarly, ovine LH contains very few sialylated structures while ovine FSH contains roughly equal amounts of sulphated and sialylated oligosaccharides. This raises the question of how different glycosylation patterns occur on LH and FSH, as both are produced by the same pituitary cell, the gonadotroph, and both have α-subunits with identical amino acid sequences. Thus the difference in glycosylation pattern may reflect the presence of the hormone specific β-subunits. Knowing the structural features and the distributions of the various types of oligosaccharide found on the gonadotropins, what are the functions of the various oligosaccharides and what effect, if any, do these carbohydrates have on biological activity?

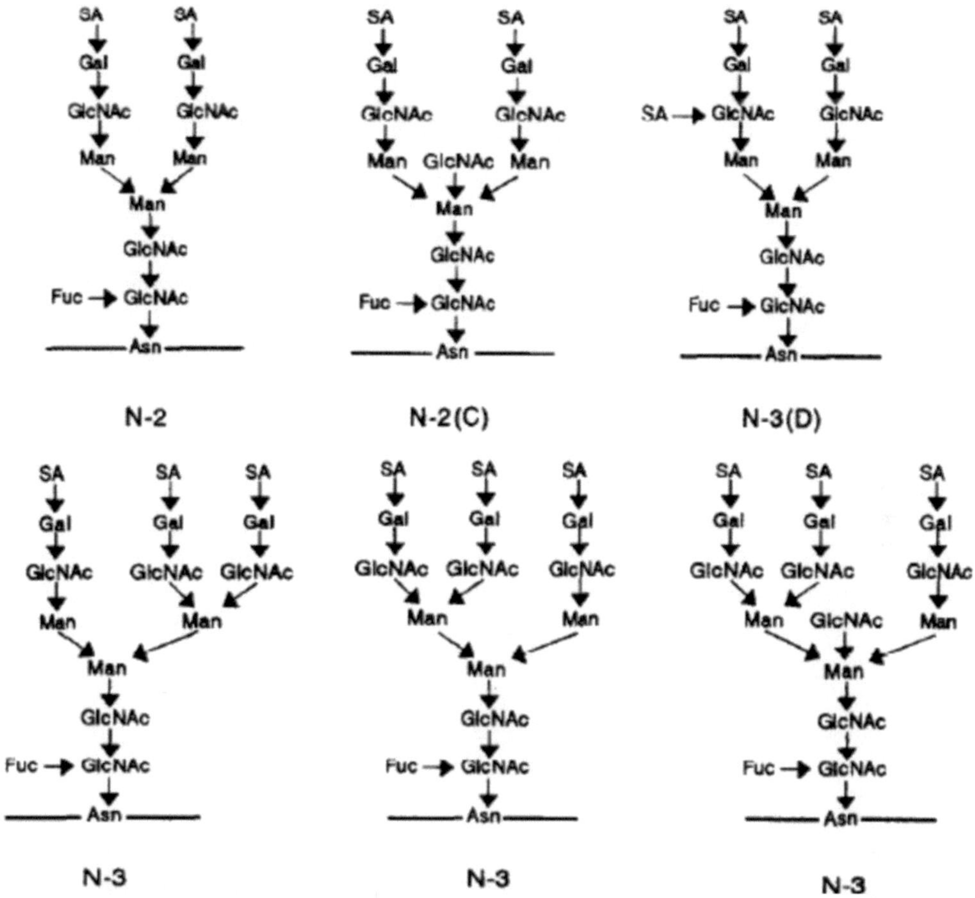

Figure 6. Structures of the sialylated dibranched and tribranched Asn-linked oligosaccharides in the pituitary glycoprotein hormones [49]. Only the highly sialylated structures are shown; see Green and Baenziger [11] for additional structures.

Gonadotrophin	Glycosylation type						
	Neutral	S-1	S-2	S-N	N-1	N-2	N-3
bLH	33	45	22	0	0	0	0
bFSH	32	11	1	1	5	39	11
bTSH	18	32	48	2	0	0	0
oLH	26	56	13	4	1	0	0
oFSH	32	14	16	10	10	11	7
hLH	16	19	7	23	19	16	0
hFSH	10	2	0	5	19	39	25
hTSH	18	25	18	21	5	12	0

Table 1. Relative distributions of neutral, sulphated, sialylated and sulphated / sialylated oligosaccharides expressed as a percentage of total oligosaccharides found in the pituitary glycoprotein hormones [12, 49].

8. Functions of the oligosaccharide residues of the gonadotropins

The overall in vivo activity of the gonadotropins is dependent upon several distinct characteristics: (i) their clearance rate from circulation, (ii) their ability to recognise the correct target cell receptor and (iii) their ability to induce cell signal transduction pathways.

The clearance rate of certain gonadotropins, for example FSH, is directly affected by the presence or absence of sialic acid. Removal of sialic acid by neuraminidase treatment decreases the in vivo biological activity of FSH due to its rapid elimination from the circulation by the hepatic asialoglycoprotein receptor [67, 68]. However, the in vitro biological response is not diminished [69, 70]. Aggarwal and Papkoff [71] examined the relationship of sialic acid residues to in vitro biological activities of the equine gonadotropins. In this study it was found that the in vitro LH activity of desialylated equine CG and equine LH was five and two times greater, respectively, than that of native hormone, as measured by the ability to stimulate steroidogenesis in rat Leydig cells. In contrast to this, Aggarwal and Papkoff [71] also showed that desialylating equine CG and equine FSH drastically reduced the ability of these hormones to stimulate CAMP production (FSH activity). So in the case of equine FSH at least, sialic acid appears to play an important role in in vitro biological activity. In agreement with Aggarwal and Papkoff, a study by West et al. [72] examined the effects of neuraminidase treated ovine pituitary FSH (reducing its acidity) in prepubertal lambs and observed an increased clearance rate and reduced ability to facilitate follicle development and maturation compared with more acidic FSH. However, most data support the hypothesis that sialic acid is present to prevent rapid clearance from circulation, and it is not essential for receptor binding or for signal transduction.

When gonadotropins are totally deglycosylated, either by chemical or enzymic means, their receptor binding ability is not diminished [73] in fact in some cases, it is increased compared with native hormone. For example, Calvo et al. [74] demonstrated a three-fold increase in the ability of deglycosylated human FSH to bind to FSH receptors of bovine testes, when compared with native hormone. Berman et al. [75] showed that the relative binding affinity of deglycosylated human TSH (while not a gonadotropin, is a structurally very similar glycoprotein hormone) was six-fold higher than that of native TSH. However, deglycosylated gonadotropins have a greatly diminished capacity for the stimulation of cAMP production by target cells [76, 77]. Hence, a deglycosylated hormone may bind to its receptor but fail to stimulate a biological response.

In apparent contrast to these findings, Cole et al. [78] has reported that significant steroidogenic activity of LH is maintained after enzymatic removal of oligosaccharides. Retention of some steroidogenic activity in the absence of CAMP production raises the possibility that deglycosylated hormones may act through alternative signal transducing systems and/or second messengers.

Deglycosylated hormones become antagonists of the native hormone in in vitro bioassays [51, 79, 80]. However, some deglycosylated hormones show poor in vivo antagonism. For example, Liu et al. [81] have shown that deglycosylated human CG is a full agonist at the

LH/CG receptor in the primate in vivo despite being a near-complete antagonist of human CG in vitro. Similarly, Patton et al. [82] showed that neither deglycosylated human CG, nor deglycosylated α-intact β-human CG, succeeded in terminating luteal cell function when administered to healthy young women during the mid-luteal phase of their menstrual cycles. This demonstrates that neither of these CG preparations exhibit antagonistic properties. In this study, it was suggested that the failure to interfere with LH maintenance of postovulatory corpora lutea is a result of residual agonist activity of the deglycosylated human CG. Experiments carried out by deglycosylating α- or β-subunits and then recombining the deglycosylated subunits with their native counterparts, support the premise that it is the oligosaccharides of the α-subunit, and not those of the β-subunit, which are essential for producing a biological response [73, 80, 83]. As stated earlier, uncombined α-subunit, which has been isolated from bovine pituitary is O-glycosylated. It is possible that such O-linked oligosaccharides may play a role in regulating dimerisation of pituitary gonadotropins [19]. Begeot et al. [84] demonstrated that uncombined α-subunit induces the development of lactotropes in the pituitary of 13-day-old rat foetuses, indicating that uncombined α-subunit may have a functional role other than that of a gonadotropin subunit. An additional role for uncombined α-subunit has been reported by Blithe et al. [85]. Using free α molecules isolated from the urine of pregnant women, as well as purified reference preparations of human CG α-subunit, Blithe et al. [85] have reported that free α-molecules stimulate the release of prolactin from human decidual cells in culture.

Hence this report suggests a novel role for free α in the paracrine regulation of decidual prolactin secretion.

The gonadotroph cells of the pituitary have the ability to segregate LH and FSH into separate secretory granules. Baenziger and Green [86] have suggested that the oligosaccharides present on LH and FSH may act as 'recognition-markers' to allow the cells to carry out this function. The presence of predominantly sialic acid residues on FSH and sulphate residues on LH may result in the targeting of these hormones to separate secretory granules.

9. Biosynthesis of gonadotropins bearing Asn-linked oligosaccharides

Biosynthesis of glycoprotein hormones involves protein biosynthesis and both co and post-translational modification by the addition of carbohydrate groups. The α- and β-subunits of the gonadotropins are synthesised by translation of their respective mRNAs. The transcription of α- and β-subunit genes is influenced by a number of factors including steroid hormones such as progesterone, estradiol and testosterone. The regulation of transcription of the gonadotropin subunit genes has been reviewed in several papers [87, 88].

Once mRNA has been produced, protein synthesis occurs on polysomes bound to the rough endoplasmic reticulum (RER). If gonadotropin subunit mRNA is subjected to translation using a cell-free translation system (i.e. ribosomes, mRNA etc., but no Golgi membrane-bound processing enzymes), then the resultant gonadotropin subunits are of slightly higher molecular weight as the signal peptide is not removed [89-91]. Glycosylation does not occur as the enzymes and oligosaccharides required for glycosylation are not present, while the increased molecular weight of the subunit is due to the presence of an N-terminal signal peptide. In vivo, this signal sequence is cleaved from the nascent polypeptide, by a signal peptidase located on the luminal surface of the RER membrane, hence it is not present on mature secreted protein. Elements of the signal hypothesis are reviewed by Jackson and Blobel [92]. Immature gonadotropin subunits containing a signal sequence are termed pre-α and pre-β subunits. Processing of pre-α and pre-β subunits to their mature forms involves two events, i.e. the cleavage of the signal peptide and glycosylation. Signal peptide cleavage occurs co-translationally [92] while glycosylation occurs both co- and post-translationally [24, 93].

Baenziger and Green [86] have proposed the synthetic pathway, outlined in Fig. 7, for the synthesis of the sulphated and sialylated Asn-linked oligosaccharides of the pituitary glycoprotein hormones. This proposed pathway was based upon the established pathway for N-linked glycosylation [41] and the structures of the oligosaccharides found in pituitary glycoprotein hormones isolated from pituitary tissue [11].

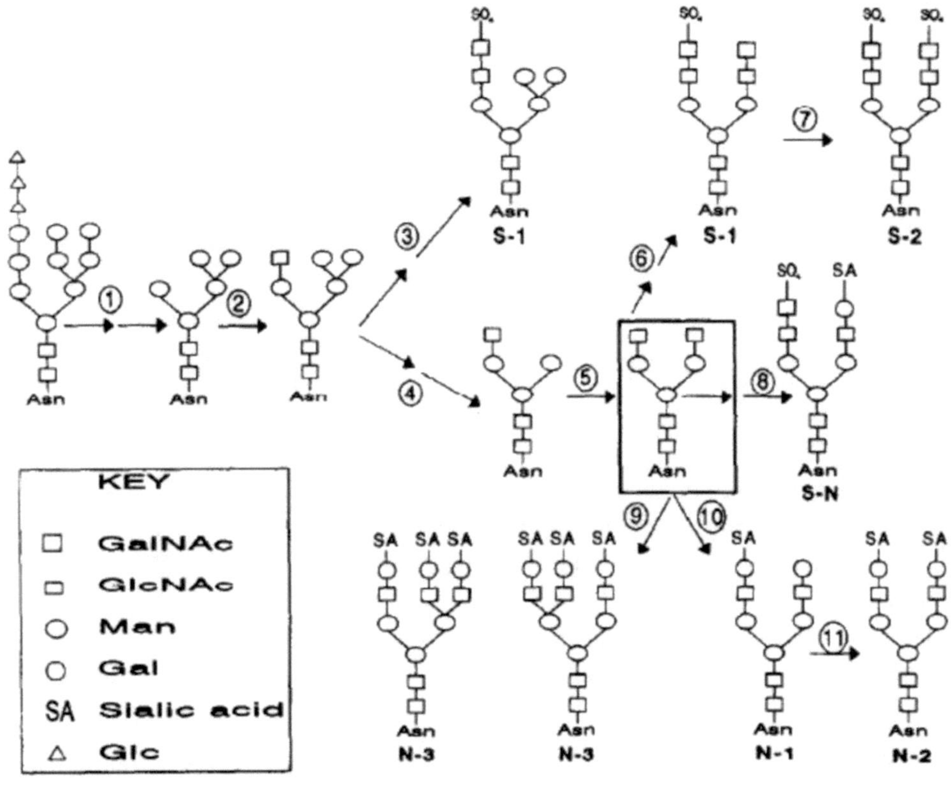

Figure 7. Proposed pathway for the biosynthesis of the sulphated and sialylated oligosaccharides in the pituitary glycoprotein hormones [49, 86].

The primary event in the process of N-linked glycosylation is the transfer of an oligosaccharide core of GlcManGlcNAc from a dolichol phosphate donor to specific Asn residues of the nascent polypeptide chain. As stated earlier, Asn must be in the sequence Asn-X-Ser/Thr in order to become glycosylated. This transfer process occurs co-translationally and is mediated by the enzyme oligosaccharyl transferase. While the glycoprotein is still in the RER, the three peripheral glucose residues are cleaved (step 1; Fig. 7). Specifically, α-glucosidase I removes the terminal glucose and α-glucosidase II cleaves the remaining two glucose residues. Different numbers of mannose residues, 0, 1, or 3 may be removed in the RER by specific glycosidases [94]. Formation of disulphide bonds and αβ-dimerisation [47, 48] is also initiated in the RER. The αβ-dimeric precursor of the mature glycoprotein is packaged into transfer vesicles and transferred from the RER to the cis-Golgi. The cis-Golgi is one of three compartmentalised areas of the organelle known as the Golgi apparatus. It is in the Golgi that vital post-translational modification events take place which play a pivotal role in determining the type of oligosaccharides which will be present in the mature glycoprotein. Hence, post-translational events in the Golgi determine, to some extent, the biological properties of the mature hormone.

In the cis-Golgi, α-1,2-mannosidase may cleave additional mannose residues yielding the ManGlcNAc intermediate (step 1; Fig. 7). This intermediate serves as substrate for the addition of GlcNAc by GlcNAc transferase I in the medial-Golgi, (step 2; Fig. 7). The resulting intermediate, GlcNAcManGlcNAc, may be converted to mono sulphated hybrid oligosaccharides (S-l(A-D)) by the sequential addition of GalNAc and sulphate (step 3; Fig. 7). Alternatively, sequential action of Golgi α-mannosidase II, which removes two mannose residues (step 4; Fig. 7) and GlcNAc transferase II which adds GlcNAc (step 5; Fig. 7) yields an intermediate from which all the remaining gonadotropin-associated Asn-linked oligosaccharides can be synthesised. This key intermediate is the GlcNAcManGlcNAc structure highlighted in Fig. 7 by a bold rectangle.

Hence this key intermediate can act as a template for the production of either sulphated, sialylated or sulphated/sialylated oligosaccharides. If galactose and sialic acid are sequentially added to this key intermediate, then sialylated oligosaccharides are formed (steps 9, 10, 11; Fig. 7). Alternatively, sequential addition of GalNAc and sulphate produces sulphated oligosaccharides (steps 6, 7; Fig. 7). Step 8 (Fig. 7) illustrates how the S-N type carbohydrates are formed, i.e. by the addition of GalNAc and sulphate as well as galactose and sialic acid.

Having discussed the nature of gonadotropin heterogeneity and the biosynthetic pathways by which such a heterogeneous population of hormones may be produced, several questions remain to be answered. For example, of all the isoforms which have been isolated and purified from pituitary extracts, which of these correspond to forms which are actually secreted into the blood and reach their target tissue? There is no doubt that the pituitary gonadotropins exist as multiple isoforms within the blood and that the isoform profile of a particular hormone in the blood does change under different physiological conditions. However, it still remains unclear what effect, if any, such a change in isoform profile has on the regulation of gonadal function. The following section deals with the factors influencing isoform profiles and suggests how the above questions may be addressed.

10. Factors influencing gonadotropin isoform profile

It is now clear that the gonadotropic hormones are secreted as multiple forms into the blood; however, to date little work has been done to characterize the patterns of gonadotropin isoforms in circulation of farm animals during different physiological states. Much of the data generated to date is based on the patterns of isoforms present in the anterior pituitary rather than in circulation or using rat sertoli or granulosa cell bioassay culture systems to determine biological activity. Thus, further work is required to address the role of gonadotropin heterogeneity in ovarian function and to resolve some of the apparent incoherencies present in the literature.

In prepubertal lambs, there is a high proportion of the more acidic (typically less biopotent) forms of FSH in serum; once lambs reach puberty, there is a shift towards the less acidic (typically more bioactive) forms of FSH in serum [95]. This is consistent with data from rats where an increase in bioactive forms of FSH within the pituitary was observed during the transition through puberty [96, 97]. However, in heifers Stumpf et al. [29] failed to detect a change in the distribution of either LH or FSH isoforms in pituitaries collected during sexual maturation.

During the estrous cycle of ewes, there was little change in the pattern of LH isoforms in the pituitary between the luteal and follicular phases [98]. However, during aestrus there was a decrease in the proportion of basic forms of oLH and a marginal increase in the acidic forms of LH [98]. This is in contrast to data on FSH. In rats, there is an increase in the less acidic (more bioactive in terms of radioreceptor assay) forms of FSH in the anterior pituitary during the pro-estrous period [99] when high concentrations of estradiol are present. Similarly in humans, there is an increase in FSH bioactivity (and the less acidic forms of FSH) during the late follicular phase of the menstrual cycle [28] thought to be associated with the pro-estrus rise in estradiol. Anobile et al. [100] also observed an association between increased estradiol and basic FSH isoforms during the menstrual cycle and concluded that changes in gonadotropin isoforms through the human menstrual cycle are related to changes in the prevailing steroid environment. In contrast, Kojima et al. [101] reported no change in FSH isoform distribution in the pituitary during the follicular phase of the estrous cycle in heifers. In agreement with this, Cooke et al. [102] also reported no changes in circulatory FSH isoforms during the first or second follicular waves in beef heifers, however, did identify greater amounts of less acidic FSH isoforms during the preovulatory gonadotropin surge which was also associated with increased estradiol concentrations. In addition, Crowe et al. [103] examined the resumption of follicular waves post partum and identified no significant differences in FSH heterogeneity between late pregnancy and the early post partum period.

Interestingly, a study by Timossi et al. [104] revealed the relationship between FSH isoform and bioactivity may also be dynamic, with naturally occurring human FSH isoforms observed exhibiting differential or even unique effects at the target cell level.

Alexander and Irvine [105] have demonstrated a significant increase in the bioactive: immunoactive (B:I) ratio of equine LH in serum before ovulation, compared with the B:I ratio after ovulation. It is suggested that the change in B:I ratio may be due to a change in the carbohydrate composition of the molecule, i.e. a change in LH isoforms. In agreement with this observation, Adams et al. [106] also observed enhanced biopotency of equine LH during the preovulatory period. Adams et al. [106] suggested that enhanced biological activity of LH may be required during the preovulatory and luteal phases of the cycle to promote ovulation and proper luteal function.

Removal of gonadal steroids by ovariectomy also demonstrates a role for steroids in controlling gonadotropin isoform secretion. Ovariectomy of heifers causes a shift towards the more basic isoforms of LH and FSH, while supplementation of ovariectomised heifers with estradiol restored the LH and FSH isoform profiles to that of intact heifers [29]. However, in a further study Kojima et al. [101] failed to detect an effect of either ovariectomy or ovariectomy with estradiol supplementation on pituitary isoforms of FSH, while effects on LH were consistent with those of Stumpf et al. [29]. Where human patients suffering with polycystic ovaries were injected with estradiol there was a decrease in immunoactive FSH but not bioactive FSH resulting in an increase in serum B:I ratio, indicating a shift towards the more basic isoforms of FSH [107, 108].

It is unclear whether the effects of estradiol are directly associated with changes in FSH heterogeneity at the anterior pituitary or whether it acts via altered GnRH secretory patterns. Treatment of young women during the mid-follicular [109] and post-menopause phases [110, 111] with a GnRH antagonist dramatically suppressed bioactive FSH concentrations but not immunoactive FSH. In contrast, attempts to alter FSH isoform profiles directly by administering GnRH pulses (2 ng kg^{-1} body weight every 2 h for 24 h and every 1 h for a further 12 h), using the nutritionally restricted ovariectomised model, were unsuccessful [112]. This suggests that in the absence of a source of steroid hormones, GnRH administration was unable to alter isoform patterns of FSH. Thus, it is possible that the effects of GnRH on gonadotropin heterogeneity are dependant on alterations in steroid concentrations (likely estradiol).

Alexander and Irvine [105] have suggested that increased secretion of equine LH forms with higher biological activity during the preovulatory period occur due to the rising concentrations of serum estradiol and increased GnRH levels which may occur at this time [113]. Similarly, Adams et al. [106] propose that elevation of serum oestrogens may modify the process of post-translational processing of equine LH to effect secretion of a more biologically potent form. Alternatively, estradiol may be acting at an extra-hypophyseal site to control enzymes involved in the removal of sialic acid residues from glycoprotein hormones. Loss of sialic acid can affect equine LH in contrasting ways; increasing in vitro biological activity [71], but reducing in vivo half-life.

Bioactive FSH in serum was reported to increase, indicating a shift towards the basic forms, during pregnancy in humans (i.e. when steroid concentrations are physiologically high) while immunoactive FSH remained low [111, 114]. However, some of this increase in FSH bioactivity has been questioned due to interference of high endogenous serum estradiol in the end point measurement in sertoli cell bioassays [115].

The following conclusions can be drawn.

1. Within a species, the α subunit is common to all the gonadotropins, while the β-subunit determines the biological specificity of the hormones.
2. A heterogenous array of oligosaccharides are found associated with the gonadotropins, and that variations in these oligosaccharide moieties generate the various isoforms of the gonadotropins.
3. Carbohydrate moieties of gonadotropins may play both a functional role in the binding of gonadotropins to their receptors but more likely play critical part in signal transduction. The precise role of the carbohydrate residues in signal transduction is not clearly understood; however in general, less acidic isoforms appear more bioactive than the more acidic isoforms with recent evidence also suggesting their bioactivity may be target specific.
4. Terminal sialic acid residues appear to be involved in increasing the circulatory half-life of the gonadotropins.
5. Estradiol concentrations are important in stimulating a shift towards bioactive forms of gonadotropin hormones during different physiological states; however the precise roles, if any, of GnRH in mediating these shifts are unclear.
6. During puberty bioactive isoforms of the gonadotropins increase.
7. There is an increase in bioactive forms of FSH during the follicular phase of the rat estrous cycle and the human menstrual cycle.
8. During pregnancy in humans there is an apparent increase in bioactive FSH concentrations in serum.

Author details

Dara J. Cooke, Michael P. Mullen* and Mark A. Crowe
School of Veterinary Medicine, University College Dublin, Ireland

11. References

[1] Moenter SM, Brand RC, Karsch FJ. Dynamics of gonadotropin-releasing hormone (GnRH) secretion during the GnRH surge: insights into the mechanism of GnRH surge induction. Endocrinology. 1992 May 1, 1992;130(5):2978-84.

[2] Sunderland SJ, Crowe MA, Boland MP, Roche JF, Ireland JJ. Selection, dominance and atresia of follicles during the estrous cycle of heifers. J Reprod Fertil. 1994 August 1, 1994;101(3):547-55.

[3] Sirois J, Fortune JE. Ovarian follicular dynamics during the estrous cycle in heifers monitored by real-time ultrasonography. Biol Reprod. 1988 September 1, 1988;39(2):308-17.

* Corresponding Author

[4] Savio JD, Keenan L, Boland MP, Roche JF. Pattern of growth of dominant follicles during the estrous cycle of heifers. J Reprod Fertil. 1988 July 1, 1988;83(2):663-71.

[5] Knopf L, Kastelic JP, Schallenberger E, Ginther OJ. Ovarian follicular dynamics in heifers: test of two-wave hypothesis by ultrasonically monitoring individual follicles. Domest Anim Endocrinol. 1989 Apr;6(2):111-9.

[6] Wilson CA, Leigh AJ, Chapman AJ. Gonadotrophin glycosylation and function. J Endocrinol. 1990 April 1, 1990;125(1):3-14.

[7] Combarnous Y. Molecular Basis of the Specificity of Binding of Glycoprotein Hormones to Their Receptors. Endocr Rev. 1992 November 1992;13(4):670-91.

[8] Stockell Hartree A, Renwick AG. Molecular structures of glycoprotein hormones and functions of their carbohydrate components. Biochem J. 1992 Nov 1;287 (Pt 3):665-79.

[9] Green ED, Boime I, Baenziger JU. Differential processing of Asn-linked oligosaccharides on pituitary glycoprotein hormones: implications for biologic function. Mol Cell Biochem. 1986;72(1):81-100.

[10] Nilsson BO, Rosen SW, Weintraub BD, Zopf DA. Differences in the Carbohydrate Moieties of the Common α-Subunits of Human Chorionic Gonadotropin, Luteinizing Hormone, Follicle-Stimulating Hormone, and Thyrotropin: Preliminary Structural Inferences from Direct Methylation Analysis. Endocrinology. 1986 December 1, 1986;119(6):2737-43.

[11] Green ED, Baenziger JU. Asparagine-linked oligosaccharides on lutropin, follitropin, and thyrotropin. I. Structural elucidation of the sulfated and sialylated oligosaccharides on bovine, ovine, and human pituitary glycoprotein hormones. J Biol Chem. 1988 January 5, 1988;263(1):25-35.

[12] Green ED, Baenziger JU. Asparagine-linked oligosaccharides on lutropin, follitropin, and thyrotropin. II. Distributions of sulfated and sialylated oligosaccharides on bovine, ovine, and human pituitary glycoprotein hormones. J Biol Chem. 1988 January 5, 1988;263(1):36-44.

[13] Van Damme MP, Robertson DM, Marana R, Ritzén EM, Diczfalusy E. A sensitive and specific in vitro bioassay method for the measurement of follicle-stimulating hormone activity. Acta Endocrinol (Copenh). 1979 June 1, 1979;91(2):224-37.

[14] Ascoli M. Characterization of Several Clonal Lines of Cultured Ley dig Tumor Cells: Gonadotropin Receptors and Steroidogenic Responses. Endocrinology. 1981 January 1, 1981;108(1):88-95.

[15] Jia X-C, Hsueh AJW. Granulosa Cell Aromatase Bioassay for Follicle-Stimulating Hormone: Validation and Application of the Method. Endocrinology. 1986 October 1, 1986;119(4):1570-7.

[16] Dahl KD, Stone MP. FSH isoforms, radioimmunoassays, bioassays, and their significance. J Androl. 1992;13(1):11-22.

[17] Ryan RJ, Keutmann HT, Charlesworth MC, McCormick DJ, Milius RP, Calvo FO, et al. Structure-function relationships of gonadotropins. Recent Prog Horm Res. 1987;43:383-429.

[18] Ryan RJ, Charlesworth MC, McCormick DJ, Milius RP, Keutmann HT. The glycoprotein hormones: recent studies of structure-function relationships. The FASEB Journal. 1988 August 1, 1988;2(11):2661-9.

[19] Combarnous Y. Structure and structure-function relationships in gonadotropins. Reprod Nutr Dev. 1988;28(2A):211-28.

[20] Gray CJ. Glycoprotein gonadotropins. Structure and synthesis. Acta Endocrinol Suppl (Copenh). 1988;288:20-7.

[21] Hirschberg CB, Snider MD. Topography of Glycosylation in The Rough Endoplasmic Reticulum and Golgi Apparatus. Annu Rev Biochem. 1987;56(1):63-87.

[22] Goodwin RG, Moncman CL, Rottman FM, Nilson JH. Characterization and nucleotide sequence of the gene for the common α subunit of the bovine pituitary glycoprotein hormones. Nucleic Acids Res. 1983 October 11, 1983;11(19):6873-82.

[23] Stewart F, Thomson JA, Leigh SEA, Warwick JM. Nucleotide (cDNA) sequence encoding the horse gonadotrophin α-subunit. J Endocrinol. 1987 November 1, 1987;115(2):341-6.

[24] Pierce JG, Parsons TF. Glycoprotein Hormones: Structure and Function. Annu Rev Biochem. 1981;50(1):465-95.

[25] Boothby M, Ruddon RW, Anderson C, McWilliams D, Boime I. A single gonadotropin alpha-subunit gene in normal tissue and tumor-derived cell lines. J Biol Chem. 1981 May 25, 1981;256(10):5121-7.

[26] Ward DN, Bousfield GR, Moore KH. Gonadotropins. In: P.T. Cupps (Editor), Reproduction in Domestic Animals, 4th edn. Academic Press, San Diego, CA, pp. 25-80.; 1991; 1991.

[27] Keel BA, Schanbacher BD, Grotjan HE. Ovine luteinizing hormone. I. Effects of castration and steroid administration on the charge heterogeneity of pituitary luteinizing hormone. Biol Reprod. 1987 June 1, 1987;36(5):1102-13.

[28] Padmanabhan V, Lang LL, Sonstein J, Kelch RP, Beitins IZ. Modulation of Serum Follicle-Stimulating Hormone Bioactivity and Isoform Distribution by Estrogenic Steroids in Normal Women and in Gonadal Dysgenesis. J Clin Endocrinol Metab. 1988 September 1, 1988;67(3):465-73.

[29] Stumpf TT, Roberson MS, Wolfe MW, Zalesky DD, Cupp AS, Werth LA, et al. A similar distribution of gonadotropin isohormones is maintained in the pituitary throughout sexual maturation in the heifer. Biol Reprod. 1992 March 1, 1992;46(3):442-50.

[30] Gharib SD, Wierman ME, Shupnik MA, Chin WW. Molecular Biology of the Pituitary Gonadotropins. Endocr Rev. 1990 February 1990;11(1):177-99.

[31] Ward DN, Boustield GR. FSH structures and their relationships to the other glycoprotein hormones. In: W.W. Chin and L. Boime (Editors), Glycoprotein hormones: structure, synthesis and biologic function. Proc. Serono Symposium, March 1989, Newport Beach, CA. Serono Symposia USA, Norwell, MA, pp. 81-95.; 1990; 1990.

[32] Ward DN, Boustield GR, Gordon WL, Sugino H. Chemistry of the peptide components of glycoprotein hormones. In: B.A. Keel and H.E. Grotjan, Jr. (Editors), Microheterogeneity of glycoprotein hormones. CRC Press, Boca Raton, FL, pp. I-21. . 1989; 1989.

[33] Cornell JS, Pierce JG. Studies on the Disulfide Bonds of Glycoprotein Hormones. J Biol Chem. 1974 July 10, 1974;249(13):4166-74.

[34] Mise T, Bahl OP. Assignment of disulfide bonds in the alpha subunit of human chorionic gonadotropin. J Biol Chem. 1980 September 25, 1980;255(18):8516-22.

[35] Strickland TW, Puett D. Contribution of Subunits to the Function of Luteinizing Hormone/Human Chorionic Gonadotropin Recombinants. Endocrinology. 1981 December 1, 1981;109(6):1933-42.

[36] Bousfield GR, Liu W-K, Ward DN. Hybrids from equine LH: alpha enhances, beta diminishes activity. Mol Cell Endocrinol. 1985;40(1):69-77.

[37] Chung D, Sairam MR, Li CH. The primary structure of ovine interstitial cell-stimulating hormone III: Disulfide bridges of the α-subunit. Arch Biochem Biophys. 1973;159(2):678-82.

[38] Combarnous Y, Hennen G. The Disulphide Bridges of Porcine Luteinizing Hormone α Subunit. Biochem Soc Trans. 1974;2:915-7.

[39] Fujiki Y, Rathnam P, Saxena BB. Studies on the disulfide bonds in human pituitary follicle-stimulating hormone. Biochimica et Biophysica Acta (BBA) - Protein Structure. 1980;624(2):428-35.

[40] Hubbard SC, Ivatt RJ. Synthesis and Processing of Asparagine-Linked Oligosaccharides. Annu Rev Biochem. 1981;50(1):555-83.

[41] Kornfeld R, Kornfeld S. Assembly of Asparagine-Linked Oligosaccharides. Annu Rev Biochem. 1985;54(1):631-64.

[42] Parsons TF, Bloomfield GA, Pierce JG. Purification of an alternate form of the alpha subunit of the glycoprotein hormones from bovine pituitaries and identification of its O-linked oligosaccharide. J Biol Chem. 1983 January 10, 1983;258(1):240-4.

[43] Corless CL, Boime I. Differential Secretion of O-Glycosylated Gonadotropin α-Subunit and Luteinizing Hormone (LH) in the Presence of LH-Releasing Hormone. Endocrinology. 1985 October 1, 1985;117(4):1699-706.

[44] Kourides IA, Landon MB, Hoffman BJ, Weintraub BD. Excess free alpha relative to beta subunits of the glycoprotein hormones in normal and abnormal human pituitary glands. Clin Endocrinol (Oxf). 1980;12(4):407-16.

[45] Fetherston J, Boime I. Synthesis of bovine lutropin in cell-free lysates containing pituitary microsomes. J Biol Chem. 1982 July 25, 1982;257(14):8143-7.

[46] Parsons TF, Pierce JG. Free alpha-like material from bovine pituitaries. Removal of its O-linked oligosaccharide permits combination with lutropin-beta. J Biol Chem. 1984 February 25, 1984;259(4):2662-6.

[47] Hoshina H, Boime I. Combination of rat lutropin subunits occurs early in the secretory pathway. Proc Natl Acad Sci U S A. 1982;79(24):7649-53.

[48] Ruddon RW, Krzesicki RF, Norton SE, Beebe JS, Peters BP, Perini F. Detection of a glycosylated, incompletely folded form of chorionic gonadotropin beta subunit that is a precursor of hormone assembly in trophoblastic cells. J Biol Chem. 1987 September 15, 1987;262(26):12533-40.

[49] Cooke DJ, Crowe MA, Roche JF, Headon DR. Gonadotrophin heterogeneity and its role in farm animal reproduction. Anim Reprod Sci. 1996;41(2):77-99.

[50] Birken S, Cranfield RE. Isolation and amino acid sequence of COOH-terminal fragments from the Â-subunit of human choriogonadotropin. J Biol Chem. 1977(252):5386-92.

[51] Keutmann HT, Johnson L, Ryan RJ. Evidence for a conformational change in deglycosylated glycoprotein hormones. FEBS Lett. 1985;185(2):333-8.

[52] Bousfield GR, Sugino H, Ward DN. Demonstration of a COOH-terminal extension on equine lutropin by means of a common acid-labile bond in equine lutropin and equine chorionic gonadotropin. J Biol Chem. 1985 August 15, 1985;260(17):9531-3.

[53] Graham MY, Otani T, Boime I, Olson MV, Carle GF, Chaplin DD. Cosmid mapping of the human chorionic gonadotropin β subunit genes by field-inversion gel elect rophoresis. Nucleic Acids Res. 1987 June 11, 1987;15(11):4437-48.

[54] Tsunasawa S, Liu W-K, Burleigh BD, Ward DN. Studies of disulfide bond location in ovine lutropin β subunit. Biochimica et Biophysica Acta (BBA) - Protein Structure. 1977;492(2):340-56.

[55] Green ED, van Halbeek H, Boime I, Baenziger JU. Structural elucidation of the disulfated oligosaccharide from bovine lutropin. J Biol Chem. 1985 December 15, 1985;260(29):15623-30.

[56] Miller C, Ulloa-Aguirre A, Hyland L, Chappel S. Pituitary follicle-stimulating hormone heterogeneity: assessment of biologic activities of each follicle-stimulating hormone form. Fertil Steril. 1983 Aug;40(2):242-7.

[57] Chappel SC, Bethea CL, Spies HG. Existence of Multiple Forms of Follicle-Stimulating Hormone within the Anterior Pituitaries of Cynomolgus Monkeys. Endocrinology. 1984 August 1, 1984;115(2):452-61.

[58] Blum WFP, Gupta D. Heterogeneity of rat FSH by chromatofocusing: studies on serum FSH, hormone released in vitro and metabolic clearance rates of its various forms [ill]. J Endocrinol. 1985 April 1, 1985;105(1):29-37.

[59] Matteri RL, Papkoff H. Microheterogeneity of equine follicle-stimulating hormone. Biol Reprod. 1988 March 1, 1988;38(2):324-31.

[60] Stanton PG, Robertson DM, Burgon PG, Schmauk-White B, Hearn MT. Isolation and physicochemical characterization of human follicle-stimulating hormone isoforms. Endocrinology. 1992 May 1, 1992;130(5):2820-32.

[61] Kessler MJ, Mise T, Ghai RD, Bahl OP. Structure and location of the O-glycosidic carbohydrate units of human chorionic gonadotropin. J Biol Chem. 1979 August 25, 1979;254(16):7909-14.

[62] Kessler MJ, Reddy MS, Shah RH, Bahl OP. Structures of N-glycosidic carbohydrate units of human chorionic gonadotropin. J Biol Chem. 1979 August 25, 1979;254(16):7901-8.

[63] Mizuochi T, Kobata A. Different asparagine-linked sugar chains on the two polypeptide chains of human chorionic gonadotropin. Biochem Biophys Res Commun. 1980;97(2):772-8.

[64] Green ED, Boime I, Baenziger JU. Biosynthesis of sulfated asparagine-linked oligosaccharides on bovine lutropin. J Biol Chem. 1986 December 15, 1986;261(35):16309-16.

[65] Sairam MR. Studies on pituitary follitropin: I. An improved procedure for the isolation of highly potent ovine hormone. Arch Biochem Biophys. 1979;194(1):63-70.

[66] Parsons TF, Pierce JG. Oligosaccharide moieties of glycoprotein hormones: bovine lutropin resists enzymatic deglycosylation because of terminal O-sulfated N-acetylhexosamines. Proc Natl Acad Sci U S A. 1980;77(12):7089-93.

[67] Ryle M, Chaplain MF, Gray CJ, Kennedy JF. In: W.R. Butt, A.C. Crooke and M. Ryle (Editors), Gonadotropins and Ovarian Development. Livingston, London, pp. 98- 106. 1970.

[68] Morell AG, Gregoriadis G, Scheinberg IH, Hickman J, Ashwell G. The Role of Sialic Acid in Determining the Survival of Glycoproteins in the Circulation. J Biol Chem. 1971 March 10, 1971;246(5):1461-7.

[69] Ulloa-Aguirre A, Miller C, Hyland L, Chappel S. Production of all follicle-stimulating hormone isohormones from a purified preparation by neuraminidase digestion. Biol Reprod. 1984 March 1, 1984;30(2):382-7.

[70] Ulloa-Aguirre A, Mejia JJ, Dominguez R, Guevara-Aguirre J, Diaz-Sánchez V, Larrea F. Microheterogeneity of anterior pituitary FSH in the male rat: isoelectric focusing pattern throughout sexual maturation. J Endocrinol. 1986 September 1, 1986;110(3):539-49.

[71] Aggarwal BB, Papkoff H. Relationship of sialic acid residues to in vitro biological and immunological activities of equine gonadotropins. Biol Reprod. 1981 Jun;24(5):1082-7.

[72] West CR, Carlson NE, Lee JS, McNeilly AS, Sharma TP, Ye W, et al. Acidic Mix of FSH Isoforms Are Better Facilitators of Ovarian Follicular Maturation and E2 Production than the Less Acidic. Endocrinology. 2002 January 1, 2002;143(1):107-16.

[73] Goverman JM, Parsons TF, Pierce JG. Enzymatic deglycosylation of the subunits of chorionic gonadotropin. Effects on formation of tertiary structure and biological activity. J Biol Chem. 1982 December 25, 1982;257(24):15059-64.

[74] Calvo FO, Keutmann HT, Bergert ER, Ryan RJ. Deglycosylated human follitropin: characterization and effects on adenosine cyclic 3',5'-phosphate production in porcine granulosa cells. Biochemistry (Mosc). 1986 Jul 1;25(13):3938-43.

[75] Berman MI, Thomas Jr CG, Manjunath P, Sairam MR, Nayfen SN. The role of the carbohydrate moiety in thyrotropin action. Biochem Biophys Res Commun. 1985;133(2):680-7.

[76] Manjunath P, Sairam MR, Sairam J. Studies on pituitary follitropin X. Biochemical, receptor binding and immunological properties of deglycosylated ovine hormone. Mol Cell Endocrinol. 1982;28(2):125-38.

[77] Sairam MR, Bhargavi GN. A role for glycosylation of the alpha subunit in transduction of biological signal in glycoprotein hormones. Science. 1985 July 5, 1985;229(4708):65-7.

[78] Cole LA, Metsch LA, Grotjan HE. Significant Steroidogenic Activity of Luteinizing Hormone is Maintained after Enzymatic Removal of Oligosaccharides. Mol Endocrinol. 1987 September 1, 1987;1(9):621-7.

[79] Sairam MR, Manjunath P. Studies on pituitary follitropin XI. Induction of hormonal antagonistic activity by chemical deglycosylation. Mol Cell Endocrinol. 1982;28(2):139-50.

[80] Liu WK, Young JD, Ward DN. Deglycosylated ovine lutropin: preparation and characterization by in vitro binding and steroidogenesis. Mol Cell Endocrinol. 1984 Aug;37(1):29-39.
[81] Liu L, Southers JL, Banks SM, Blithe DL, Wehmann RE, Brown JH, et al. Stimulation of Testosterone Production in the Cynomolgus Monkey in Vivo by Deglycosylated and Desialylated Human Choriogonadotropin. Endocrinology. 1989 January 1, 1989;124(1):175-80.
[82] Patton PE, Calvo FO, Fujimoto VY, Bergert ER, Kempers RD, Ryan RJ. The effect of deglycosylated human chorionic gonadotropin on corpora luteal function in healthy women. Fertil Steril. 1988;49(4):620-5.
[83] Sairam MR. Deglycosylation of ovine pituitary lutropin subunits: Effects on subunit interaction and hormone activity. Arch Biochem Biophys. 1980;204(1):199-206.
[84] Begeot M, Hemming FJ, Dubois PM, Combarnous Y, Dubois MP, Aubert ML. Induction of pituitary lactotrope differentiation by luteinizing hormone alpha subunit. Science. 1984 November 2, 1984;226(4674):566-8.
[85] Blithe DL, Richards RG, Skarulis MC. Free alpha molecules from pregnancy stimulate secretion of prolactin from human decidual cells: a novel function for free alpha in pregnancy. Endocrinology. 1991 October 1, 1991;129(4):2257-9.
[86] Baenziger JU, Green ED. Pituitary glycoprotein hormone oligosaccharides: Structure, synthesis and function of the asparagine-linked oligosaccharides on lutropin, follitropin and thyrotropin. Biochimica et Biophysica Acta (BBA) - Reviews on Biomembranes. 1988;947(2):287-306.
[87] Habner JF. Molecular Cloning of Hormone Genes. Humana Press, Clifton Press, NJ. 1987.
[88] Chin WW, Boime JW. Glycoprotein Hormones: Structure, Synthesis and Biologic Function. Plenum Press, New York. 1990.
[89] Giudice LC, Waxdal MJ, Weintraub BD. Comparison of bovine and mouse pituitary glycoprotein hormone pre-alpha subunits synthesized in vitro. Proc Natl Acad Sci U S A. 1979 Oct;76(10):4798-802.
[90] Landefeld TD. Identification of in vitro synthesized pituitary glycoprotein alpha subunit. Translation of a possible precursor. J Biol Chem. 1979 May 25, 1979;254(10):3685-8.
[91] Godine JE, Chin WW, Habener JF. Cell-free synthesis and processing of the precursors to the subunits of luteinizing hormone. J Biol Chem. 1981 March 10, 1981;256(5):2475-9.
[92] Jackson RC, Blobel G. Post-translational processing of full-length presecretory proteins with canine pancreatic signal peptidase. Ann N Y Acad Sci. 1980;343(1):391-404.
[93] Weintraub BD, Stannard BS, Linnekin D, Marshall M. Relationship of glycosylation to de novo thyroid-stimulating hormone biosynthesis and secretion by mouse pituitary tumor cells. J Biol Chem. 1980 June 25, 1980;255(12):5715-23.
[94] Lodish HF. Transport of secretory and membrane glycoproteins from the rough endoplasmic reticulum to the Golgi. A rate-limiting step in protein maturation and secretion. J Biol Chem. 1988 February 15, 1988;263(5):2107-10.

[95] Padmanabhan V, Mieher CD, Borondy M, I'Anson H, Wood RI, Landefeld TD, et al. Circulating bioactive follicle-stimulating hormone and less acidic follicle-stimulating hormone isoforms increase during experimental induction of puberty in the female lamb. Endocrinology. 1992 July 1, 1992;131(1):213-20.

[96] Chappel SC, Ulloa-Aguirre A, Ramaley JA. Sexual maturation in female rats: time-related changes in the isoelectric focusing pattern of anterior pituitary follicle-stimulating hormone. Biol Reprod. 1983 February 1, 1983;28(1):196-205.

[97] Chappel SC, Ramaley JA. Changes in the isoelectric focusing profile of pituitary follicle-stimulating hormone in the developing male rat. Biol Reprod. 1985 April 1, 1985;32(3):567-73.

[98] Zalesky DD, Nett TM, Grotjan HE. Ovine luteinizing hormone: isoforms in the pituitary during the follicular and luteal phases of the estrous cycle and during anestrus. J Anim Sci. 1992 December 1, 1992;70(12):3851-6.

[99] Ulloa-Aguirre A, Espinoza R, Damian-Matsumura P, Larrea F, Flores A, Morales L, et al. Studies on the microheterogeneity of anterior pituitary follicle-stimulating hormone in the female rat. Isoelectric focusing pattern throughout the estrous cycle. Biol Reprod. 1988 February 1, 1988;38(1):70-8.

[100] Anobile CJ, Talbot JA, McCann SJ, Padmanabhan V, Robertson WR. Glycoform composition of serum gonadotrophins through the normal menstrual cycle and in the post-menopausal state. Mol Hum Reprod. 1998 July 1, 1998;4(7):631-9.

[101] Kojima FN, Cupp AS, Stumpf TT, Zalesky DD, Roberson MS, Werth LA, et al. Effects of 17 beta-estradiol on distribution of pituitary isoforms of luteinizing hormone and follicle-stimulating hormone during the follicular phase of the bovine estrous cycle. Biol Reprod. 1995 February 1, 1995;52(2):297-304.

[102] Cooke DJ, Crowe MA, Roche JF. Circulating FSH isoform patterns during recurrent increases in FSH throughout the estrous cycle of heifers. J Reprod Fertil. 1997 July 1, 1997;110(2):339-45.

[103] Crowe MA, Padmanabhan V, Mihm M, Beitins IZ, Roche JF. Resumption of follicular waves in beef cows is not associated with periparturient changes in follicle-stimulating hormone heterogeneity despite major changes in steroid and luteinizing hormone concentrations. Biol Reprod. 1998 June 1, 1998;58(6):1445-50.

[104] Timossi CM, Barrios-de-Tomasi J, Gonzalez-Suarez R, Arranz MC, Padmanabhan V, Conn PM, et al. Differential effects of the charge variants of human follicle-stimulating hormone. J Endocrinol. 2000 May 1, 2000;165(2):193-205.

[105] Alexander S, Irvine CH. Radioimmunoassay and in-vitro bioassay of serum LH throughout the equine estrous cycle. J Reprod Fertil Suppl. 1982;32:253-60.

[106] Adams TE, Horton MB, Watson JG, Adams BM. Biological activity of Luteinizing Hormone (LH) during the estrous cycle of mares. Domest Anim Endocrinol. 1986;3(2):69-77.

[107] Padmanabhan V, Christman GM, Zawacki CM, Kelch RP, Randolf J, J.F.,, Beitins IZ. Regulation of bioactive FSH in women with polycystic ovarian disease. 72nd Annual Meeting of the Endocrine Society, 20-23 June 1990, Atlanta, GA, Abstr 1369, p 367; 1990; 1990.

[108] Beitins IZ, Kletter GB, Padmanabhan V. Clinical applications of FSH bioassays In: M.L. Dufau, A. Fabbri and A. Isidori (Editors) Cell and Molecular Biology of the Testes. Ares Serono Symposia Series. Frontiers in Endocrinol., 5: 99- 114. 1993.

[109] Kessel B, Dahl KD, Kazer RR, Liu CH, Rivier J, Vale W, et al. The Dependency of Bioactive Follicle-Stimulating Hormone Secretion on Gonadotropin-Releasing Hormone in Hypogonadal and Cycling Women. J Clin Endocrinol Metab. 1988 February 1, 1988;66(2):361-6.

[110] Matikainen T, Ding YQ, Vergara M, Huhtaniemi I, Couzinet B, Schaison G. Differing responses of plasma bioactive and immunoreactive follicle-stimulating hormone and luteinizing hormone to gonadotropin-releasing hormone antagonist and agonist treatments in postmenopausal women. J Clin Endocrinol Metab. 1992 September 1, 1992;75(3):820-5.

[111] Padmanabhan V, Sonstein J, Olton PL, Nippoldt T, Menon KMJ, Marshall JC, et al. Serum Bioactive Follicle-Stimulating Hormone-Like Activity Increases during Pregnancy. J Clin Endocrinol Metab. 1989 November 1, 1989;69(5):968-77.

[112] Hassing JM, Kletter GB, I'Anson H, Wood RI, Beitins IZ, Foster DL, et al. Pulsatile administration of gonadotropin-releasing hormone does not alter the follicle-stimulating hormone (FSH) isoform distribution pattern of pituitary or circulating FSH in nutritionally growth-restricted ovariectomized lambs. Endocrinology. 1993 April 1, 1993;132(4):1527-36.

[113] Irvine CHG. Endocrinology of the estrous cycle of the mare: Applications to embryo transfer. Theriogenology. 1981;15(1):85-104.

[114] Simoni M, Khan SA, De Geyter C, Nieschlag E. Stimulatory and inhibitory influences of serum from pregnant women on aromatase activity of immature rat Sertoli cells. Acta Endocrinol (Copenh). 1989 August 1, 1989;121(2):265-9.

[115] Simoni M, Nieschlag E. In vitro bioassays of follicle-stimulating hormone: methods and clinical applications. J Endocrinol Invest. 1991 Dec;14(11):983-97.